Hormonal Regulation of Fluid and Electrolytes

Environmental Effects

Hormonal Regulation of Fluid and Electrolytes

Environmental Effects

Edited by
John R. Claybaugh
Tripler Army Medical Center, Hawaii
and
Charles E. Wade
Letterman Army Institute of Research
San Francisco, California

Plenum Press • New York and London

Library of Congress Cataloging-in-Publication Data

Hormonal regulation of fluid and electrolytes : environmental effects / edited by John R. Claybaugh and Charles E. Wade.
p. cm.
"Proceedings of a Federation of American Societies for Experimental Biology Conference on Hormonal Regulation of Fluid and Electrolytes: Environmental Effects, held April 1-3, 1987, in Washington, D.C."--T.p. verso.
Includes bibliographical references.
ISBN 0-306-43488-1
1. Water-electrolyte balance (Physiology)--Endocrine aspects--Congresses. 2. Water-electrolyte balance (Physiology)--Environmental aspects--Congresses. 3. Hormones--Physiological effect--Congresses. I. Claybaugh, John R. II. Wade, Charles E. III. Federation of American Societies for Experimental Biology. IV. Federation of American Societies for Experimental Biology Conference on Hormonal Regulation of Fluid and Electrolytes: Environmental Effects (1987 : Washington, D.C.)
QP90.4.H67 1989
612'.01522--dc20 89-77900
CIP

Proceedings of a Federation of American Societies of Experimental Biology Conference on Hormonal Regulation of Fluid and Electrolytes: Environmental Effects, held April 1-3, 1987, in Washington, D.C.

A Division of Plenum Publishing Corporation
233 Spring Street, New York, N.Y. 10013

Printed in the United States of America

PREFACE

The concept of this book has developed over the past fifteen years as interest in the water and electrolyte disturbances associated with most environmental settings moved from a research area of descriptive discovery to one dealing with the mechanisms responsible for the previously observed disturbances. Most of the contributing authors have been involved in both aspects of this evolution of research, focusing on those problems associated with body fluid and electrolyte balance and searching for hormonal explanations. What did not accompany this transition, however, was a source of information encompassing the area of interest. Instead, the previous format of environmentally focused symposia, reviews, and books continued to be the only sources available. For instance, various books deal with the physiology of high altitude, space, or exercise but do not necessarily provide adequate coverage of water and electrolyte disturbances.

To our knowledge, the format of this book is unique. We have made the central focus water and electrolyte physiology with an emphasis on endocrinology and tried to comprehensively cover this area of physiology in some of the more heavily studied environments. This book too, then, will have its limitations in coverage. For instance, in-depth coverage of the respiratory and cardiovascular responses to the high altitude environment will not be found, but since these areas are so integrally associated with water and electrolyte regulation they are not ignored.

In addition to a reference text, hopefully this book will be used for some advanced graduate courses in environmental physiology, providing a starting point for future work. The editors would appreciate any comments on the utility of this book either as a reference or as a course text.

The editors are indebted to Dr. Linda Kullama whose scientific knowledge of the field and editorial knowledge were invaluable assets in the completion of the final draft of this book. We would also like to take this opportunity to acknowledge and thank our editor at Plenum Publishing Corporation, Patricia Vann, for her encouragement, advice, patience, and sense of humor in completing this project.

John R. Claybaugh
Charles E. Wade

CONTENTS

Chapter 1

FLUID AND ELECTROLYTE HOMEOSTASIS DURING AND FOLLOWING EXERCISE: HORMONAL AND NON-HORMONAL FACTORS

C.E. Wade, B.J. Freund, and J.R. Claybaugh

Chapter 2

HORMONAL REGULATION OF FLUID AND ELECTROLYTES: EFFECTS OF HEAT EXPOSURE AND EXERCISE IN THE HEAT

R.P. Francesconi, M.N. Sawka, R.W. Hubbard and K.B. Pandolf

Chapter 4

HORMONAL AND RENAL RESPONSES TO HYPERBARIA

S.K. Hong and J.R. Claybaugh

Chapter 5

HEAD-OUT WATER IMMERSION: A CRITICAL EVALUATION OF THE GAUER-HENRY HYPOTHESIS

J.A. Krasney, G. Hajduczok, K. Miki, J.R. Claybaugh, J.L. Sondeen, D.R. Pendergast and S.K. Hong

Chapter 6

FLUID AND ELECTROLYTE BALANCE AND HORMONAL RESPONSE TO THE HYPOXIC ENVIRONMENT

J.R. Claybaugh, C.E. Wade and S.A. Cucinell

1

FLUID AND ELECTROLYTE HOMEOSTASIS DURING AND FOLLOWING EXERCISE: HORMONAL AND NON-HORMONAL FACTORS

Charles E. Wade[1], Beau J. Freund[2], and John R. Claybaugh[2]

[1]Letterman Army Institute of Research
Division of Military Trauma Research
Presidio of San Francisco, CA 94129-6800

[2]Department of Clinical Investigation
Tripler Army Medical Center
TAMC, H.I. 96859-5000

INTRODUCTION

Precise control of fluid and electrolyte homeostasis is essential for the survival of man. The performance of exercise results in a significant disturbance of water and electrolyte homeostasis. These alterations during exercise are due to the loss of fluids and electrolytes primarily in sweat and to voluntary dehydration associated with an inappropriate suppression of thirst. During the performance of exercise, as well as during recovery, compensatory measures occur to rectify these changes. A variety of hormones are important in the compensatory responses to correct water and electrolyte disturbances. The goal of this chapter is to describe the changes in water and electrolyte homeostasis resulting from exercise and the responses, regulation, and actions of the hormones important in correcting these imbalances.

NON-HORMONAL EFFECTS OF EXERCISE

Water and Electrolyte Balance during Exercise

During exercise there is an increase in metabolism with an accompanying increase in heat production. The increase in body heat stores is usually maintained within tolerable limits because sweating is initiated. Sweat rate during the performance of long duration moderate intensity exercise is on the order of 1000 to 1500 ml per hour (24,39,69,114) and can represent a two to

TABLE 1. Electrolyte concentrations (mEq/l of sweat and plasma) (162).

	Na^{+}	K^{+}	Ca^{++}	Mg^{++}	Cl^{-}
Sweat	60	8.8	3.4	1.2	46
Plasma	135-145	3.5-5.0	4.3-5.3	1.5-2.5	96-106

three percent decrease in total body water. The rate of sweating may be further increased in individuals who are adapted/acclimated to the exercise-induced increase in heat stores and to hot environments (24,35,87,115). Sweating represents not only a loss of water but also of electrolytes. The concentration of solutes in sweat is less than that of plasma (i.e., hypotonic) (Table 1) (87,143,162); however, this loss of solutes can result in a significant reduction in total body solute content. For example, one hour of exercise producing one liter of sweat with a sodium concentration of 60 mEq/l represents a 2% reduction in total body sodium (19,174). This net loss applies to all electrolytes that are contained in sweat.

The increase in metabolism during exercise necessitates an increase in respiration. Respiratory water loss is a function of the intensity of exercise (111). An increase in respiratory water loss on the order of 120 to 300 ml/hr occurs during heavy exercise (111). However, this route contributes only a fraction of the total water loss occurring during exercise.

Water and electrolytes are also lost in the urine during exercise, though the rate is reduced compared to resting levels (see below). The continued renal excretion during exercise is necessary to eliminate biological waste materials, which if not excreted would be toxic. This process is especially important during exercise since the increase in metabolism increases the production of by-products. The urine flow rate during exercise is on the order of 30 ml/hr (47,133,134), but is dependent upon several factors such as the intensity and duration of the exercise as well as the hydration status of the subjects. Thus, during exercise, though there is a net decrease in the renal excretion of water and electrolytes, a loss in the urine occurs.

On the other hand, water is produced by the increase in metabolism during exercise via glycogen and oxidative processes. The metabolism of one gram of glycogen releases a calculated 3 to 4 ml of water (123). During heavy exercise by well trained individuals, this metabolic water may contribute 300 to 500 ml/hr (94,143). Though this is a source for an increase in body water, there is still a net decrease as losses exceed this metabolic production.

Another more obvious source of water gain during exercise is by fluid intake. The amount of water provided through drinking is dependent upon a variety of factors, but during long duration exercise typically ranges from 250 to 400 ml/hr (7,20,114). This rate of intake does not prevent losses during exercise. The net loss of water during the course of exercise is reflected in a reduction in body weight (Table 2). Of note is the consistency of the decrease in weight during exercise even with free access to fluids. The decrease in weight is on the order of 400 to 900 grams per hour (20,114,167). Fig. 1 shows the change in body weight of eight male subjects undertaking daily long distance runs of 1.5 to 3 hours in duration (167). Access to fluids was provided throughout the period of exercise. There did not appear to be a thirst or drinking adaptation to the daily exercise, as a consistent degree of voluntary dehydration was tolerated. Also of interest is that on the next day, 20 hours post exercise, body weight had returned to control values. This represents a rectification of the fluid losses that were incurred over the exercise. Urine flow rate also has attained control levels at this time (167,168). Consequently, while there is a net loss of fluids during exercise, primarily due to sweating, compensatory mechanisms correct the deficit within 24 hours. The compensatory mechanisms involved must entail the conservation of water by the kidneys as well as an increase in fluid intake associated with an increase in thirst.

TABLE 2. Representative fluid balance during exercise in ml/hr. Parentheses denote positive fluid factor.

1250	sweat
300	respiratory
30	renal
1580	total loss
(300)	metabolic production
(300)	fluid intake
930	net loss*

*The net loss is presumed to be reflected by the decrease in body weight.

The loss of electrolytes during the performance of daily exercise is not so readily corrected. Though plasma concentrations are decreased or maintained, the excretion of electrolytes by the kidneys is still decreased for up to 24 hours after the completion of exercise (40,101,167,168). Further, there is a tendency for certain electrolytes such as potassium to be reduced in the plasma and to have an increased loss in the urine as well. The correction of the losses in electrolytes incurred during daily exercise may not be complete within 24 hours.

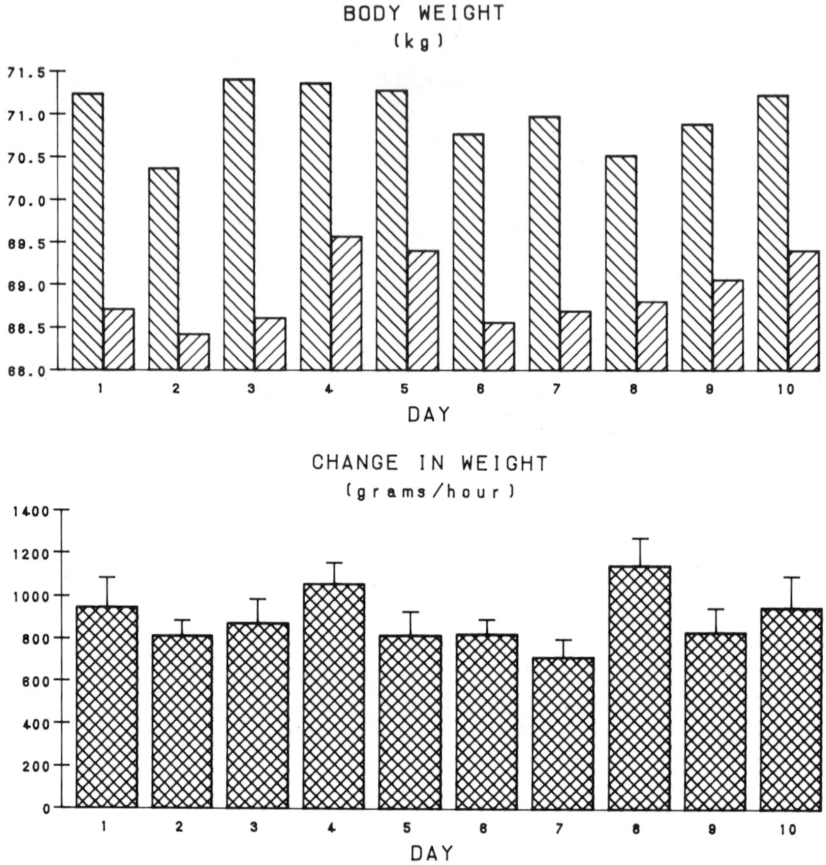

Fig. 1. Body weight pre (first bar - downsloping diagonal) and post (second bar - upsloping diagonal) exercise and the change in body weight per hour in eight male subjects undertaking daily long distance runs 1.5 to 3 hours in duration. Access to fluids was provided throughout the period of exercise. (Drawn from data obtained during previous studies by Wade et al. (167).

This deficit in total body electrolytes may be further accentuated by the losses incurred if the exercise is repeated the next day (101,167,168).

Thirst and Fluid Intake

In response to exercise there is an increase in plasma osmolality and a decrease in blood volume (57,166,173,174). Both of these factors are primary regulators of thirst and subsequently fluid intake (2,4,152,153). Thirst is the strong motivation to seek water and thus is a subjective sensation which can only be defined in man. However, the amount of fluid intake is inferred to be indicative of the sensation of thirst if satiation is achieved. During exercise there is voluntary dehydration in that even with free access to fluids a net water loss and hemoconcentration are observed (69,76,114,168). Exercising subjects will replace only one to two thirds of the fluid loss by drinking (20,114). This inappropriate thirst resulting in voluntary dehydration during exercise is paradoxical and the factors involved are not known. The quantity of fluid consumed during and following exercise is influenced by a variety of factors such as the temperature of the fluid, the time of ingestion in relation to the last meal, and taste (2,4,76,152).

Following exercise, the role of drinking in fluid replacement is not well studied (76). Though fluid losses can be replaced within 24 hours after the completion of exercise, the contribution of voluntary intake is unclear. With fluid deprivation alone, Rolls and coworker (138) found that only 65% of the volume loss was voluntarily replaced within 2 to 3 minutes. Thereafter there was a marked reduction in the rate of fluid intake. The reduction in the rate of fluid intake was initially associated with the feeling of stomach fullness and subsequently with the fall in plasma osmolality and expansion of blood volume after 12 minutes. Similar factors may play a role in the modulation of drinking after exercise. Nose et al. (118-120) recently reported that following mild exercise in the heat only 68% of the fluid loss was replaced over three hours of recovery with free access to water. When the subjects were provided with a salt solution (0.45% NaCl), 82% of the water loss was replaced over the same time period. The difference in rate of rehydration between the two fluids appeared to be related to the degree of suppression of plasma renin activity and aldosterone concentration. Suppression of these hormones would be associated with a decrease in the plasma levels of angiotensin II, a powerful dipsogen (135). Nose et al. (118-120) concluded that the delay in rehydration after exercise/heat-induced dehydration results from removal of osmotic and volume stimuli of thirst, as well as a decrease of the hormones responsible for the maintenance of sodium homeostasis due to the act of drinking. Similar findings have been noted in animals during rehydration following a period of fluid restriction (159). The rectification of total body water after exercise may ultimately be a function of the proportional distribution of the ingested fluid and electrolytes among the various body compartments. That is, rapid rehydration with water after exercise while expanding plasma volume reduces electrolyte concentrations. The retention of water in the vascular compartment before complete distribution removes the volume and osmotic drives of thirst. These stimuli are reinstated only after this water is moved out of the vascular space. Following these fluid shifts thirst would again be stimulated.

The replacement of the deficit in electrolytes induced during exercise is also unclear. Salt appetite, while identified in animals, has not been clearly defined in man (45). For instance, the study of sodium intake and its role in replacement following exercise is hampered in that in most studies, available intake far exceeds requirements. Further, in studies in which sodium intake is restricted, the kidneys conserve sodium, thus maintaining total body content. In animals, the replacement of fluid loss is isotonic if salt water is provided as well as water (2,45,153). The animals tend to drink amounts of each fluid such that plasma osmolality and volume are replaced concomitantly. Additionally, hormonal mechanisms are altered to maintain this equilibrium by regulating renal sodium reabsorption (159). In man, however, there is a lag in this response. Even with the ingestion of a salt solution, the replacement is incomplete (119). Hence, the role of electrolyte intake in the rectification of the electrolyte deficit following exercise at present is unclear.

Renal Responses to Exercise

Exercise results in a decrease in urine flow rate (Table 3) (128,129). The degree of the antidiuresis following exercise is dependent on a variety of factors. Prior fluid ingestion may attenuate or potentiate the change in flow rate dependent upon when the intake of fluids occurred in relation to the exercise. For instance, in some studies attempts are made to hydrate the subjects to guarantee an adequate urine flow, yet a non-exercise control is often not performed to evaluate the effect of the waterload alone. The renal responses to a waterload in the absence of exercise would normally present as an increase in flow rate with a subsequent fall over time. This response could mask the response to exercise. The intensity of exercise may also affect the response of urine flow rate to exercise. As the work load is increased, the flow is reduced more (81,166). Of interest is that at low work intensities, less than 35% of maximum, urine flow may be increased (81,82,166). Above this intensity of exercise the rate of urine flow is reduced. The decrease in flow rate also persists through a period post exercise. Following an acute exercise (2 min of maximal work load) in hyperhydrated subjects, pre-exercise urine flow rates were not attained within 80 min post exercise, even if the hydration status was maintained (129). Thus, during and following exercise there is a reduction in urine output facilitating the conservation of fluids and electrolytes.

The ability of the kidneys to conserve fluid and electrolytes is the product of the amount filtered and the net volume reabsorbed. The amount filtered is a function of the rate of renal blood flow. During exercise of light to moderate intensities there may be a slight increase in renal blood flow. However, if the exercise intensity is increased or the duration prolonged, renal blood flow is reduced (Fig. 2). The decrease in renal blood flow is enough to result in a reduction in glomerular filtration rate (GFR) (Table 3). Castenfors (21,28) noted that during heavy exercise of short duration, in the supine posture, renal blood flow was inversely related to the intensity of the exercise. The decrease in renal blood flow results from glomerular afferent arteriole vasoconstriction modulated by a combination of sympathetic nervous activity and circulating catecholamines (12,28). Further, the decrease in renal blood flow is accompanied by a reduction in GFR that is not a one to one relationship. The filtration fraction, the ratio of GFR to renal plasma flow, is increased from 15 to 25% (29). The increase in the filtration fraction is attributed to an increase in efferent glomerular arteriole resistance, possibly mediated by an increase in the circulating levels of angiotensin II (12). Maximal exercise results in a 40% reduction in GFR (166). During a 85 km cross country ski race, the reduction in GFR was about 30% (133,134). The decrease in GFR during the race was correlated with the reduction in urine flow rate. That is, the decrease in fluid delivered to the kidney, due to a decrease in renal blood flow, resulted in a proportional decrease in water loss via urine. However, this relationship may be altered in subjects who are well hydrated (27).

The change in the GFR, besides reducing the loss of water and solutes directly, possibly affects the tubular handling of water and solutes during exercise (121,171). Normally, 65% of the filtered sodium and water is reabsorbed in the proximal tubule (171). The active reabsorption of sodium and accompanying passive reabsorption of water in the proximal tubule are a function of the peritubular capillary oncotic pressure which could be expected

TABLE 3. Renal Function - Pre and Post Exercise

Type of Exercise	Duration (min)	Work load+	GFR (ml/min) Pre	GFR (ml/min) Post	V (ml/min) Pre	V (ml/min) Post	C_{osm} (ml/min) Pre	C_{osm} (ml/min) Post	C_{H_2O} (ml/min) Pre	C_{H_2O} (ml/min) Post	Reference
Running	30	---	135	91	0.5	0.2	1.9	0.5	-1.4	-0.4	(131)
Running		100 km	116	60	1.0	0.4					(43)
Bicycle Erg.	57	80%*			1.7	1.0	3.2	1.8	-1.5	-0.8	(110)
Bicycle Erg.	60	60%	134	112	2.7	1.2	3.5	2.4	-0.9	-1.1	(130)
Bicycle Erg.	45	119 W	188	172	15.0	8.0	4.6	3.1	10.4	4.9	(28)(h,s)
Bicycle Erg.	30	150 W	118	156	0.8	1.1					(163)
		200 W	132	140	0.7	0.9					(h)
Treadmill	60	35%	138	145	0.8	0.8	2.4	2.3	-1.6	-1.5	(166)
	60	70%	159	101	0.8	0.5	2.5	1.4	-1.7	-0.9	
	20	100%	154	88	0.7	0.4	2.3	1.3	-1.6	-0.8	
		100%	160	89	2.2	1.3	3.3	1.8	-1.1	-0.5	
Treadmill	60	5.6 km	142	165	1.1	4.9	2.0	2.3	-0.9	2.6	(81)(h)
	60	8.0 km	144	144	1.0	1.4	2.1	2.1	-1.1	-0.7	
	60	10.5 km	133	83	1.3	0.6	2.3	0.9	-1.0	-0.3	
Treadmill	30	70%			1.2	0.5	2.8	1.2	-1.6	-0.7	(178)
	30	70%			4.8	1.0	3.9	1.3	0.9	0.3	(178)
Treadmill	15	70%	98	80	1.0	0.7	2.3	1.5	-1.3	-0.8	(47)
	299	42 km		43		0.4		0.5		-0.1	
Treadmill	60	60%			1.2	0.4	3.2	1.0	-2.0	-0.6	(40)
Treadmill	15	100%	150	96	0.7	0.6					(169)
Skiing	436	85 km	121	87	0.7	0.5	2.2	1.6	-1.5	-1.1	(29)
Skiing	330	70 km	130	94	0.6	0.4					(133)

(h) Supplemental fluids provided
(s) exercise performed in the supine position
* percent of maximal oxygen consumption
\+ workload or distance (kilometers)
W = watts

to be increased as a result of the increased filtration fraction (171). This would result in an increased proportion of sodium and water reabsorption also contributing to the conservation of both solutes and water.

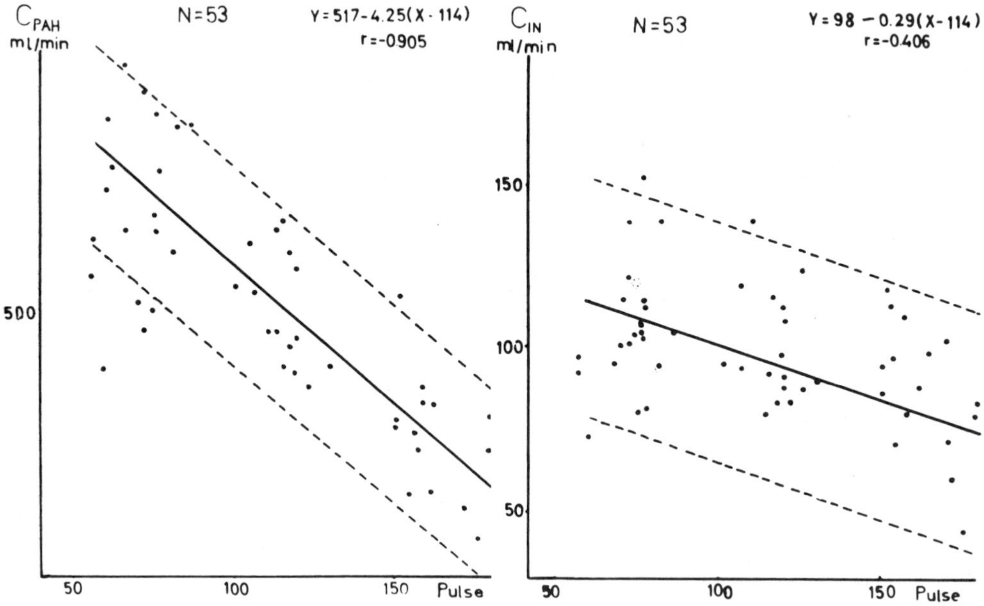

Fig. 2. Renal blood blow determined by PAH clearance and glomerular filtration rate measured by inulin clearance in relationship to heart rate in male subjects performing short heavy exercise on a bicycle ergometer in the supine position. (Reproduced with permission, reference 29)

Exercise results in an antidiuresis which, in addition to alterations in GFR, is purported to be caused by an increase in the plasma concentration of the antidiuretic hormone vasopressin (AVP). Increased AVP would be expected to produce a concentrated urine, via an increased reabsorption of water (Table 3, Fig. 3) (128,129). However, Refsum and Stromme (133,134) have suggested that prolonged exercise causes an impairment of the renal concentrating mechanism. In subjects participating in a 70 km cross-country ski race of 4.5 to 6.5 hours in duration, they found urine flow rate to be decreased from 0.6 to 0.4 ml/min and the urine osmolality to be decreased to 621 mOsm/kg H_2O compared to the value at the start of the race, 911 mOsm/kg H_2O. The decrease in urinary solute concentration accompanying a reduction in urine flow rate and in GFR suggested a decline in urinary concentrating ability. In a subsequent study (134) they confirmed this finding and reported a decline in the urine to plasma

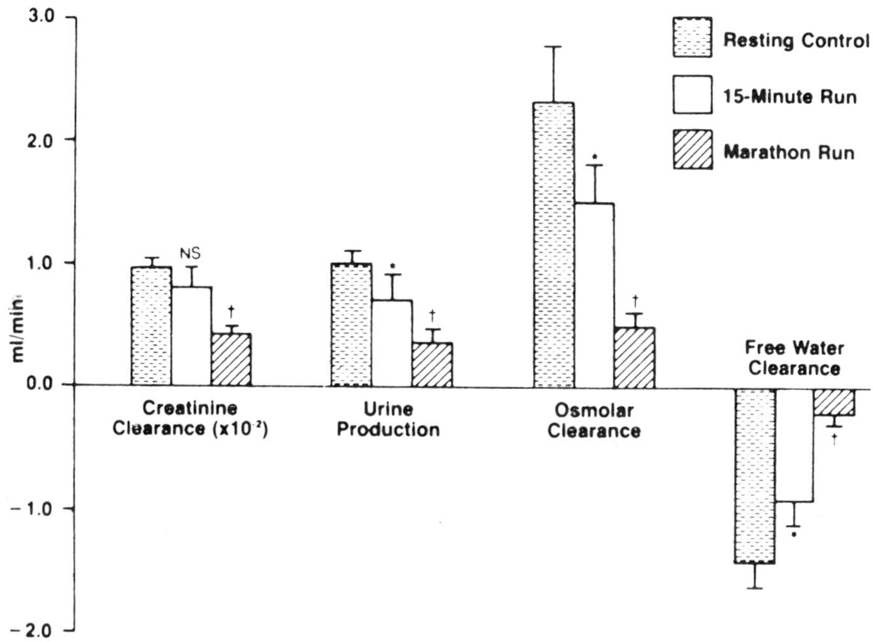

*Fig. 3. Renal function during treadmill running for 15 min and a marathon running for an average of 299 min. The running was performed at similar intensities, approximately 70% of maximum oxygen uptake. The subjects were five trained individuals with diagnosed coronary heart disease who showed no difference from a control population. * different from control; + different from control and 15-min run ($P < 0.05$). (Reproduced with permission, reference 47)*

osmolality ratio as well. Kachadorian and Johnson (81,82) report that moderate exercise results in a concentrated urine production, while heavy exercise impairs the concentrating mechanism. The inability to maximize the renal concentrating mechanism, and thus maximally conserve water during heavy exercise when the loss of water through other routes would presumably be greater, is paradoxical.

The antidiuresis during exercise is often attributed to a concentrated urine when in fact, in relation to plasma osmolality, which increases during exercise, urinary osmolality is decreased (146,166). This results in a reduction in the urine to plasma ratio as mentioned previously. The decrease in this ratio and in the rate of urine flow results in a reduction in the calculated osmotic clearance rate (Table 3, Fig. 3). That is, there is an increase in solute reabsorption during exercise reflected in a decrease in the percent of filtered osmotic load excreted. An example of the decrease in the percent of the filtered load excreted for various solutes is shown in Fig. 4 during short and prolonged exercise. Similar findings are noted by other investigators (101,133,164). The increase in reabsorption of solutes may in part be due to the combination of decreased GFR and increased filtration fraction as mentioned above. The increase in reabsorption leads to a decrease in osmotic clearance and thus to a decrease in urine flow rate. In Fig. 5 the relationship of urine flow rate to osmotic clearance is shown. The difference between the osmotic clearance and urine flow rate is due to water reabsorption in the collecting duct. The rate of water reabsorption (TC_{H_2O}) is the deviation of the relationship of osmotic clearance to urine flow from the line of identity. Thus, as urine flow is reduced during exercise less water is reabsorbed (134,146,166). Another way of expressing this is by the use of the term free water clearance (C_{H_2O}), which is the difference between urine flow rate and osmotic clearance or the negative

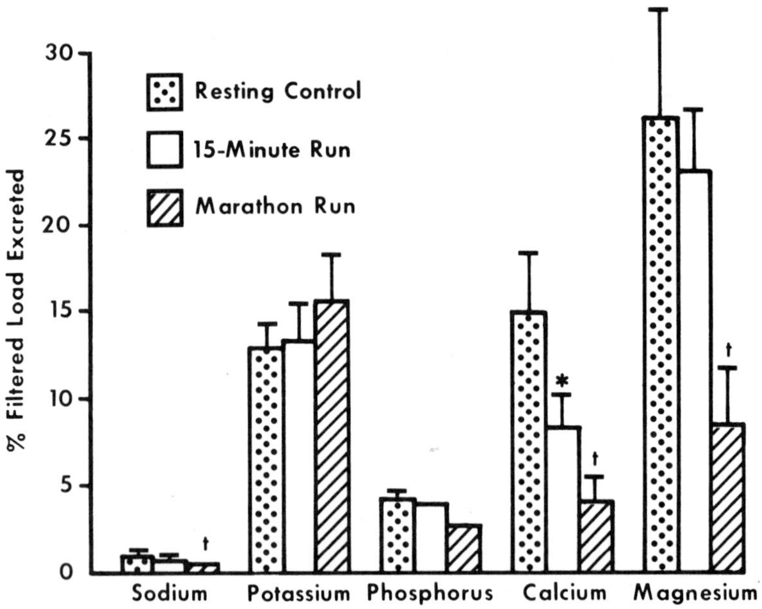

*Fig. 4. Fractional excretion rates of filtered electrolytes at rest, after a 15 min treadmill run and a marathon run, 299 min in duration. Values were determined in five subjects with the running intensities being approximately 70% of maximum oxygen uptake for both tests. * and + see Fig. 3 legend. (Reproduced with permission, reference 47)*

value of tubular water reabsorption. Since some degree of tubular water reabsorption is usually occurring, free water clearance is a negative number. The negativity of free water clearance has led to some confusion. That is, as free water clearance becomes less negative the urine is less concentrated due to a reduced tubular reabsorption. This is the case during exercise (Table 3, Fig. 3). Though urine flow rate is decreased during exercise, the reduction in osmotic clearance is greater. This difference in the degree of the decreases in urine flow rate and the rate of osmotic clearance results in a calculated increase in free water clearance or a reduction in tubular water reabsorption.

At the end of the ascending loop of Henle the filtrate is hypoosmotic. The ability to produce a concentrated urine from the end of distal tubule to the end of the collecting duct is dependent upon: a) the tonicity of the interstitial fluid of the renal medulla; b) sufficient delivery of urea to the collecting duct; c) the presence of AVP and d) the ability of the distal tubule and collecting duct cells to respond to AVP. As previously alluded to, the concentrating ability of the kidneys is compromised during exercise and alterations of each of the above parameters has been offered as an explanation (134,146,166).

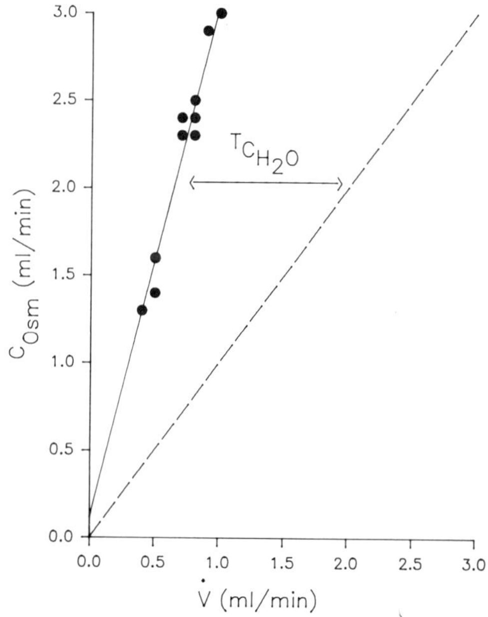

Fig. 5. The relationship of osmotic clearance (C_{osm}) and urine flow rate (V) during exercise. The isosmotic state that the dashed line represents is a urine osmolality equal to plasma osmolality. The shift of the relationship of C_{osm} to V to the left indicates a concentrated urine. The difference between the two lines is the rate of tubular water reabsorption (TC_{H_2O}). During exercise, as urine flow rate is decreased, C_{osm} and TC_{H_2O} are reduced, that is, the urine is then less concentrated. (Drawn from data in reference 166)

The tonicity of the renal medullary interstitial fluid is dependent upon the reabsorption of sodium in excess of water in the ascending loop of Henle (161). Exercise produces a decrease in GFR and an increase in proximal tubular reabsorption of sodium. This results in a decrease in the delivery to the ascending loop of Henle and results in a reduction in the medullary concentration gradient. The gradient could also be decreased by an increase in medullary capillary blood flow which is dependent on arterial pressure. During exercise there is an increase in arterial blood pressure and a redistribution of renal blood flow from the renal cortex to the medulla which could result in the "washing out" of the medullary concentration gradient.

The medullary recycling of urea is important in maintaining the concentration gradient (6,96,99,161). Exercise reduces the filtered load of urea, as GFR is decreased. The passive reabsorption of urea in the proximal tubule may also be increased. The net result is a decrease in urea delivery to the loop of Henle collecting duct. This could result in a decrease in the amount of urea available for the development of the medullary gradient.

At rest, plasma AVP concentration is directly related to the urine to plasma osmolality ratio (9,13,161,172). That is, as the plasma levels increase a more concentrated urine is produced due to an increase in the reabsorption of water in the collecting duct. During exercise this relationship is not observed (166). AVP levels are increased during exercise (see below), yet the urine concentration is reduced and tubular water reabsorption is decreased. It has been suggested that the action on the collecting duct of AVP may be inhibited during exercise. Prostaglandins are effective blockers of the actions of AVP and are elevated during exercise (3,50,177). However, the dilution of urine may be induced even at rest in the presence of adequate AVP levels and no change in prostaglandin concentrations if there is a decrease in GFR of 30% or more (98-100,121). At workloads greater than 70% of maximum, GFR is decreased by more than 30% and is accompanied by an increase in free water clearance even though AVP levels are increased. Therefore, a decrease in urinary concentrating ability during exercise may occur despite elevated levels of plasma AVP.

The impairment of the renal concentrating ability during exercise appears to be primarily a function of the reduction in GFR. Refsum and Stromme (134) found the change in GFR to be related to the decrease in urine concentration. However, within minutes following exercise the GFR is returned to resting levels yet an increase in tubular water reabsorption is often not observed, possibly reflecting the time necessary to reestablish the renal medullary concentration gradient (166).

Even if the fluids and food provided offer adequate water intake, they may not rectify the electrolyte losses incurred during exercise. Following heavy daily exercise there is a reduction in the percent of filtered sodium excreted, indicative of an increased tubular reabsorption and conservation. This conservation may persist over 48 hours even if the diet is adequate and salt is provided ad libitum (55,86,167,168). Thus, renal mechanisms play a role in rectification of the loss of electrolytes that occurred during exercise. This conservation of sodium has led to speculation that there may be a potassium deficit following heavy exercise since potassium is exchanged for sodium in the distal tubule of the kidney in the presence of aldosterone (90). Sodium is actively reabsorbed and potassium secreted to maintain electroneutrality. This loss of potassium coupled with the losses due to sweating have raised concern as to the maintenance of potassium homeostasis with heavy exercise (90).

Summary of Fluid and Electrolyte Homeostasis During Exercise

Exercise results in the loss of water and electrolytes, primarily due to sweating. The correction of this water loss following exercise is predominately by an increase in fluid intake. However, the water loss is not fully rectified within the first four hours after exercise, apparently due to voluntary dehydration due to an inappropriate or incomplete sensation of thirst. Water balance is restored within 24 hours. Renal conservation of water occurs during and following exercise passively as it is primarily due to reabsorption accompanying the increased reabsorption of solutes to rectify their loss. There does not appear to be an increase specifically in water reabsorption, and in fact it may decrease during exercise. Though electrolyte reabsorption by the kidneys is increased and adequate quantities are available from consumption in the diet, the losses incurred during exercise may not be corrected within 48 hours. A variety of hormonal systems play roles in these corrections of losses of water and electrolytes resulting from exercise.

HORMONAL EFFECTS OF EXERCISE

Exercise produces increases in the circulating concentrations of a variety of hormones. To be discussed here are those thought to impact on the maintenance of fluid and electrolyte homeostasis. The hormones of particular interest are AVP, atrial natriuretic peptide and aldosterone (149). These hormones are progressively increased during exercise (Fig. 6) and have been shown at rest to modify the loss of fluids and electrolytes from the kidneys or in sweat. Further, the role of these hormones and the renin-angiotensin system in thirst and the subsequent restoration of fluid loss by drinking will also be considered.

In considering the activities of hormones, plasma concentration is assumed to be the determining factor. The concentration of a hormone in the plasma is a function of the rate of release and of the rate of metabolism. In the following discussions the rate of release in response to exercise has been concentrated upon; however, the metabolism of the various hormones may also be altered. The possibility of a change in the rate of metabolic clearance during exercise is likely as blood flow is redistributed away from organs such as the liver and kidney (139). Changes in the clearance, due to exercise, of the hormones to be discussed have not specifically been investigated. A change in the number of receptors for the hormones may also occur during exercise and therefore affect the activity of the hormones.

Vasopressin

The neurohypophyseal hormone AVP is increased during exercise (Table 4) (165). The reported basal levels of AVP are variable, from 1 to 4 pg/ml. These differences are due to different assay procedures and the hydration status of the subjects. Despite these differences, if the same type of maximal exercise is performed, the response of AVP is similar. For instance, after a maximal treadmill exercise, a six to eight fold increase in AVP levels is observed independent of the investigator performing the study. Maximal bicycle ergometer exercise produces a 4 to 6 fold increase (Table 4). The response to maximal exercise is not altered due to the training status of the subjects (35,38,60,61,65,110) and is similar in males and females (105).

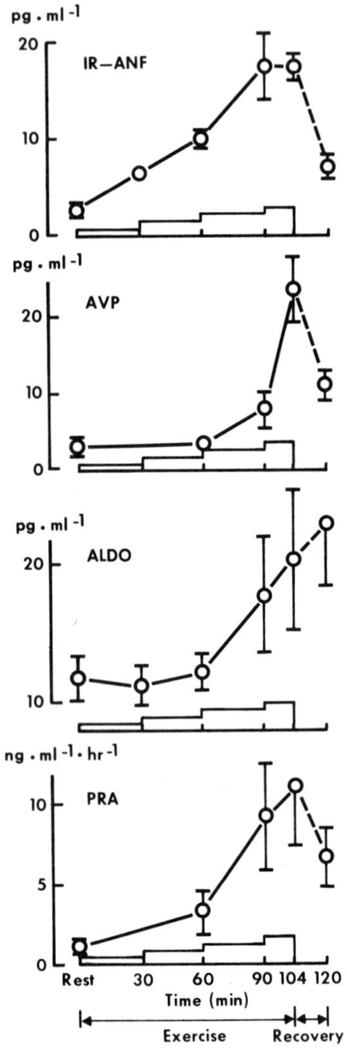

Fig. 6. Hormonal responses to exercise of five subjects performing exercise on a bicycle ergometer at 50, 100, 150 and 196 watts or 32.6, 49.4, 71.4, and 88% of maximum oxygen uptake. The dashed line represents the value at 15 min post exercise. (Reproduced with permission, reference 155)

Table 4. Plasma vasopressin levels in response to exercise

Exercise	Workload	PAVP (pg/ml) Pre	PAVP (pg/ml) Post	Reference
Bicycle Erg.	65%	1.0	8.3	(35)
Bicycle Erg.	100 W	1.5	2.2	(37) (c)
	175 W		7.1	
	225 W		20.5	
Bicycle Erg.	100 W(50%)	1.0	1.0	(38) (c)
	175 W(75%)		3.4	
	225 W(90%)		7.9	
Bicycle Erg.	80%	3.0	14.4	(110) (c)
Bicycle Erg.	87%	3.6	5.1	(65)
Bicycle Erg.	49%	3.3	3.5	(155) (c)
	71%		7.7	
	88%		25.0	
Bicycle Erg.	85 W	4.7	8.5	(23) (h)
	85 W	4.7	4.5	
Treadmill	35%	2.8	3.2	(166) (c)
	70%	2.0	5.3	
	100%	2.2	6.8	
Treadmill	100%	1.2	5.1	(169) (c)
Treadmill	100%	1.6	24.5	(60) (c)
Treadmill	100%	3.8	15.8	(105)
Treadmill	1 mph	2.8	2.2	(108)

(c) calculated from figures; (h) hydrated

Of note is that the response of AVP to exercise is variable between subjects but remarkably reproducible within an individual. As an example, Maresh et al. (105), in a study of women performing maximal treadmill exercise, found that the individual responses ranged from 3 to 50 pg/ml but the response was very repeatable within an individual. Further, following training at a similar relative workload, the AVP response to exercise is the same.

The increase in AVP levels in response to submaximal work is variable. In response to an increasing work load, plasma AVP concentrations show a threshold response (Fig. 6). That is, above a workload of 70% of maximum oxygen consumption, an increase is observed (38,155). However, this response is dependent upon the duration of the exercise. At a workload of 70% of maximum oxygen consumption, AVP concentrations were not altered after 20 minutes but were increased after 60 minutes (166). On a bicycle ergometer at a workload of 65% of maximum for two hours, an 88% increase in plasma levels of AVP was observed (36). At a similar work load, six minutes of exercise failed to produce a change (38). Thus, the response of AVP to exercise is modulated by the intensity, duration, and mode of exercise. Following maximal exercise, resting AVP levels are attained within one hour (60,166,169). Daily exercise does not alter the basal plasma levels or the urinary excretion rate of AVP (167). Further, there is no difference in basal levels in trained subjects compared to controls (60,61). In longitudinal studies, resting AVP levels are not altered after training in males (35,36,38,65,110); however, in females basal values were decreased (105). The reason for this difference in the studies of Maresh et al. (105) may be related to the initial levels in the females being high, 3.8 pg/ml, compared to normal levels.

Regulation. AVP is modulated by a variety of factors, many of which are altered during exercise (13,145,149). Of primary interest are the increase in plasma osmolality and reduction in blood volume which occur during exercise (57,165). AVP is released in response to an increase in plasma osmolality as sensed by a cerebral osmoreceptor. The AVP response to changes in plasma osmolality is linear when threshold values are exceeded (13,137). During maximal exercise, plasma osmolality is increased by 10 to 20 mOsm/kg H_2O (38,155,166,169). At rest this would induce an increase in plasma AVP on the order of 3 to 6 pg/ml (13,71,137). This increase, while less than that incurred during exercise, would still account for the majority of the increase. A variety of investigators have demonstrated a relationship between the change in plasma osmolality and AVP concentration during exercise and this would appear to be the primary mediator of release (35,166).

The reduction in blood volume during exercise could mediate the release of AVP during exercise (13,145,148). The performance of exercise results in a decrease in plasma volume directly related to the intensity (166,173). Maximal exercise results in a decrease on the order of 14% (166,173). Reduction of the plasma volume by hemorrhage or dehydration to the same degree as that observed during exercise results in a significant increase in plasma AVP levels (31,149). The increase in plasma AVP concentration is exponentially related to the decrease in blood volume, and is sensed by low and high pressure baroreceptors. However, exercise produces an increase in mean arterial pressure, thus negating a role of high pressure baroreceptors in the increase in AVP (155,166). The increase in mean arterial pressure could in fact provide a negative input. Further, the role of the low pressure cardiopulmonary baroreceptors is questionable in that the response of central venous pressure is transient (139). At the onset of exercise central venous pressure is increased with a reduction occurring during prolonged exercise as "cardiovascular drift" occurs. This may in part explain the differential response due to exercise duration. That is, initially the increase in central venous pressure suppresses AVP while later the decrease facilitates the release. In conclusion, while exercise may induce a decrease in calculated or measured blood volume, the effective blood volume as sensed by the high and low baroreceptors may actually be increased and thus would blunt the release of AVP.

A variety of other factors (165) are suggested to play a role in the release of AVP during exercise including: angiotensin II (132,135), body temperature (33,72), hydration status (166), psychological factors (140), metabolism, and peripheral nerve stimulation. These factors appear to modulate the response of AVP release to the primary regulator during exercise, i.e., the increase in plasma osmolality.

Actions. An increase in plasma AVP level is normally associated with renal conservation of fluids induced by an increase in water reabsorption in the collecting duct (13,172). The increased water reabsorption in the collecting tubule results in a more concentrated urine. In resting subjects changes in plasma AVP concentrations on the order of 5 to 7 pg/ml result in a maximally concentrated urine (13). This change in plasma levels is similar to that induced during heavy exercise; however, a decrease in urine concentration is noted rather than the expected increase (133,134,166). This is indicative of a reduction in the reabsorption of water in the collecting duct even though AVP is increased. This increase in free water clearance in the presence of an elevation of plasma AVP levels may be due to the physical properties of water reabsorption in the kidneys as we have previously discussed. However, the blockade of the actions of AVP on the collecting duct is a possible explanation for the kidneys' inability to produce a concentrated urine. If the decrease in GFR during exercise exceeds 30%, the actions of AVP may be negated (98,100). However, following recovery from heavy long duration exercise when the decrease in GFR has been rectified and AVP levels are still elevated, the increase in free water clearance (a reduction in tubular water reabsorption) persists (166). Prostaglandins are effective blockers of the action of AVP on the collecting duct and are increased during exercise (177). The increase in free water clearance could be attributed in part to the inhibition of the actions of AVP by prostaglandins (3). Zambraski et al. (178) evaluated the possible role of prostaglandins in the increase in free water clearance in euhydrated and dehydrated subjects. The prostaglandins were inhibited by the administration of aspirin for three days before testing. The exercise was 30 min of treadmill running at 70% of maximum oxygen uptake. The blockade of prostaglandin synthesis did not alter the changes in free water clearance during exercise in either hydrated or dehydrated subjects. Therefore, the reason for the decrease in tubular water reabsorption in the presence of an increase in plasma AVP following exercise is unclear but appears to be independent of the increase in prostaglandin levels and the physical properties involved in renal function.

Changes in plasma AVP levels during exercise have been implicated in the modulation of plasma volume, specifically the increase associated with training (35). Following training, plasma concentrations of AVP are not altered at rest or during exercise even though plasma volume may be expanded (35,60,65,110). The absence of a change in plasma levels does not negate a possible role of

AVP in the expansion of plasma volume in that receptor sensitivity may be increased. Following exercise, trained subjects have been reported to expand plasma volume during recovery from exercise, and to better defend plasma volume in response to maneuvers such as postural changes or immersion (32,60,176). This better maintenance of plasma volume in trained subjects has in part been attributed to AVP (35) but other mechanisms must be involved. As yet, the exact role of AVP in the modulation of plasma volume during and following exercise is not defined.

AVP is suggested to decrease extrarenal water loss (144). The increase in plasma AVP during exercise is also suggested to play a role in the secretion rate and composition of sweat (52,66). Subcutaneous injection of AVP decreases the rate of secretion and concentration of sweat induced by thermal stimulation at the local site (52). However, a relationship has not been demonstrated between plasma level of AVP and the rate of secretion or concentration of sweat. In trained individuals in whom the rate of sweating is increased and the electrolyte concentration decreased, the plasma AVP levels would not be different than that of untrained subjects at a similar relative workload (35,36). Thus, AVP does not appear to play a role in the regulation of sweating induced during exercise or in the alterations due to training. AVP has been implicated in the regulation of thirst (2). However, the response is acute and has only been demonstrated in animals. It does not appear that AVP modulates thirst during exercise.

Atrial Natriuretic Peptide

Atrial natriuretic peptide (also called atrial natriuretic factor, ANF), is released from the atria in response to distention induced by pressure or other mechanical manipulations (68). ANF is believed to modulate the excretion of sodium with an accompanying loss of water. Thus, an increase in ANF during exercise would result in an additional loss of both water and salt.

In fact, a variety of investigators have demonstrated ANF to be increased during acute exercise (Table 5) (62). With maximal exercise, the increase in ANF is on the order of 500%, from resting values of 10 to 30 pg/ml to those at the end of exercise, 50 to 90 pg/ml. Of note is the consistency of this observation between investigators and the independence from the mode of exercise (treadmill vs cycle ergometer). The response to acute exercise demonstrates a relationship with exercise intensity (Fig. 6). However, whether the relationship is a function of relative or absolute workload has not been specifically investigated. It appears however that relative workload is the primary modulator in the acute response in that at maximal work (100%) there is no difference observed between trained and untrained subjects despite the absolute workload being much greater in the trained subjects (60,61). Following completion of heavy exercise, basal levels are attained within 60 minutes (56,60).

The duration of exercise may also play a role in the response of ANF. As the duration of exercise increases, the concentration of ANF may decrease. Freund et al. (59) found ANF levels to be increased in the initial phase of a

Table 5. Atrial Natriuretic Factor Responses to Exercise.

Type of Exercise	Level of Exercise	Baseline ANF Values (pg/ml)	Exercise ANF Values (pg/ml)	Reference
Treadmill	100%	12.7	87.5	(60)
	100%	15.0	77.8	
Cycle Ergometry	50 W	97.0	106.0	(63)(b,c)
	100 W		122.0	
	150 W		165.0	
	200 W		176.0	
Treadmill	Stages I-IV of Bruce Protocol	20.4	82.0	(75)
Cycle Ergometry	50 W	42.0	40.5(c)	(85) (c,e)
	100 W		51.0(c)	
	150 W		55.5(c)	
	200 W		81.0(c)	
Treadmill	Stages I-IV of Bruce Protocol	25.5	98.1	(122)
Cycle Ergometry	75 W	36.0	42.0	(126) (c)
	100%		90.0	
Cycle Ergometry	20%	39.0	39.6	(142) (s)
	40%	46.5	95.4	
Cycle Ergometry	100 W	14.1	22.2	(150)
	100%		50.1	
Cycle Ergometry	30%	2.6	6.5	(155)
	50%		10.0	
	70%		17.4	
	90%		17.2	

(continued)

Table 5. (continued)

Type of Exercise	Level of Exercise	Baseline ANF Values (pg/ml)	Exercise ANF Values (pg/ml)	Reference
Cycle Ergometry	50 W	54.0	51.0	(156) (c)
	100 W		55.5	
	150 W		60.0	
	200 W		87.0	
Cycle Ergometry	50 W	51.5	42.0	(157) (c)
	100 W		54.5	
	150 W		61.5	
	200 W		92.1	

All values for ANF have been converted to pg/ml and unless indicated, were on extracted plasma.

(b) indicates ANF levels were determined on unextracted plasma.
(c) indicates values were estimated from figure in manuscript.
(e) indicates it is unknown if ANF levels were determined on extracted or unextracted plasma.
(%) percent of maximum oxygen consumption
(s) supine exercise

marathon race. At the end of the race, values were still increased compared to control levels, but were reduced compared to those during the initial phase of the race. Chan and coworkers (30) observed a decrease in the concentration of ANF at the end of a marathon though initial values were high. The duration of the exercise thus appears to play an important role in the response of ANF to exercise.

Resting levels of ANF are increased with age (127). Freund et al. (59) compared the ANF levels of young and middle aged men during the first 10 km of a marathon race. Though no significant difference was observed at rest, the response to exercise was greater in the older subjects, 124 pg/ml compared to 55 pg/ml. The response of ANF to exercise appears to be accentuated in older subjects.

Regulation. ANF has been proposed to be released in response to tachycardia (62). Since exercise is associated with an increase in heart rate, it has been speculated that this increase contributes in part to the elevation of ANF levels during exercise (48,63). In fact, the rise during exercise has been correlated with the increase in heart rate (142,150). However, others have not observed a relationship (116,117,156,157). Thamsborg et al. (156,157) provide evidence that ANF is not modulated by heart rate. In subjects performing exercise after beta-1 adrenoreceptor blockade the increase in ANF was greater than that without blockade even though the rise in heart rate was markedly reduced. Even more convincing is the report by Walsh et al. (170) in which atrial pacing was performed in dogs both with and without atrial pressure being held constant via balloon occlusion of the inferior vena cava. Their results clearly demonstrate that the release of ANF during tachycardia is primarily dependent on increased atrial pressure and not heart rate. Therefore the increase in heart rate during exercise does not appear to be a major modulator in the increase in ANF.

Increases in atrial stretch or pressure provide the most significant input into the stimulation of ANF release (107,130). The changes in ANF associated with heart rate and mean arterial pressure may well be the result of concomitant changes in atrial pressure. Exercise increases atrial pressure but this response can be transitory if the exercise is prolonged and the thermal load is significant. This is due to the phenomena of "cardiovascular drift" (139). At the onset of exercise, the increase is larger compared to late in exercise when blood volume is redistributed to compensate for the increase in heat stores. Late in exercise, as venous return is reduced and atrial pressure is reduced, ANF levels may also decrease. This may provide an explanation for the transient response of ANF during a marathon run (30,59). During the beginning of the race atrial pressures are increased, resulting in the release of ANF. Late in the race, when blood flow is redistributed and atrial pressure decreased, ANF levels fall and could be decreased below resting values. Of interest is the recent study of cardiac transplant patients showing an increase in ANF in response to exercise (42). This suggests that despite denervation, exercise stimulated the release of ANF, presumably by direct mechanostimulation. Increases in atrial pressure or stretch are the primary mediator of plasma ANF concentrations at rest and appear to be the predominant regulators during exercise as well.

Actions. The injection of ANF at pharmacological doses produces a diuresis and a natriuresis. Manipulation increasing plasma ANF concentrations also results in an increase in urine flow with an accompanying natriuresis (63,68,113,141). Though the increase in ANF and alterations in urine function occur concomitantly, a direct relationship has been questioned (68,95). Further, during heavy acute exercise in the presence of an increase in ANF an antidiuresis and conservation of sodium occurs.

The renal response to low intensity exercise could be mediated by ANF. At low intensity exercise a natriuresis and a diuresis may occur (10,81,82,163). These changes in renal function may be the result of an increase in ANF levels that occurs prior to the increase in other hormones and the reduction in GFR. Tanaka et al. (155) found ANF levels to be increased at a workload of 35% of maximum, well below the exercise intensity necessary to increase plasma AVP or aldosterone concentrations. Unfortunately, measurements of renal function were not obtained during this study. Virvidakis et al. (163) found low intensity exercise (bicycle ergometer 100/150 W) at a workload similar to that in the study of Tanaka et al. (155) to increase urine flow rate from 0.8 to 1.1 ml/min and sodium excretion rate from 115 to 154 umol/min after one hour. These changes accompanied an increase in glomerular filtration rate from 118 to 156 ml/min in the absence of a change in plasma concentration of sodium. Kachadorian and Johnson (81,82) note similar changes during moderate treadmill exercise. Thus, the diuresis and natriuresis reported with low intensity exercise could in part be due to an increase in plasma ANF concentrations.

Release of ANF can modulate the release of other hormones important in the maintenance of fluid and electrolyte homeostasis. These hormones have actions antagonistic to those of ANF. The release of AVP in response to a decrease in blood volume or osmotic stimulation is attenuated by the infusion of ANF. The administration of ANF to a human subject reduces resting PRA and aldosterone levels (41). However, the doses infused to elicit changes in these other hormones would produce plasma concentrations far in excess of those attained during exercise (16). Therefore, the role of ANF in the regulation of these hormones during exercise is not yet defined.

The actions of ANF in the modulation of thirst during exercise or on the secretion of water and electrolytes from sweat glands have yet to be investigated. It is possible that ANF may have a role in these functions, but during exercise the observed responses would be opposed to the actions of ANF. Januszewicz et al. (79) have found ANF to decrease with water deprivation in rats. Within three minutes of rehydration basal values were attained. These data suggest ANF may be modulated by an oropharyngeal reflex similar to that of AVP (64,158). Further, other investigators (77,78,83,106) suggest that ANF may have antidipsogenic actions. Others (160) have suggested ANF may also regulate salt appetite in animals. Thus, the plasma concentrations of ANF could inhibit thirst and rapidly be altered in response to fluid intake following exercise.

Renin-angiotensin System

Renin is released from the juxtaglomerular apparatus in the kidney and converts angiotensinogen to angiotensin I. In the lung angiotensin I is converted to angiotensin II, which modulates the release of aldosterone from the adrenal cortex and is a powerful dipsogen (135,136). This cascade is potentiated during exercise and subsequently plays an important role in the regulation of fluid and electrolyte homeostasis.

Exercise increases plasma renin activity (PRA; Table 6). With increasing workloads a progressive rise in PRA is observed above a threshold which occurs at about 70% of maximum oxygen consumption (Fig. 6). Gleim and coworkers (67) equated this increase with attainment of the anaerobic threshold, that point during progressive exercise at which there is an abrupt increase in plasma lactate, minute ventilation, and CO_2 production. The percent change in PRA was correlated with the change in blood lactate. This hypothesis was further evaluated by the performance of isokinetic leg exercises which increased plasma lactate levels in the absence of some of the hemodynamic changes associated with bicycle ergometer exercise. The increase in PRA in response to the isokinetic exercise was also correlated with the rise in blood lactate. It thus appears that the increase in PRA during exercise is somehow related to the

Table 6. Plasma renin activity and angiotensin II levels in response to exercise

Exercise	Workload	PRA (ng AI/ml/hr)		AII (ng/L)		Reference
		Pre	Post	Pre	Post	
Bicycle Erg.	65%	1.6	12.3			(35)
Bicycle Erg.	100 W	2.0	3.4			(37) (c)
	175 W		5.1			
	225 W		7.5			
Bicycle Erg.	100 W(50%)	2.0	3.9			(38) (c)
	175 W(75%)		6.5			
	225 W(90%)		15.1			
Bicycle Erg.	80%	0.6	2.8			(110) (c)
Bicycle Erg.	87%	1.6	6.0			(65)
Bicycle Erg.	50 W	1.3	1.6			(49)
	110 W		1.9			
	124 W		2.7			
Bicycle Erg.	45%	5.9	9.2	43	94	(103) (c)
	75%		16.1		168	
Bicycle Erg.	100%	0.5	1.5	17	61	(51) (c)
Bicycle Erg.	39%	1.0	1.1	20	22	(50)
	83%		2.0		51	
	100%		2.7		123	
Bicycle Erg.	49%	1.2	3.4			(155) (c)
	71%		9.2			
	88%		11.1			
Bicycle Erg.	85 W	4.7	18.1			(23)
	85 W		3.4			(h)
Bicycle Erg.	100-120 W	2.5	4.1			(175)
	100-120 W	2.1	2.7			
Bicycle Erg.	40%	1.0	1.2			(93)
	70%		2.8			
	100%		3.5			

(continued)

Table 6. (continued)

Exercise	Workload	PRA (ng AI/ml/hr) Pre	PRA (ng AI/ml/hr) Post	AII (ng/L) Pre	AII (ng/L) Post	Reference
Bicycle Erg.	30%	0.9	1.2	25	26	(151)
	60%		1.8		41	
	100%		3.1		146	
Treadmill	35%	0.3	0.8			(166) (c)
	70%	0.4	2.6			
	100%	0.3	2.5			
Treadmill	60%	0.9	2.8	14	54	(40) (c)
Treadmill	100%	1.4	5.6			(169) (c)
Treadmill	100%	2.5	8.9			(60) (c)
Treadmill	1 mph	3.3	2.4			(108)
Treadmill	100%	4.4	24.9			(70)
Swimming	100%	3.7	12.5			
Treadmill	100%	1.6	6.8			(105)
Running	Marathon	1.6	4.9			(20)
Running	3x300 m	2.4	4.1	22	93	(91)
Running	3x300 ml	2.3	4.0	23	94	(1) (c)
Skiing	85 km	1.7	6.6			(22)

(c) calculated from figures; (h) hydrated;
(%)= % of maximal oxygen consumption

onset of anaerobiosis during exercise. Though PRA is closely related to the intensity of exercise, the response may be modulated due to a variety of factors such as mode of exercise, diet or body position (see below).

Exercise duration affects PRA in that at exercise workloads below the threshold, an increase may be elicited. Wade and Claybaugh (166) noted an increase in PRA after one hour of exercise at 35% while after 20 min an increase was not observed. At a workload of 70%, PRA was increased at 20 min and further elevated at 60 min. The performance of long duration exercise may increase PRA to values that exceed those observed following acute maximal exercise. Freund et al. (59) found maximal exercise to increase PRA to 9 ng AI/ml/hr while at the end of a marathon race the levels were 12 ng AI/ml/hr. This difference in the PRA response due to exercise duration demonstrates that lactate concentration is not the sole determinate of the increase in that at the end of a marathon, levels were lower, 2.5 mM (20) compared to levels attained at the end of acute maximal exercise, 7 mM (166). Other factors besides those associated with the onset of anaerobiosis must contribute to the increase in PRA during long duration exercise.

Information as to the effect of training on PRA at rest and during exercise is conflicting. Fagard et al. (50), comparing runners and nonathletes, found resting concentrations to be lower in the runners, yet the rate of change in response to exercise was similar. M'Buyamba-Kabangu et al. (102) reported a negative relationship between peak oxygen consumption and resting PRA, while Geyssant et al. (65) found both resting and exercise levels of PRA to be decreased with training. Convertino et al. (35,38) studied the PRA response to exercise before and after a short period of intense training. Though an increase in peak oxygen consumption was induced, resting PRA and the response to the relative workload were not altered. Other investigators, using both longitudinal and cross sectional studies, do not observe a difference in resting or exercise PRA (60,61,105,110). Therefore, the exact effect of training on PRA regulation at rest and during exercise is still unclear.

The increase in PRA during exercise is correlated with the increase in angiotensin II (151). Infusion of renin at rest results in an increase in angiotensin II, while the infusion of angiotensin II reduces PRA (136). Thus, it is inferred that the increase in angiotensin II during exercise is due to the rise in PRA. During exercise, angiotensin II levels are increased exhibiting effects of intensity and duration similar to those of PRA (Table 6). Training, however, results in a slightly different response. Fagard et al. (50) found resting angiotensin II levels not to be altered in trained subjects but the response to exercise was attenuated. This is surprising in light of the lower resting PRA and similar response to exercise as noted earlier. The reason for this disparity is not clear but the relationship of PRA to angiotensin II may be dissociated by a variety of factors (see below).

Regulation. The release of renin from the juxtaglomerular cells in the kidney is altered by a variety of physical, neural, and hormonal factors. The degree of stretch of the renal arterioles by hydrostatic pressure modulates renin release (136). The elevation of blood pressure during exercise would provide a negative input into the release of renin; however, renal arterioles are constricted as indicated by a decrease in renal blood flow. Therefore, the reduction in renal blood flow due to neural inputs may facilitate the release of renin during exercise. In dogs, which do not have a change in renal blood flow during exercise, renin is still increased, suggesting other mechanisms of regulation at least in this species (179).

Sympathetic nerve activity is increased during exercise, as are circulating levels of catecholamines (154). An increase in sympathetic nerve activity stimulates the release of renin. A number of investigators have studied the role of sympathetic nerves in the regulation of the increase in renin during exercise by using blocking agents (21,97,104). These studies are complicated by the fact that sympathetic nerve activity also modulates renal blood flow. Hence, the relative roles of changes in sympathetic nerve activity versus renal blood flow could not be clearly delineated. Zambraski and coworkers (179) were able to separate the role of the change in renal blood flow and sympathetic nerve activity by using dogs, a species in which renal blood flow is not changed during exercise. These studies clearly demonstrate that in exercising dogs the increase in renin release is due to the increase in sympathetic nerve activity independent of the change in renal blood flow. Beta-1 receptors were specifically implicated in the response as blockade of these receptors eliminated the increase in renin during exercise. This study also demonstrated that the release of renin during exercise was independent of alterations in renal prostaglandin synthesis. Subsequent study of human subjects supports the finding that beta-1 receptors modulate the PRA response to exercise (73).

The increase in plasma angiotensin II levels during exercise may provide a negative feedback on the release of renin. Fagard et al. (51) infused angiotensin II in subjects during maximal exercise and attenuated the renin increase. The circulating levels of angiotensin II attained during the infusion, 161 pg/ml, far exceeded the level observed during exercise, 60 pg/ml. Further, the infusion of angiotensin II increased blood pressure which may have altered renal perfusion pressure and subsequently renin release. Renin release is also inhibited by AVP which is increased during exercise (135,136). The role of AVP in the regulation of renin release during exercise has not specifically been investigated. The release of renin in response to exercise may be modulated by negative feedback from angiotensin II and/or AVP.

Renin secretion is increased when there is a decrease in the sodium chloride reabsorption across the macula densa of the glomerulus. The rate of reabsorption is dependent upon the activity of the cells and the concentration of sodium delivered to the cells. During exercise, the decrease in glomerular filtration rate and probable increase in sodium reabsorption in the proximal tubule would result in a reduction in delivery of sodium and chloride to the macula densa, thus decreasing the quantity of sodium reabsorbed. This decrease in reabsorption could facilitate the release of renin during exercise. Castenfors (28) blocked sodium reabsorption in the ascending loop of Henle, thus increasing delivery to the macula densa, and did not markedly change the PRA response to exercise. Thus, the role of sodium delivery to the macula densa in the PRA response to exercise appears to be of minor importance.

Renin converts angiotensinogen to angiotensin I which is subsequently converted in the lungs to angiotensin II. The increase in angiotensin II during exercise is highly correlated with the increase in plasma renin activity (151). However, other factors appear to play a role. In comparing trained and untrained subjects Fagard et al. (50) noted differences in resting PRA values in the absence of a difference in angiotensin II levels. Further, in response to exercise similar changes in PRA were observed but the trained subjects had an attenuated angiotensin II response. Though renin is the primary regulator of angiotensin II production during exercise, it appears other factors may play a role.

Renin substrate, or angiotensinogen, can be a rate limiting step in the cascade of the renin-angiotensin system during prolonged stimulation. Thus, the rate of angiotensin II production would be influenced by changes in the plasma level of angiotensinogen. Angiotensinogen is synthesized in the liver. Liver blood flow is reduced during exercise but does not appear to affect the availability of angiotensinogen. The production of angiotensinogen is stimulated by glucocorticoids and estrogens, which may be altered by exercise. Angiotensin II also provides positive feedback on the production of angiotensinogen. Modulation of the synthesis of angiotensinogen could limit the production of angiotensin II during exercise but does not appear to be a factor.

In summary, the rate of formation of angiotensin II during exercise depends primarily on the rate of secretion of renin. The secretion of renin appears to be predominately controlled by the increase in sympathetic nerve activity during exercise. The production of angiotensinogen, although a possible rate limiting step in the formation of angiotensin II, does not appear to be affected by exercise.

Actions. The renin angiotensin system is implicated in a variety of functions. Activation of the system stimulates the release of AVP, ACTH, and aldosterone; increases blood pressure, and stimulates drinking. The increase in AVP during exercise was attributed to the increase in angiotensin II as the rise in AVP is correlated with the increase in PRA. Recent work by Wade et al. (169) found the opposite. Blockade of the production of angiotensin II failed to alter the increases in AVP, ACTH, and aldosterone to exercise. Further, the inhibition of the renin-angiotensin system, while attenuating the increase in blood pressure during maximal exercise, did not affect the change in GFR or the renal handling of water or solutes. Thus the role of the renin-angiotensin system in the stimulation of AVP, ACTH, and aldosterone is unclear.

Angiotensin II may play a role in the rate and degree of rehydration following exercise. Angiotensin II is a powerful dipsogen in animals (2,4,45,135,153). The recent studies by Nose et al. (118-120) would suggest a possible role of angiotensin II in the replacement of fluid loss following exercise in that PRA was related to the change in plasma volume which was a function of the degree of rehydration. This data may be interpreted two ways: that PRA is a function of plasma volume or that thirst is a function of PRA (the renin-angiotensin system). In favor of the first interpretation is that ingestion of an isotonic saline solution, which decreased PRA, resulted in a greater degree of rehydration compared to the drinking of water which did not alter PRA to the same extent. The role of the renin-angiotensin system in thirst and voluntary intake during exercise is open for further investigation.

Aldosterone

With exercise there is an increase in the plasma concentrations of the mineralocorticoid aldosterone (Table 7). Aldosterone is produced in the adrenal

Table 7. Plasma aldosterone in response to exercise

Exercise	Workload	Aldo (ng/dl) Pre	Post	Reference
Bicycle Erg.	80%	28	364	(110)
Bicycle Erg.	87%	66	345	(65)
Bicycle Erg.	45%	23	32	(103) (c)
	75%		48	
Bicycle Erg.	100%	7	19	(51)
Bicycle Erg.	49%	11.8	12.2	(155) (c)
	71%		17.8	
	88%		20.3	
Bicycle Erg.	85 W	32	70	(23) (h)
	85 W	24	48	
Bicycle Erg.	100-120 W	20	38	(175) (s)
	100-120 W		26	
Bicycle Erg.	30%	9	12	(151)
	60%		7	
	100%		24	
Treadmill	100%	10	45	(105)
Treadmill	60%	14	54	(40) (c)
Treadmill	100%	13	21	(169) (c)
Treadmill	100%	13.3	25.2	(60) (c)
Treadmill	1 mph	7	3	(108)
Treadmill	100%	11	23	(70)
Swimming	100%	10	20	
Running	3x300 m	3	12	(91)
Running	Marathon	12	34	(20)
Running	3x300 ml	3	12	(1)

(c) calculated from figures; (h) hydrated; (s) supine

cortex and modulates the renal reabsorption of sodium. Resting aldosterone levels are highly variable, being influenced by factors such as sodium intake, time of day, and plasma ACTH concentration. These factors also modulate the aldosterone response to exercise. Acute maximal exercise was found to increase plasma aldosterone concentration from 7 to 19 ng/ml (169). The increase in aldosterone occurs above a threshold workload and increases progressively thereafter (Fig. 6). In normal subjects the response of aldosterone to exercise mirrors those of PRA and angiotensin II to exercise.

Exercise duration affects the response of plasma aldosterone. Costill et al. (40) had subjects perform exercise at 60% of maximal oxygen consumption for 60 min and aldosterone was increased by 386%. Further, a 24 hr endurance race as well as a 10 hr triathalon both produced a 300% rise (55). These increases are similar to the increase induced by maximal exercise, 270% (60,169). Of note is that the increase in aldosterone during exercise is highly consistent with the increase being a function of the initial concentration.

Aldosterone is unique in its response to exercise in that resting values are not attained within the first hour or two of recovery from exercise. Following heavy exercise, plasma concentrations may be increased for days (86,167,168). Costill and coworker (40) reported the plasma level after a single 60 min exercise to be increased compared to resting values for six hours, while following a ten hour triathalon race, Fellmann et al. (55) found concentrations to remain elevated for 24 hr. Additional daily bouts of exercise may result in a persistently elevated plasma aldosterone concentration. Wade et al. (167,168) found exercise to result in an increase in aldosterone that was still observed the next day at the onset of additional exercise. This led to a progressive increase in urinary aldosterone excretion over ten days with daily exercise which would be indicative of an increase in plasma levels. Further, Kosunen et al. (92) observed an increase in resting aldosterone levels over the course of a track season with the increase greatest during the most intense period of training. However, in trained subjects, resting aldosterone concentrations are not altered compared to untrained controls (60,61,65,110) nor is the response to similar relative loads of exercise different (60,65,110). The continued increase in plasma aldosterone levels therefore appears to be a function of performing heavy exercise in excess to that to which the individual is trained.

Regulation. The renin-angiotensin system is the major regulator of aldosterone secretion (135,136). Angiotensin II not only stimulates the release of aldosterone but facilitates its production as well (136). During exercise the increase in plasma aldosterone levels has been correlated with changes in the renin-angiotensin system (60,91,118). Recently though, the increase in aldosterone has been suggested to involve additional factors besides the renin-angiotensin system (51,169). With the infusion of angiotensin II, which elevated levels to three times peak exercise values, the performance of maximal exercise still produced an increase in plasma aldosterone (51). Blockade of the production of angiotensin II by the administration of a converting enzyme inhibitor reduced resting aldosterone concentrations but failed to alter the response to exercise (169). Though correlated with the increase in the renin-angiotensin system during exercise, it appears other factors modulate the release of aldosterone during exercise.

Aldosterone secretion is normally stimulated by an increase in ACTH, an increase in plasma potassium concentration, or by a reduction in plasma sodium levels, as well as an increase in angiotensin II (136). Plasma sodium concentrations are increased during the course of exercise and would therefore suppress aldosterone release (166,168,169). Plasma potassium levels are unchanged or increased during maximal exercise and could stimulate the release of aldosterone (166,168,169). Exercise also stimulates the release of ACTH which is a powerful stimulator of aldosterone release and production (25,89,109,169). The integration of these factors in the regulation of aldosterone during exercise has yet to be clearly defined.

Actions. Aldosterone modulates the reabsorption of sodium in the distal tubule of the nephron (112,136). This reabsorption is important in the maintenance of sodium balance and, indirectly, potassium homeostasis. The increase in plasma aldosterone during exercise and the persistence of the increase following exercise is closely related to the reabsorption of sodium by the kidneys (168). It must also be remembered that the reabsorption of sodium is coupled to the passive reabsorption of water and the secretion of potassium. During exercise and especially following long duration exercise, aldosterone appears to play a major role in the correction of fluid and electrolyte homeostasis.

The increase in aldosterone may also decrease the loss of sodium in the sweat. Injection of aldosterone decreases the secretion of sodium in sweat (34). Conversely, Kirby and Convertino (87) recently reported the sweat sodium concentration to be increased in the presence of an increase in plasma aldosterone concentration during exercise in a hot environment. Nevertheless, the role of aldosterone in the modulation of sodium loss in sweat during exercise is still unclear.

Other Hormones

Plasma catecholamines are increased during exercise, reflecting an increase in sympathetic nervous activity and increased release from the adrenal medulla (70,93,154). Plasma catecholamines are progressively increased with increasing work intensities and are affected by both exercise duration and mode (70,154). The increase in catecholamines plays a role in minimizing the fluid and electrolyte losses during exercise by regulating (or reflecting the sympathetic nervous system regulation of) renal blood flow, the release of renin, and shifting blood flow distribution. This reduction of renal blood flow resulting in a decreased GFR during exercise allows the conservation of both fluids and electrolytes (12,46,171).

Plasma prolactin levels are increased, unchanged, or decreased during exercise (80,147). Prolactin has been implicated in the modulation of renal hemodynamics, but infusion to plasma concentrations greater than those attained during exercise does not alter renal blood flow (14). Further, sodium excretion was not changed during these infusions. Prolactin has also been suggested to result in an antidiuresis. This conclusion was based upon data obtained during infusions. Subsequently, it has been reported that the prolactin preparations were contaminated with AVP which would account for the conservation of water (84). Thus, the changes in prolactin that are sometimes observed during exercise do not appear to play a role in the conservation of fluids or electrolytes.

Prostaglandins are increased during exercise (44,50,88) and have been suggested to modulate the responses and actions of hormones important in the regulation of fluid and electrolyte homeostasis during exercise (15,177). Prostaglandins may also have a direct action on the renal handling of sodium independent of aldosterone (17,18). Zambraski et al. (178) found that blockade of the synthesis of prostaglandins did not affect the renal responses to exercise.

Factors Modulating Hormonal Responses to Exercise

A variety of factors may modulate the hormonal responses to exercise. In this section some of these factors and studies of their influence are presented. It must be emphasized that not all of the hormonal systems will be presented and that other chapters in this book contain detailed discussions of specific effects of environmental manipulations on the responses to exercise.

Mode of exercise. The mode of exercise can greatly impact on the hormonal responses. In a comparison of maximal swimming and running, Guezennec et al. (70) found differential hormone responses. The change in PRA, however, was significant with the value attained after running, 20.9 ng AI/ml/hr, being greater than that after swimming, 8.7 ng AI/ml/hr. The peak aldosterone concentration with running was 12.3 ng/dl compared to 10.2 ng/dl during swimming with no significant difference between the types of exercise. The differential hormone responses and dissociation of hormone interactions induced by the two types of exercise may be the result of differences in posture, immersion, heat load, or other factors. Thus the mode of exercise may influence hormone responses.

Posture. Changes in body posture result in a variety of compensatory actions, such as vascular volume shifts (5,74). Wolf et al. (175) compared the responses of PRA and aldosterone during upright and supine bicycle ergometer exercise. The exercise was performed for 20 minutes at 40 to 50% of the maximum workload determined in that body position. In the upright posture, exercise increased PRA by 66% and aldosterone levels by 90%. Performance of the exercise in the supine posture increased PRA by 18% and aldosterone by 49%. Thus, the posture in which exercise is performed may influence the hormonal responses.

Diet. The deprivation of food and the lack of sleep affect the responses of aldosterone and PRA to exercise. Opstad et al. (124) evaluated the PRA and aldosterone responses to maximal exercise in subjects provided minimal food and sleep over three days. The increase in PRA during exercise was accentuated from 0.7 to 4.3 nmol AI/ml/hr. In the control experiments, exercise increased aldosterone concentrations 2-fold. After the period of food and sleep deprivation the increase was 4-fold. Even with adequate caloric intake responses to exercise may be modified. Leenen et al. (97) assessed the effects of varying sodium intake on the response of PRA to submaximal bicycle ergometer exercise. Though the resting PRA levels were increased by dietary sodium restriction the absolute response was not altered. Aurell and Vikgren (11) found salt-loading to attenuate the response of PRA to exercise while salt deprivation resulted in a potentiation. Thus, manipulation of diet may modify the hormonal responses to exercise.

Hydration Status. The hydration status of the subjects alters the response of several hormones to exercise. Hypohydration, reducing plasma volume and increasing plasma osmolality potentiates the responses of hormones to exercise (23,26). The performance of moderate exercise on a treadmill (25% of maximum oxygen consumption) in a hot environment did not alter aldosterone concentration when the subjects were euhydrated but hypohydration resulted in an increase (58). Prior ingestion of water can also attenuate the response of AVP to exercise. The intake of 300 ml of water 30 min before the performance of maximal treadmill exercise reduces the increase induced in plasma AVP by 65% (166). This occurs without significant differences in the changes in plasma osmolality or volume being noted. This reduction in the response of AVP to exercise may be due to a oralpharyngeal input into the regulation of AVP release (64,158). Hydration status of the subjects may modify the hormonal responses to exercise and might affect the actions of hormones as well (8).

Environment. The environment in which exercise is performed can affect the hormonal responses. In other chapters in this book these alterations are discussed in greater detail. For example Maher and colleagues (103) studied the change in the renin-angiotensin system during exercise at sea level and at altitude. On the first day at altitude resting PRA was decreased, but angiotensin II levels were not altered. In response to exercise the PRA increase was attenuated while the increase in angiotensin II remained unchanged. Heat exposure may also alter the response of the renin angiotensin system to exercise with acclimatization inducing further changes. Therefore, the environment in which exercise is performed as well as the environment to which the subjects are adapted will influence the hormonal responses.

Disease. A variety of diseases modify the hormonal responses to exercise. In patients with cardiac disease, Petzl et al. (126) found the ANF response to exercise to be exaggerated. Fasola and coworkers (53,54) reported the response of PRA to exercise in hypertensive patients to be decreased, while Pedersen et al. (125) found no difference in the response between normotensive and hypertensive patients. These findings emphasize that underlying diseases may affect the response of the hormones to exercise, and that further studies are warranted.

Training. As mentioned previously, training may alter the hormonal response to exercise at similar absolute submaximal workloads. However, an alteration is not produced at similar relative workloads nor with maximal exercise. Convertino et al. (38) assessed the changes in PRA and AVP in four subjects before and after eight days of intensive training. At submaximal workloads the increases in PRA and AVP were decreased. When the data were expressed as a function of maximal exercise, the changes were a function of the relative workload. Thus, at absolute workloads the hormonal responses may be altered by the degree of training of the subjects, while the response to similar relative workloads is unaltered.

Summary

The hormonal responses to exercise are affected by a diversity of factors. These factors must be considered when interpreting and comparing the results from various studies. It is imperative that control of as many of the factors as possible be emphasized when designing studies investigating the hormonal regulation of fluid and electrolyte homeostasis during and following exercise.

CONCLUSION

In this review we have attempted to present the factors important in the regulation of fluid and electrolyte homeostasis during exercise and the responses, regulation and actions of the hormones suggested to be important in this process. In the performance of exercise there is a loss of both fluid and electrolytes. The loss of fluid is compounded by an inappropriate thirst which leads to a voluntary dehydration. This voluntary dehydration is associated with an increase in plasma osmolality and a decrease in blood volume, both of which are important stimulators of thirst, AVP release, and activation of the renin-angiotensin II-aldosterone axis. The degree of response of the various hormonal systems is a function of the intensity, duration and type of exercise as well as other confounding factors. Following exercise, thirst results in voluntary fluid intake which, though not initially complete, assists in the rectification of fluid balance within 24 hours. The correction of the losses in electrolytes, however, may require up to 72 hours.

The conservation of fluid and electrolytes by the kidneys is predominately due to physical factors associated with a decrease in renal blood flow and thus glomerular filtration. These changes are in part due to increases in catecholamines and angiotensin II. During exercise there is a decrease in the urine flow rate due to an increase in solute reabsorption with accompanying passive reabsorption of water. The increase in plasma aldosterone during exercise and the continued elevation of levels following exercise is in part responsible for the increase in renal reabsorption of sodium. The excretion of free water is actually increased during exercise in the presence of an increase in AVP. The reason for the failure of an increase in AVP to produce a concentrated urine during exercise is not clear, but may be the result of alterations in renal blood flow during exercise as well as a potential "washing out" of the concentration gradient in the kidneys. Finally, ANF is transiently increased during exercise and may explain the increase in urine flow rate reported with light intensity exercise. The increase in ANF does not appear to be important in the regulation of solute excretion during moderate to high intensity exercise in that reabsorption is facilitated to a greater degree by an increase in aldosterone. Thus, the renin-angiotensin-aldosterone axis appears to be the primary modulator of the renal handling of fluid and electrolytes during exercise.

The conservation of fluid and electrolytes in sweat during exercise does not appear to be mediated by hormones classically associated with this function. In fact, the changes in sweat rate and composition appear primarily oriented towards the dissipation of heat rather than conservation of water and electrolytes.

The hormonal regulation of thirst associated with exercise is not clear. However, recent work suggests that a balance between plasma volume and sodium concentration is required to facilitate thirst and that these factors are in part affected by (or affect) the renin-angiotensin system. ANF, on the other hand, may suppress drinking and may prove to account for the unexplained voluntary dehydration during exercise. The regulation of thirst during exercise by hormonal systems will prove to be an interesting area in the future.

In summary, numerous hormonal systems appear to play roles in the maintenance of fluid and electrolyte balance during and following exercise. Of primary importance appears to be the modulation and conservation of solutes by the kidneys, as well as thirst stimulating the intake of fluids.

The opinions or assertions contained herein are the private views of the authors and are not to be construed as official or as reflecting the views of the Department of the Army or the Department of Defense.

REFERENCES

1. Adlercreutz, H., Haerkoenen, M., Kuoppasalmi, K., Kosunen, K., Naeveri, H. and Rehunen, S. Physical activity and hormones. Adv Cardiol 18:144-157, 1976.
2. Adolph, E.F. Regulation of water intake in relation to body water content. In: Handbook of Physiology: Alimentary Canal. Food and Water Intake, edited by Washington, DC: American Physiology Society, 1967, p. 163-172.
3. Anderson, R.J., Berl, T., McDonald, K.M. and Schrier, R. Evidence for an in vivo antagonism between vasopressin and prostaglandin in the mammalian kidney. J Clin Invest 56:420-426, 1975.
4. Andersson, B. Regulation of water intake. American Physiological Society 58:582-603, 1978.
5. Annat, G., Guell, A., Gauquelin, G., Vincent, M., Mayet, M.H., Bizollon, Ch.A., Legros, J.J., Potter, M. and Gharib, C. Plasma vasopressin, neurophysin, renin and aldosterone during a 4-day head-down bed rest with and without exercise. Eur J Applied Physiol 55:59-63, 1986.
6. Armsen, T. and Reinhardt, H.W. Transtubular movement of urea at different degrees of water diuresis. Pflugers Arch 326:270-280, 1971.

7. Astrand, P. and Saltin, B. Plasma and red cell volume after prolonged severe exercise. J Appl Physiol 19:829-832, 1964.
8. Atherton, J.C., Evans, J.A., Green, R. and Thomas, S. Influence of variations in hydration and in solute excretion on the effects of lysine-vasopressin infusion on urinary and renal tissue composition in the conscious rat. J Physiol 213:311-327, 1971.
9. Atherton, J.C., Green, R. and Thomas, S. Influence of lysine-vasopressin dosage on the time course of changes in renal tissue and urinary composition in the conscious rat. J Physiol 213:291-309, 1971.
10. Aurell, M., Carlsson, M., Grimby, G. and Hood, B. Plasma concentration and urinary excretion of certain electrolytes during supine work. J Appl Physiol 22:633-638, 1967.
11. Aurell, M. and Vikgren, P. Plasma renin activity in supine muscular exercise. J Appl Physiol 31(6):839-841, 1971.
12. Baer, P.G. and McGiff, J.C. Hormonal systems and renal hemodynamics. Ann Rev Physiol 42:589-601, 1980.
13. Baylis, P.H. Osmoregulation and control of vasopressin secretion in healthy humans. Am J Physiol 253:R671-R678, 1987.
14. Berl, T., Brautnar, N., Ben-David, N., Czaczkes, W. and Kleeman, C. Osmotic control of prolactin release and its effect on renal water excretion in man. Kidney International 10:158-163, 1976.
15. Berl, T., Raz, A., Wald, H., Horowitz, J. and Czaczkes, W. Prostaglandin synthesis inhibition and the action of vasopressin: studies in man and rat. Am J Physiol 232(6):F529-F537, 1977.
16. Bie, P., Wang, C., Leadley, J.Jr. and Goetz, K. Hemodynamic and renal effects of low-dose infusions of atrial peptide in awake dogs. Am J Physiol 254:R161-R169, 1988.
17. Bolger, P.M., Eisner, G.M., Ramwell, P.W. and Slotkoff, L.M. Effect of prostaglandin synthesis on renal function and renin in the dog. Nature 259:244-245, 1976.
18. Bolger, P.M., Eisner, G.M., Ramwell, P.W., Slotkoff, L.M. and Corey, E.J. Renal actions of prostacyclin. Nature 271:467-469, 1978.
19. Boling, E.A. and Lipkind, J.B. Body composition and serum electrolyte concentrations. J Appl Physiol 18(5):943-949, 1963.
20. Boudou, P., Fiet, J., Laureaux, C., Patricot, M.C., Guezennec, C.Y., Foglietti, M.J., Villette, J.M., Friemel, F. and Haag, J.C. Variations of a few plasmas and urinary components in marathon runners. Ann Biol Clin 45:37-45, 1987.
21. Bozovic, L. and Castenfors, J. Effect of dihydralazine on plasma renin activity and renal function during supine exercise in normal subjects. Acta Physiol Scand 70:281-289, 1967.
22. Bozovic, L., Castenfors, J. and Piscator, M. Effect of prolonged, heavy exercise on urinary protein excretion and plasma renin activity. Acta Physiol Scand 70:143-146, 1967.
23. Brandenberger, G., Candas, V., Follenius, M., Libert, J.P. and Kahn, J.M. Vascular fluid shifts and endocrine responses to exercise in the heat. Eur J Applied Physiol 55:123-129, 1986.
24. Buono, M.J. and Sjoholm, N.T. Effect of physical training on peripheral sweat production. J Appl Physiol 65(2):811-814, 1988.

25. Buono, M.J., Yeager, J.E. and Sucec, A.A. Effect of aerobic training on the plasma ACTH response to exercise. J Appl Physiol 63:2499-2501, 1987.
26. Candas, V., Libert, J.P., Brandenberger, G., Sagot, J.C., Amoros, C. and Kahn, J.M. Hydration during exercise. Eur J Applied Physiol 55:113-122, 1986.
27. Castenfors, J. Renal function during exercise. Acta Physiol Scand 70(suppl. 293):1-44, 1967.
28. Castenfors, J. Effect of ethacrynic acid on plasma renin activity during supine exercise in normal subjects. Acta Physiol Scand 70:215-220, 1967.
29. Castenfors, J. Renal function during prolonged exercise. Ann NY Acad Sci 301:151-159, 1978.
30. Chan, K., Pipe, A. and DeBold, A.J. Atrial natriuretic hormone in marathon running. Medicine and Science in Sports 20(2):S39-S39, 1988.(Abstract)
31. Claybaugh, J. and Share, L. Vasopressin, renin, and cardiovascular responses to continuous slow hemorrhage. Am J Physiol 24:519-523, 1973.
32. Claybaugh, J.R., Pendergast, D.R., Davis, J.E., Akiba, C., Pazik, M. and Hong, S.K. Fluid conservation in athletes: responses to water intake, supine posture, and immersion. J Appl Physiol 61:7-15, 1986.
33. Collins, K. and Weiner, J. Endocrinological aspects of exposure to high environmental temperatures. Physiol Rev 48:785-859, 1968.
34. Collins, K.J. Action of exogenous aldosterone on the secretion and composition of drug-induced sweat. Clin Sci 30:207-213, 1969.
35. Convertino, V.A., Brock, P.J., Keil, L.C., Bernauer, E.M. and Greenleaf, J.E. Exercise training-induced hypervolemia: role of plasma albumin, renin, and vasopressin. J Appl Physiol 48:665-669, 1980.
36. Convertino, V.A., Greenleaf, J.E. and Bernauer, E.M. Role of thermal and exercise factors in the mechanism of hypervolemia. J Appl Physiol 48:657-664, 1980.
37. Convertino, V.A., Keil, L.C. and Bernauer, E.M. Plasma volume, osmolality, vasopressin, and renin activity during graded exercise in man. J Appl Physiol 50:123-128, 1981.
38. Convertino, V.A., Keil, L.C. and Greenleaf, J.E. Plasma volume, renin and vasopressin responses to graded exercise after training. J Appl Physiol 54:508-514, 1983.
39. Costill, D.L. Water and electrolyte requirements during exercise. Clinics in Sports Medicine 3:639-648, 1984.
40. Costill, D.L., Branam, G., Fink, W. and Nelson, R. Exercise induced sodium conservation: changes in plasma renin and aldosterone. Medicine and Science in Sports 8:209-213, 1976.
41. Cuneo, R.C., Espiner, E.A., Nicholls, M.G., Yandle, T.G., Joyce, S.L. and Gilchrist, N.L. Renal, hemodynamic, and hormonal responses to atrial natriuretic peptide infusions in normal man, and effect of sodium intake. J Clin Endocrinol Metab 63:946-953, 1986.
42. Cushner, H.M., Mulrow, J.P., Copley, J.B., Latham, R.L., Bailey, S. and Fried, T.A. Atrial natriuretic peptide (ANP) response to physiologic maneuvers in cardiac transplant patients. Kidney International 33:259-259, 1988.(Abstract)
43. Decombaz, J., Reinhardt, P., Anantharaman, K. and Glutz, G.V. Biochemical changes in a 100 km run: free amino acids, urea, and creatinine. Eur J Applied Physiol 41:61-72, 1979.

44. Demers, L.M., Harrison, T.S., Halbert, D.R. and Santen, R.J. Effect of prolonged exercise on plasma prostaglandin levels. Prostaglandins and Medicine 6:413-418, 1981.
45. Denton, D.A. Salt appetite. In: Handbook of Physiology: Alimentary Canal. Food and Water Intake, edited by Washington, DC: American Physiology Society, 1967, p. 433-459.
46. DiBona, G.F. Neural mechanisms in body fluid homeostasis. Fed Proc 45:2871-2877, 1986.
47. Dressendorfer, R.H., Wade, C.E. and Scaff, J.H. Renal function during short-term and prolonged strenuous exercise in coronary heart disease patients. J Cardiac Rehabil 3:575-582, 1983.
48. Espiner, E.A., Nicholls, M.G., Yandle, T.G., Crozier, I.G., Cuneo, R.C., McCormick, D. and Ikram, H. Studies on the secretion, metabolism and action of atrial natriuretic peptide in man. J Hypertension 4 (Supplement 2):S85-S91, 1986.
49. Fagard, R., Amery, A., Reybrouck, T., Lijnen, P., Moerman, E., Bogaert, M. and De Schaepdryver, A. Effects of angiotensin antagonism on hemodynamics, renin, and catecholamines during exercise. J Appl Physiol 43:440-444, 1977.
50. Fagard, R., Grauwels, R., Groeseneken, D., Lijnen, P., Staessen, J., Vanhees, L. and Amery, A. Plasma levels of renin, angiotensin II, and 6-ketoprostaglandin F1a in endurance athletes. J Appl Physiol 59:947-952, 1985.
51. Fagard, R., Lijnen, P. and Amery, A. Effects of angiotensin II on arterial pressure, renin and aldosterone during exercise. Eur J Applied Physiol 54:254-261, 1985.
52. Fasciolo, J.C., Totel, G.L. and Johnson, R.E. Antidiuretic hormone and human eccrine sweating. J Appl Physiol 27:303-307, 1969.
53. Fasola, A.F., Martz, B.L. and Helmer, O.M. Renin activity during supine exercise in normotensives and hypertensives. J Appl Physiol 21(6):1709-1712, 1966.
54. Fasola, A.F., Martz, B.L. and Helmer, O.M. Plasma renin activity during supine exercise in offspring of hypertensive parents. J Appl Physiol 25(4):410-415, 1968.
55. Fellman, N., Sagnol, M., Bedu, M., Falgairette, G., Van Praagh, E., Gaillard, G., Jouanel, P. and Coudert, J. Enzymatic and hormonal responses following a 24 h endurance run and a 10 h triathlon race. Eur J Applied Physiol 57:545-553, 1988.
56. Follenius, M. and Brandenberger, G. Increase in atrial natriuretic peptide in response to physical exercise. Eur J Applied Physiol 57:159-162, 1988.
57. Fortney, S.M., Vroman, N.B., Beckett, W.S., Permutt, S. and LaFrance, N.D. Effect of exercise hemoconcentration and hyperosmolality on exercise responses. J Appl Physiol 65(2):519-524, 1988.
58. Francesconi, R.P., Sawka, M.N., Pandolf, K.B., Hubbard, R.W., Young, A.J. and Muza, S. Plasma hormonal responses at graded hypohydration levels during exercise-heat stress. J Appl Physiol 59:1855-1860, 1985.
59. Freund, B., Hashiro, G., Buono, M., Claybaugh, J. and Chrisney, S. Endocrine and electrolyte responses during and following a marathon in young versus middle aged runners. Medicine and Science in Sports 20(2):1988.(Abstract)

60. Freund, B.J., Claybaugh, J.R., Dice, M.S. and Hashiro, G.M. Hormonal and vascular fluid responses to maximal exercise in trained and untrained males. J Appl Physiol 63:669-675, 1987.
61. Freund, B.J., Claybaugh, J.R., Hashiro, G.M. and Dice, M.S. Hormonal and renal responses to water drinking in moderately trained and untrained humans. Am J Physiol 254:R417-R423, 1988.
62. Freund, B.J., Wade, C.E. and Claybaugh, J.R. Effects of exercise on atrial natriuretic factor: implications to fluid homeostasis. Sports Medicine 6:364-376, 1988.
63. Fyhrquist, F., Tikkanen, I., Toetterman, K.J., Hynynen, M., Tikkanen, T. and Andersson, S. Plasma atrial natriuretic peptide in health and disease. Eur Heart J 8 (Supplement B):117-122, 1987.
64. Geelen, G., Keil, L.C., Kravik, S.E., Wade, C.E., Thrasher, T.N., Barnes, P.R., Pyka, G., Nesvig, C. and Greenleaf, J.E. Inhibition of plasma vasopressin after drinking in dehydrated humans. Am J Physiol 247:R968-R971, 1984.
65. Geyssant, A., Geelen, G. and Denis, C.H. Plasma vasopressin, renin activity, and aldosterone: Effect of exercise training. Eur J Applied Physiol 6:21-30, 1981.
66. Gibiniski, K., Kozbowski, S., Chwalbinska-Moneta, J., Giec, L., Zmudzinski, J. and Markiewicz, A. ADH and thermal sweating. Eur J Applied Physiol 42:1-13, 1979.
67. Gleim, G.W., Zabetakis, P.M., DePasquale, E.E., Michelis, M.F. and Nicholas, J.A. Plasma osmolality, volume, and renin activity at the "anaerobic threshold". J Appl Physiol 56:57-63, 1984.
68. Goetz, K.L. Physiology and pathophysiology of atrial peptides. Am J Physiol 254:E1-E15, 1988.
69. Greenleaf, J.E. and Sargent, F.II. Voluntary dehydration in man. J Appl Physiol 20(4):719-724, 1965.
70. Guezennec, C.Y., Defer, G., Cazorla, G., Sabathier, C. and Lhoste, F. Plasma renin activity, aldosterone and catecholamine levels when swimming and running. Eur J Applied Physiol 54:632-637, 1986.
71. Hammer, M., Ladefoged, J. and Olgaard, K. Relationship between plamsa osmolality and plasma vasopressin in human subjects. Am J Physiol 238:E313-E317, 1980.
72. Hellman, K. and Weiner, J. Antidiuretic substance in urine following exposure to high temperatures. J Appl Physiol 6:194-198, 1953.
73. Hespel, P., Lijnen, P., Vanhees, L., Fagard, R. and Amery, A. Beta-adrenoceptors and the regulation of blood pressure and plasma renin during exercise. J Appl Physiol 60:108-113, 1986.
74. Hinghofer-Szalkay, H., Kravik, S.E. and Greenleaf, J.E. Effect of lower-body positive pressure on postural fluid shifts in men. Eur J Applied Physiol 57:49-54, 1988.
75. Hodsman, G.P., Phillips, P.A., Ogawa, K. and Johnston, C.I. Atrial natriuretic factor in normal man: effects of tilt, posture, exercise and haemorrhage. J Hypertension 4 (Supplement 6):S502-S505, 1986.
76. Hubbard, R.W., Sandick, B.L., Matthew, W.T., Francesconi, R., Sampson, J.B., Durkot, M.J., Maller, O. and Engell, D.B. Voluntary dehydration and alliesthesia for water. J Appl Physiol 57:868-875, 1984.

77. Itoh, H., Nakao, K., Katsuura, G., Morii, N., Shino, s., Yamada, T., Sugawara, A., Saito, Yl, Watanabe, K., Igano, K., Inouye, K. and Imura, H. Atrial natriuretic polypeptides: structure-activity relationship in the central action - a comparison of their antidipsogenic actions. Neuroscience Letters 74:102-106, 1987.
78. Januszewicz, P., Gutkowska, J., Thibault, G., Garcia, R., Mercure, C., Jolicoeur, F., Genest, J. and Cantin, M. Dehydration-induced changes in the secretion of atrial natriuretic factor in Brattleboro rats: effect of water-drinking. Neuroscience Letters 67:203-207, 1986.
79. Januszewicz, P., Thibault, G., Gutkowska, J., Garcia, R., Mercure, C., Jolicoeur, F., Genest, J. and Cantin, M. Atrial natriuretic factor and vasopressin during dehydration and rehydration in rats. Am J Physiol 251:E497-E501, 1986.
80. Johansson, G., Uusitupa, M., Haerkoenen, M., Siitonen, O., Aro, A. and Korhonen, T. Hormonal effects of beta-receptor blockade during exercise. Acta Endocrinol 104:10-14, 1983.
81. Kachadorian, W.A. and Johnson, R.E. Renal responses to various rates of exercise. J Appl Physiol 28:748-752, 1970.
82. Kachadorian, W.A. and Johnson, R.E. The effect of exercise on some clinical measures of renal function. Am Heart J 82:278-280, 1971.
83. Katsuura, G., Nakamura, M., Inouye, K., Kono, M., Nakao, K. and Imura, H. Regulatory role of atrial natriuretic polypeptide in water drinking in rats. European J. Pharmacol. 121:285-287, 1986.
84. Keeler, R. and Wilson, N. Vasopressin contamination as a cause of some apparent renal actions of prolactin. Can. J. Physiol. Pharmacol. 54:887-890, 1976.
85. Keller, N., Moller, T., Sykulski, R., Storm, T.L. and Thamsborg, G.M. Effect of alpha-1 adrenoreceptor blockade on plasma levels of atrial natriuretic peptide during dynamic exercise in normal man. Horm Metabol Res 19:344-344, 1987.
86. Keul, J., Kohler, B., Von Glutz, G., Luethi, U., Berg, A. and Howald, H. Biochemical changes in a 100 km run: carbohydrates, lipids, and hormones in serum. Eur J Applied Physiol 47:181-189, 1981.
87. Kirby, C.R. and Convertino, V.A. Plasma aldosterone and sweat sodium concentrations after exercise and heat acclimation. J Appl Physiol 61:967-970, 1986.
88. Kiyonaga, A., Arakawa, K., Tanaka, H. and Shindo, M. Blood pressure and hormonal responses to aerobic exercise. Hypertension 7:125-131, 1985.
89. Kjaer, M., Bangsbo, J., Lortie, G. and Galbo, H. Hormonal response to exercise in humans: influence of hypoxia and physical training. Am J Physiol 254:R197-R203, 1988.
90. Knochel, J., Dotin, L. and Hamburger, R. Pathophysiology of intense physical conditioning in a hot climate. I. Mechanisms of potassium depletion. J Clin Invest 51:242-255, 1972.
91. Kosunen, K. and Pakarinen, A. Plasma renin, angiotensin II, and plasma and urinary aldosterone in running exercise. J Appl Physiol 41:26-29, 1976.

92. Kosunen, K., Pakarinen, A., Kuoppasalmi, K., Naveri, H., Rehunen, S., Standerskjold-Nordenstam, C.G., Harkonen, M. and Aldercreutz, H. Cardiovascular function and the renin-angiotensin-aldosterone system in long-distance runners during various training periods. Scand J Clin Lab Invest 40:429-435, 1980.
93. Kotchen, T., Hartley, L., Rice, T.W., Mougey, E., Jones, L. and Mason, J. Renin, norepinephrine and epinephrine responses to graded exercise. J Appl Physiol 31:178-184, 1975.
94. Kozlowski, S. and Saltin, B. Effect of sweat loss on body fluids. J Appl Physiol 19:1119-1124, 1964.
95. Kurosawa, T., Sakamoto, H., Katoh, Y. and Marumo, F. Atrial natriuretic peptide is only a minor diuretic factor in dehydrated subjects immersed to the neck in water. Eur J Applied Physiol 57:10-14, 1988.
96. Lassiter, W.E., Gottschalk, C.W. and Mylle, M. Micropuncture study of net transtubular movement of water and urea in nondiuretic mammalian kidney. Am J Physiol 200:1139-1146, 1961.
97. Leenen, F.H., Boer, P. and Geyskes, G.G. Sodium intake and the effects of isoproterenol and exercise on plasma renin in man. J Appl Physiol 45:870-874, 1978.
98. Levinsky, N., Davidson, D.G. and Berliner, R.W. Effects of reduced glomerular filtration on urine concentration in the presence of antidiuretic hormone. Am J Physiol 196:451-456, 1959.
99. Levinsky, N.G. and Berliner, R.W. The role of urea in the urine concentrating mechanism. J Clin Invest 38:741-748, 1959.
100. Levinsky, N.G., Davidson, D.G. and Berliner, R.W. Effects of reduced glomerular filtration on urine concentration in the presence of antidiuretic hormone. J Clin Invest 38:730-740, 1959.
101. Lijnen, P., Hespel, P., Eynde, E.V. and Amery, A. Urinary excretion of electrolytes during prolonged physical activity in normal man. Eur J Applied Physiol 53:317-321, 1985.
102. M'Buyamba-Kabangu, J., Fagard, R., Lijnen, P. and Amery, A. Relationship between plasma renin activity and physical fitness in normal subjects. Eur J Applied Physiol 53:304-307, 1985.
103. Maher, J.T., Jones, L.G., Hartley, H., Williams, G.H. and Rose, L.I. Aldosterone dynamics during graded exercise at sea level and high altitude. J Appl Physiol 39:18-22, 1975.
104. Manhem, P. and Hoekfelt, B. Prolonged clonidine treatment: catecholamines, renin activity and aldosterone following exercise in hypertensives. Acta Med Scand 209:253-260, 1981.
105. Maresh, C.M., Wang, B.C. and Goetz, K.L. Plasma vasopressin, renin activity, and aldosterone responses to maximal exercise in active college females. Eur J Applied Physiol 54:398-403, 1985.
106. Masotto, C. and Negro-Vilar, A. Inhibition of spontaneous or angiotensin II-stimulated water intake by atrial natriuretic factor. Brain Res Bull 15:523-526, 1985.
107. Matsubara, H., Nishikawa, M., Umeda, Y., Taniguchi, T., Iwasaka, T., Kurimoto, T., Yamane, Y. and Inada, M. The role of atrial pressure in secreting atrial natriuretic polypeptides. Am Heart J 113:1457-1462, 1987.
108. Meehan, R.T. Renin, aldosterone, and vasopressin responses to hypoxia during 6 hours of mild exercise. Aviat Space Environ Med 57:960-965, 1986.

109. Meirleir, K.D., Naaktgeboren, N., Steirteghem, A.V., Gorus, F., Olbrecht, J. and Block, P. Beta-endorphin and ACTH levels in peripheral blood during and after aerobic and anaerobic exercise. Eur J Applied Physiol 55:5-8, 1986.
110. Melin, B., Eclache, J.P. and Geelen, G. Plasma AVP, neurophysin, renin activity, and aldosterone during submaximal exercise performed until exhaustion in trained and untrained men. Eur J Applied Physiol 44:141-151, 1980.
111. Mitchell, J.W., Nadel, E.R. and Stolwijk, J.A. Respiratory weight losses during exercise. J Appl Physiol 32(4):474-476, 1972.
112. Morris, D.J. The Metabolism and Mechanism of Action of Aldosterone. Endocrine Reviews 234-247, 1981.
113. Mueller, F.B., Erne, P., Raine, A.E., Bolli, P., Linder, L., Resink, T.J., Cottier, C. and Buhler, F.R. Atrial antipressor natriuretic peptide: release mechanisms and vascular action in man. J Hypertension 4 (Supplement 2):S109-S114, 1986.
114. Myhre, L.G., Hartung, G.H. and Tucker, D.M. Plasma volume and blood metabolites in middle-aged runners during a warm-weather marathon. Eur J Applied Physiol 48:227-240, 1982.
115. Nadel, E.R., Pandolf, K.B., Roberts, M.R. and Stolwijk, J.A. Mechanism of thermal acclimitization to exercise and heat. J Appl Physiol 37:515-520, 1974.
116. Nishikimi, T., Kohno, M., Matsuura, T., Akioka, K., Teragaki, M., Yasuda, M., Oku, H., Takeuchi, K. and Takeda, T. Effect of exercise on circulating atrial natriuretic polypeptide in valvular heart disease. American Journal of Cardiology 58:1119-1120, 1986.
117. Nishikimi, T., Kohno, M., Matsuura, T., Kanayama, Y., Kaname, A., Teragaki, M., Yasuda, M., Oku, H., Takeuchi, K. and Takeda, T. Circulating atrial natriuretic polypeptide during exercise in patients with essential hypertension. J Hypertension 4 (Supplement 6):S546-S549, 1986.
118. Nose, H., Mack, G.W., Shi, X. and Nadel, E.R. Involvement of sodium retention hormones during rehydration in humans. J Appl Physiol 65(1):332-336, 1988.
119. Nose, H., Mack, G.W., Shi, X. and Nadel, E.R. Role of osmolality and plasma volume during rehydration in humans. J Appl Physiol 65 (1): 325-331, 1988.
120. Nose, H., Mack, G.W., Shi, X. and Nadel, E.R. Shift in body fluid compartments after dehydration in humans. J Appl Physiol 65(1):318-324, 1988.
121. Ochwadt, B. Relation of renal blood supply to diuresis. Prog Cardiovasc Dis 3:501-510, 1961.
122. Ogawa, K., Smith, A.I., Hodsman, G.P., Jackson, B., Woodcock, E.A. and Johnston, C.I. Plasma atrial natriuretic peptide: concentrations and circulating forms in normal man and patients with chronic renal failure. Clin Exp Pharm Physiol 14:95-102, 1987.
123. Olsson, K.E. and Saltin, B. Variation in total body water with muscle glycogen changes in man. Acta Physiol Scand 80:11-18, 1970.
124. Opstad, P.K., Oktedalen, O., Aakvaag, A., Fonnum, F. and Lund, P.K. Plasma renin activity and serum aldosterone during prolonged physical strain. Eur J Applied Physiol 54:1-6, 1985.

125. Pedersen, E.B., Kornerup, H.J. and Larsen, J.S. Responsiveness of the renin-aldosterone system during exercise in young patients with essential hypertension. Eur J Clin Invest 11:403-408, 1981.
126. Petzl, D.H., Hartter, E., Osterode, W., Boehm, H. and Woloszczuk, W. Atrial natriuretic peptide release due to physical exercise in healthy persons and in cardiac patients. Klin Wochenschr 65:194-196, 1987.
127. Poortmans, J.R. Effect of exercise on the renal clearance of amylase and lysozyme in humans. Clin Sci 43:115-120, 1972.
128. Poortmans, J.R. Exercise and renal function. Exercise and Sports Science Reviews 5:255-294, 1977.
129. Poortmans, J.R. Exercise and renal function. Sports Medicine 1:125-153, 1984.
130. Raine, A.E., Phil, D., Erne, P., Burgisser, E., Muller, F.B., Bolli, Pl, Burkart, F. and Buhler, F.R. Atrial natriuretic peptide and atrial pressure in patients with congestive heart failure. N Engl J Med 315:533-537, 1986.
131. Raisz, L.G., Au, W.Y. and Scheer, R.L. Studies on the renal concentrating mechanism. III. Effect of heavy exercise. J Clin Invest 39:8-13, 1959.
132. Ramsey, D., Keil, L., Sharpe, M. and Shinsako, J. Angiotensin II infusion increases vasopressin, ACTH, and 11-hydroxycorticosteroid secretion. Am J Physiol 234:R66-R71, 1978.
133. Refsum, H.E. and Stromme, S.B. Relationship between urine flow, glomerular filtration, and urine solute concentrations during prolonged heavy exercise. Scand J Clin Lab Invest 35:775-780, 1975.
134. Refsum, H.E. and Stromme, S.B. Renal osmol clearance during prolonged heavy exercise. Scand J Clin Lab Invest 38:19-22, 1977.
135. Reid, I.A. Actions of angiotensin II on the brain: mechanisms and physiologic role. Am J Physiol 246:F533-F543, 1984.
136. Reid, I.A. and Ganong, W.F. Control of aldosterone secretion. In: Hypertension: Pathophysiology and Treatment, edited by Genest, J., Koiw, E. and Kuchel, O. New York: McGraw-Hill, 1977, p. 265-292.
137. Robertson, G.L., Mahr, E.A., Athar, S. and Sinha, T. Development and clinical application of a new method for the radioimmunoassay of arginine vasopressin in human plasma. J Clin Invest 52:2340-2352, 1973.
138. Rolls, B.J., Wood, R.J., Rolls, E.T., Lind, H., Lind, W. and Ledingham, J.G. Thirst following water deprivation in humans. Am J Physiol 239: R476-R482, 1980.
139. Rowell, L.B. Human cardiovascular adjustments to exercise and thermal stress. Physiol Rev 54:75-159, 1974.
140. Rydin, H. and Verney, E.B. The inhibition of water diuresis by emotional stress and by muscular exercise. Q J Exp Physiol 27:343-374, 1938.
141. Sagnella, G.A., Markandu, N.D., Shore, A.C. and MacGregor, G.A. Changes in plasma immunoreactive atrial natriuretic peptide in response to saline infusion or to alterations in dietary sodium intake in normal subjects. J Hypertension 4 (Supplement 2):S115-S118, 1986.
142. Saito, Y., Nakao, K., Sugawara, A., Nishimura, K., Sakamoto, M., Narito, M., Yamada, T., Itoh, H., Shiono, S., Kuriyama, T., Hirai, M., Ohi, M., Toshihiko, B. and Imura, H. Atrial natriuretic polypeptide during exercise in healthy man. Acta Endocrinologica (Copenh) 116:59-65, 1987.
143. Saltin, B. Aerobic work capacity and circulation at exercise in man. Acta Physiol Scand 62 (Supplement 230):1-52, 1964.

144. Schlein, E.M., Spooner, G.R., Day, C., Pickering, M. and Cade, R. Extrarenal water loss and antidiuretic hormone. J Appl Physiol 31(4):569-572, 1971.
145. Schrier, R.W., Berl, T. and Anderson, R.J. Osmotic and nonosmotic control of vasopressin release. Am J Physiol 236:F321-F332, 1979.
146. Schrier, R.W., Keller, H.I., Gilliland, P.F. and Teschan, P.E. Renal, metabolic, and circulatory responses to heat and exercise. Ann Intern Med 73:213-223, 1970.
147. Shangold, M.M., Gatz, M.L. and Thysen, B. Acute effects of exercise on plasma concentrations of prolactin and testosterone in recreational women runners. Fertility and Sterility 35:699-702, 1981.
148. Share, L. Blood pressure, blood volume, and the release of vasopressin. In: Handbook of Physiology, edited by Knobil, E. and Sawyer, W. Washington, DC: American Physiological Society, 1974, p. 243-252.
149. Share, L. and Claybaugh, J. Regulation of body fluids. Ann Rev Physiol 34:235-260, 1972.
150. Somers, V.K., Anderson, J.V., Conway, J., Sleight, P. and Bloom, S.R. Atrial natriuretic peptide is released by dynamic exercise in man. Horm Metabol Res 18:871-872, 1986.
151. Staessen, J., Fagard, R., Hespel, P., Lijnen, P., Vanhees, L. and Amery, A. Plasma renin system during exercise in normal men. J Appl Physiol 63:188-194, 1987.
152. Stevenson, J.A. Central mechanisms controlling water intake. In: Handbook of Physiology: Alimentary Canal. Food and Water Intake, edited by Washington,DC: American Physiology Society, 1967, p. 173-187.
153. Stricker, E.M. and Verbalis, J.G. Hormones and behavior: the biology of thirst and sodium appetite. Am. Scientist 76:261-267, 1988.
154. Svedenhag, J. The sympatho-adrenal system in physical conditioning. Acta Physiol Scand 125 (Supplement 543):3-73, 1985.
155. Tanaka, H., Shindo, M., Gutkowska, J., Kinoshita, A., Urata, H., Ikeda, M. and Arakawa, K. Effect of acute exercise on plasma immunoreactive - atrial natriuretic factor. Life Sciences 39:1685-1693, 1986.
156. Thamsborg, G., Storm, T., Keller, N., Sykulski, R. and Larsen, J. Changes in plasma atrial natriuretic peptide during exercise in healthy volunteers. Acta Med Scand 221:441-444, 1987.
157. Thamsborg, G., Sykulski, R., Larsen, J., Storm, T. and Keller, N. Effect of Beta-1 adrenoreceptor blockade on plasma levels of atrial natriuretic peptide during exercise in normal man. Clin Physiol 7:313-318, 1987.
158. Thrasher, T.N., Nistal-Herrera, J.F., Keil, L.C. and Ramsay, D.J. Satiety and inhibition of vasopressin secretion after drinking in dehydrated dogs. Am J Physiol 240:E394-E401, 1981.
159. Thrasher, T.N., Wade, C.E., Keil, L.C. and Ramsay, D.J. Sodium balance and aldosterone during dehydration and rehydration in the dog. Am J Physiol 247:R76-R83, 1984.
160. Toth, E., Stelfox, J. and Kaufman, S. Cardiac control of salt appetite. Am J Physiol 252:R925-R929, 1987.
161. Ullrich, K.J., Kramer, K. and Boylan, J.W. Present knowledge of the counter-current system in the mammalian kidney. Prog Cardiovasc Dis 3:395-431, 1961.

162. Verde, T., Shephard, J., Corey, P. and Moore, R. Sweat composition in exercise and in heat. J Appl Physiol 53:1540-1545, 1982.
163. Virvidakis, C., Loukas, A., Symvoulidou, D.M. and Mountokalakis, T. Renal responses to bicycle exercise in trained athletes: influence of exercise intensity. Int J Sports Med 7:86-88, 1986.
164. Vlcek, J., Stemberk, V. and Koupil, P. Renal excretion of amino acids at submaximum exertion. Cas Lek ces 126:147-149, 1987.
165. Wade, C.E. Response, regulation, and actions of vasopressin during exercise: a review. Medicine and Science in Sports and Exercise 16:506-511, 1984.
166. Wade, C.E. and Claybaugh, J. Plasma renin activity, vasopressin concentration, and urinary excretory responses to exercise in men. J Appl Physiol 49:930-936, 1980.
167. Wade, C.E., Dressendorfer, R.H., O'Brien, J.C. and Claybaugh, J.R. Renal function, aldosterone, and vasopressin excretion following repeated long distance running. J Appl Physiol 50:709-712, 1981.
168. Wade, C.E., Hill, L.C., Hunt, M.M. and Dressendorfer, R.H. Plasma aldosterone and renal function in runners during a 20-day road race. Eur J Applied Physiol 54:456-460, 1985.
169. Wade, C.E., Ramee, S.R., Hunt, M.M. and White, C.J. Hormonal and renal responses to converting enzyme inhibition during maximal exercise. J Appl Physiol 63:1796-1800, 1987.
170. Walsh, K.P., Williams, T.D.M., Pitts, S.E., Lightman, S.L. and Sutton, R. Role of atrial pressure and rate release of atrial natriuretic peptide. Am J Physiol 254:R607-R610, 1988.
171. Wardener, D. and Hugh, E. The control of sodium excretion. Am J Physiol 235:F163-F173, 1978.
172. Weitzman, R. and Kleeman, C.R. Water metabolism and neurohypophyseal hormones. In: Clinical Disorders of Fluid and Electrolyte Metabolism, edited by Maxwell, M.H. and Kleeman, C.R. New York: McGraw-Hill Book Co., 1980, p. 531-645.
173. Wilkerson, J., Gutin, B. and Horvath, S.M. Exercise-induced changes in blood, red cell, and plasma volumes in man. Med Sci Sports 9:155-158, 1977.
174. Wilkerson, J.E., Horvath, S.M., Gutin, B., Molnar, S. and Diaz, F.J. Plasma electrolyte content and concentration during treadmill exercise in humans. J Appl Physiol 53:1529-1539, 1982.
175. Wolf, J.P., Nguyen, N.U., Dumoulin, G. and Berthelay, S. Plasma renin and aldosterone changes during twenty minutes' moderate exercise. Eur J Applied Physiol 54:602-607, 1986.
176. Wyndham, C., Benade, A., Williams, C., Strydon, N., Goldin, A. and Heyns, A. Changes in central circulation and body fluid spaces during acclimatization to heat. J Appl Physiol 25:586-593, 1968.
177. Zambraski, E. and Dunn, M. Renal prostaglandin (PG) secretion and excretion in exercising dogs. Fed Proc 38:893-893, 1979.
178. Zambraski, E., Rofrano, T. and Ciccone, C. Effects of aspirin treatment on kidney function in exercising man. Med Sci Sports Exerc 14:419-423, 1982.
179. Zambraski, E.J., Tucker, M.S., Lakas, C.S., Grassl, S.M. and Scanes, C.G. Mechanism of renin release in exercising dog. Am J Physiol 246:E71-E76, 1984.

2

HORMONAL REGULATION OF FLUID AND ELECTROLYTES: EFFECTS OF HEAT EXPOSURE AND EXERCISE IN THE HEAT

R.P. Francesconi, M.N. Sawka, R.W. Hubbard and K.B. Pandolf

US Army Research Institute of Environmental Medicine
Natick, Massachusetts 01760-5007

INTRODUCTION

A review of the endocrine factors which subserve fluid and electrolyte regulation during acute or chronic sedentary heat exposure or during exercise in the heat necessarily focuses on two target organs - the sweat gland and the kidney. While the acquisition of heat acclimation in humans is partially characterized by a striking ability to secrete increased quantities of a more dilute sweat (3,121,131), there are relatively few studies in the scientific literature describing the direct hormonal control of sweat secretory rate, composition, or total output. Further, studies which have reported these direct effects of exogenously administered hormones (e.g. aldosterone, angiotensin I or II, antidiuretic hormone or vasopressin) on sweat gland activity provided, at best, inconsistent results with various investigators reporting increased, decreased, or no effects on sweat secretion.

Effects of Exogenous Hormones

In an attempt to confirm the responsiveness of the eccrine sweat gland to antidiuretic hormone (vasopressin, AVP) stimulation, Fasciolo et al. (48) injected AVP subdermally at 3 sites (forearm, abdomen, thigh) in 6 male volunteers and collected sweat samples for three 40 min periods at each site and the contralateral control area. Sweating was induced by heat exposure or Mecholyl administration, and the results indicated that, indeed, sweat secretion was generally reduced by AVP treatment; moreover, the sodium (Na^+) concentration of the sweat was increased, and these investigators concluded that AVP had a direct effect on sweat duct permeability and water reabsorption.

In a very early experiment Ladell (109) injected deoxycorticosterone acetate intramuscularly in acclimated subjects and collected forearm sweat during work in a hot environment. The results indicated that the hormone, acting directly on sweat gland secretion, elicited a 30% reduction in the sodium chloride (NaCl) content of the sweat. At approximately the same time Conn et al. (29) also administered deoxycorticosterone acetate to men before, during, and after acclimation to heat, and reported that the concentration of NaCl lost in sweat was significantly lowered and that cessation of hormonal administration promptly resulted in increased salt losses even in acclimated subjects. In fact, they concluded that the exogenous administration of hormone repressed endogenous mineralocorticoid secretion, and full recovery from this hyposecretory activity required several days.

Twenty years later Collins (24) administered d-aldosterone at 6 h intervals and induced sweating by intradermal injection of methacholine. He reported that between 12-30 h following the first aldosterone injection, the sodium/potassium ratio was maximally depressed, urine flow and sweat secretion were both attenuated, and 2 days were necessary for these variables to return to normal levels after the final injection of aldosterone. These studies led Braun et al. (18) to administer d-aldosterone exogenously to young, healthy volunteers in an attempt to accelerate the acquisition of heat acclimation. They concluded (18) that while the total time necessary for full acclimation was not reduced, performance time was increased while mean rectal temperature and heart rate were reduced during the first several days of exercise in the heat.

In other related studies Gibinski et al. (69) administered 1.25 mg aldosterone acetate or 0.5 and 1.0 g Aldactone (spironolactone) before exposure to a hot, wet ($48^o/40^oC$, db/wb) environment and measured several sweat variables during the heat exposure. They (69) observed no effects of either intervention on sweat chloride, sodium, and potassium. While urinary Na/K ratios were decreased by heat exposure and heat exposure plus aldosterone administration, the antagonistic effects of Aldactone on aldosterone prevented Na conservation and urinary Na/K ratios were unaffected (70) in this trial. Since Aldactone affected urinary sodium conservation while sweat sodium concentrations were unaffected by this treatment, these workers concluded that the mechanisms of action in the sweat glands and kidneys "differ entirely".

When Zgoda et al. (168) exposed 10 test subjects to 49^oC for 2 h/d for 5 d and administered AVP intranasally to 5 subjects daily, they reported that the AVP-treated group manifested decreased rectal temperature (T_{re}) and heart rate during the heat exposure. In a related paper (11) a 10 min work interval was added at the conclusion of the 2 h heat exposure, and they observed no effects on sweat rate while "psychophysiological" improvement was noted in subjects receiving the peptide. Senay and van Beaumont (153) injected vasopressin (Pitressin) intramuscularly before a final hour of heat exposure with water replenishment and observed no effects of AVP administration on evaporative water loss while urinary water loss was reduced in both subjects. Ratner and Dobson (127) had earlier reported that AVP administration and heat exposure elicited a marked increase in urinary osmolality with no changes in sweat osmolality. In a more recent paper Gibinski et al. (71) also administered AVP to a group of volunteers and observed no effects on sweat rate, osmolality, and electrolytes. In the latter experiments (71) no effects on urine osmolality were reported. Thus, despite a significant number of investigations, uncertainties persist with respect to the effects of exogenously administered hormones on the volume and chemical composition of both sweat and urine.

Clearly, these sometimes divergent observations, especially with respect to exogenous AVP, underscore the fact that the control of fluid and electrolyte balance in higher organisms is an extremely complex and exquisitely controlled system involving certainly not only hormonal, but also neural and other physiological factors (106). This topic has been the subject of frequent and extensive reviews and is well beyond the scope and intent of the current paper (for general reviews see: 9,13,81,97,128). In addition, there are several earlier reviews available which readers might wish to consult concerning water and electrolyte balance and metabolism during sedentary or active exposure to hot environments (23,28,46,80,112,166). Although Doucet (40) has recently noted that there are over 20 hormones controlling kidney function and regulation, most of these have not been investigated for their potential impact in controlling fluid and electrolyte balance during heat exposure.

Generally, it has been concluded that sedentary exposure to or exercise in a hot environment for at least 1 h by non-acclimated individuals without fluid replenishment is usually accompanied by a reduction of the interstitial and plasma volumes (56) and a significant loss of Na^+ in sweat (100). Additionally,

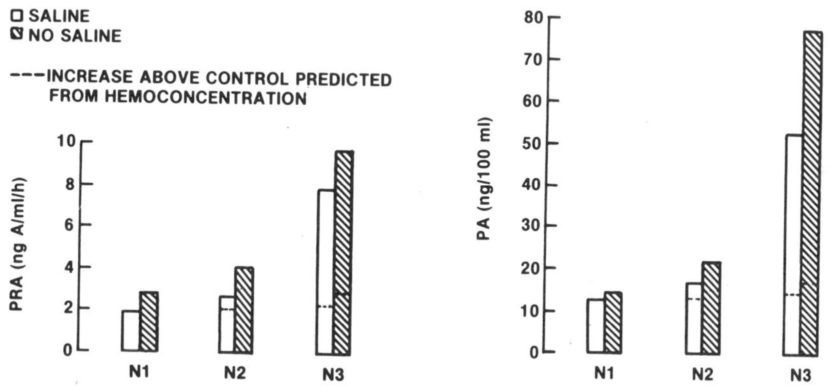

FIGURE 1. Effects of consumption of 0.75 liters of 1% saline on plasma renin activity and plasma aldosterone levels during a heat acclimation regimen. The N1 sample was taken after 25 min rest at 40°C., the second (N2) sample 5 min after 30 min intermittent exposure to a hot bath (40°C.), and the final sample (N3) during the final minute of 10 min continuous exercise on a bicycle ergometer (40°C., 75W). The rest interval, hot bath, and exercise period were contiguous. The blood samples were taken on alternate days during an 11 d heat acclimation program. Mean values for 6 young adult males are depicted. Results of this study emphasize the importance of exercise (N3), with its concurrent diversion of blood flow from the viscera, in stimulating the biosynthesis and reducing the clearance of PRA and PA. (Redrawn from: Davies et al., J. Appl. Physiol., 50; 605, 1981 with permission of the publisher).

blood flow is redistributed from the visceral circulation (135,136) to the exercising muscles or skin surface for heat dissipation. The early decrements in plasma volume (83) and renal blood flow (143) stimulate the activity of the renin-angiotensin system (47,52) as well as the synthesis and release of aldosterone (34,37) (Fig.1). If a heat/exercise regimen is maintained for at least several consecutive days, stimulated aldosterone (A) and vasopressin (AVP) secretion will effect precipitous declines in urinary volumes (23,46) in euhydrated and, especially, hypohydrated individuals and Na^+ excretion in the urine (62) followed soon thereafter by significant decrements in sweat Na^+ (12). Because of the marked reductions in sweat and urinary Na^+ loss, Na^+ balance may be rapidly re-established even in the presence of only moderate levels of Na^+ consumption, and this may contribute to the beginnings of plasma volume (PV) expansion associated with heat acclimation.

If daily exercise in a hot environment persists, water and electrolyte equilibrium is usually fully re-established after approximately 1 week of the exercise/heat regimen (6) as long as fluid and electrolyte replacement is adequate. Certainly by this time sweat and urinary Na^+ losses have been minimized even while sweat volume has been significantly increased (160), urinary output is adequate but attenuated, and resting PV may be expanded over a broadly reported range, e.g. 7% (15), 15% (85), and 23% (147) while total body water may be expanded by approximately 6% (32). The magnitude of the hormonal responses and adjustments which help to maintain fluid and electrolyte balance during acute or recurrent sedentary heat exposure or exercise in the heat may be affected by the acclimation (or training) status of the individual, the hydrational status, the nutritional status (especially with respect to electrolytes), the duration and intensity of the stress, as well as additional variables which may be introduced by the actual experimental scenario. In this chapter we will attempt to consider each of the important factors relevant to the hormonal control of or the hormonal response to electrolyte and fluid perturbations during sedentary or active exposure to heat stress.

SEDENTARY HEAT EXPOSURE

Perhaps the most rapid sedentary exposure to heat stress eliciting significant alterations in hormones controlling plasma volume was reported by a Helsinki group using conditions "typical of a Finnish sauna bath". Kosunen et al. (108) and Adlerkreutz et al. (2) reported the hormonal responses of experienced sauna users to 20 min exposure at 85-90°C. Their results indicated that just 10 min after exposure to the intense heat stress, levels of plasma renin activity (PRA) and angiotensin II were significantly increased; increments in plasma aldosterone (PA) levels were delayed until 20 min after exposure with even greater elevations observed 0.5 h after completion of the heat stress. Generally, hormonal levels had returned to control ranges 6 h following heat exposure (Fig. 2).

These extremely rapid hormonal responses suggest that fluid shifts and shifts in blood flow-cardiac output distribution are stimulatory to endocrinological responses in the absence of notable fluid loss. Rowell (134)

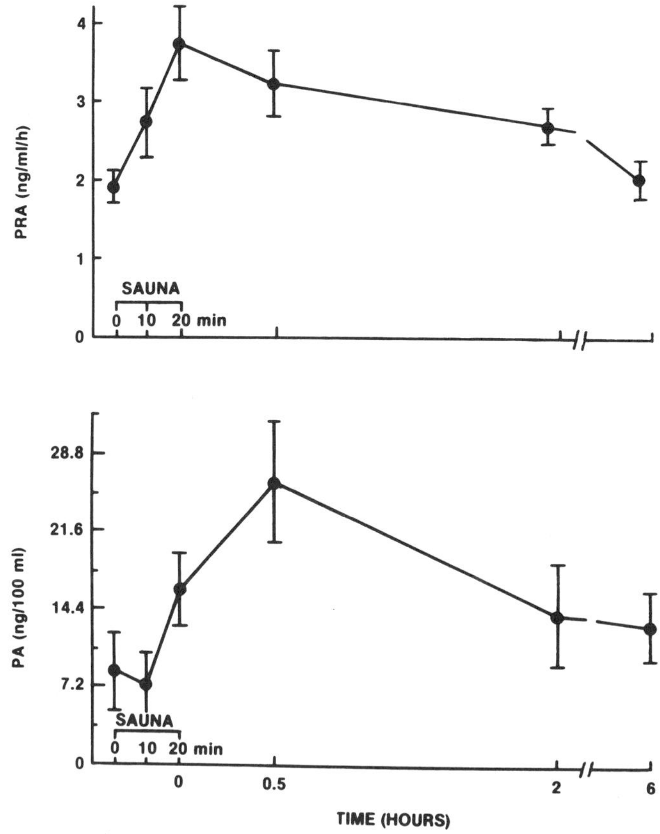

FIGURE 2. Effects of intense heat (85-90°C.) on plasma renin activity and aldosterone levels in 6 healthy adult males who were experienced sauna users. Mean values ±SEM are depicted. Venous blood samples were taken at the times noted while subjects remained sedentary. The rapidity of the PRA response may indicate the importance of diversion of blood flow from the renal bed in increasing PRA; the greater (4X) response of PA may implicate the generalized adrenocorticotrophic effect. (Redrawn from: Kosunen et al., J. Appl. Physiol., 41; 323, 1976 with permission of the publisher).

has estimated that skin blood flow can be increased to 7-8 L/min during severe heat stress, and concluded that splanchnic vasoconstriction was initiated primarily by the sympathetic nervous system since increments in PRA occur concomitantly with elevations in heart rate and plasma norepinephrine levels. Baroreceptors may be initially involved followed by the activation of volume, osmo-, and thermoreceptors as the stress persists, eliciting plasma volume decrements, osmolality increments, and elevations in core temperature.

Dumoulin et al. (41) used an 80°C environment and 20 min exposure time to effect significant elevations in both PRA and PA. In their earlier report Kosunen et al. (108) indicated that no changes occurred in PV as estimated from hematocrit, hemoglobin, and plasma protein (PP) values. The rapidity of the hormonal changes in these studies is noteworthy; just 10 min after intense heat exposure, circulating indices of fluid and electrolyte conservation and splanchnic and renal vasoconstriction were evident. The spontaneity of these responses suggests that increased circulating hormonal levels can be elicited by reduced hepatic and renal clearance in addition to accelerated biosynthesis of these hormones. Collins et al. (26) have reported that the metabolic clearance rate of aldosterone was reduced from 77 L/h to 57 L/h when deep body temperature was raised by 1.08^{o}C. The effects of acclimation on the clearance of fluid and electrolyte regulatory hormones have not been assessed (25).

Rocker et al. (132) extended the heat exposure (70-75°C) to 4 h with a 10 min interval at 19-21°C during each hour. With no fluid replenishment this test scenario effected a dehydration of 2.4 kg or 3.4% of pre-exposure body weight. In addition to observing a 100% elevation of plasma vasopressin (PVP) at the end of the heat exposure, which was further increased to approximately 160% 90 min later, they also reported significant increments in plasma osmolality and concomitant decrements in plasma volume, thus emphasizing the importance of the duration of the stress in affecting physiological responses and the impact of fluid loss in addition to fluid shifts in eliciting marked hormonal elevations. Earlier, these workers had employed the same experimental protocol (133) to show that untrained women manifested smaller reductions in plasma volume than men.

While sedentary exposure to sauna temperatures thus elicited rapid and intense alterations in circulating hormone levels when large shifts in fluid volumes and blood flow distribution were occurring, much of the experimental work in humans as well as higher animals has been accomplished under much lower ambient conditions. Szczepanska-Sadowska (161) used pre-implanted thermodes near the pre-optic area of dog forebrain to raise brain temperature by 1.5^{o}C in the absence of generalized heat stress and remarkably observed 10-fold elevations in circulating AVP levels just 10 min after heating. Eisman and Rowell (43) exposed 6 male baboons to environmental temperatures ranging from 42-49°C and observed 24% reductions in renal blood flow per ^{o}C rise in core temperature giving rise to 98% increments in PRA per ^{o}C elevation. This same group of investigators would later (47) use human subjects in water- perfused suits to show that raising T_{re} by 1°C elicited increases in PRA of 135% and in splanchnic vascular resistance of 73%. Beta-blockade, induced by propranolol administration, reduced PRA, but elevations in splanchnic vascular resistance were less affected. These investigators speculated (47) that while PRA is effective in eliciting visceral vasoconstriction when heat stress is mild, increased stress intensity may stimulate sympathetic nervous system- induced vasoconstriction. Rowell (134) later hypothesized that angiotensin II may have more marked effects on the renal versus the splanchnic circulation.

Thus, in the absence of exercise, exposure to heat stress is accompanied by reduced urinary fluid and electrolyte loss partially under the influence of increased PRA (43,47,49) and aldosterone (49,55). Simultaneously, cutaneous vasodilation, occurring in humans generally over the entire surface of the body from the lower extremities to the cheek and ear region (148), permits the increased peripheral blood flow provided by the enormous increments in cardiac output which results in similarly increased evaporative, radiative, and convective heat loss under appropriate conditions. Of course, in the passive mode the absence of increased metabolic heat production from muscular activity results in comparably lower sweat rates to maintain thermal equilibrium under specified conditions of ambient temperature and duration of exposure.

Elizondo et al. (44) used an environmental temperature of 36-40^oC to induce sweat rates of up to 0.65 $mg/cm^2/min$, and reported that while sodium concentration increased with increasing sweat rate, the potassium concentration of the sweat was reduced. These investigators (44) used local skin heating (to 42^oC) and arterial occlusion to increase or decrease, respectively, sweat output, but did not speculate on the control of electrolyte loss in the sweat. Harrison (82) investigated the effects of 2 h sedentary exposure to 48^oC, and observed that while plasma Na^+ and K^+ were unaffected, a linear decrease of water from the intravascular space occurred which could be correlated with either increasing hematocrit or protein concentration. Additionally, van Beaumont et al. (164) used similar conditions (sedentary, 45^oC, 3 h) to demonstrate that thermal dehydration (1.9% loss in body weight, bw) was accompanied by proportionately greater reductions in plasma volume (5.9%) than heat stress alone. These investigators (164) concluded that the dynamics of hemodilution and hemoconcentration during sedentary heat exposure may be related to the onset of sweating, initial sweat rate, and total sweat loss.

To this point, the results from studies using initially euhydrated human subjects in climatic chambers, sedentary exposure to heat ranging from moderate to intense, and durations ranging from a fraction of an hour to several hours indicated that hormonal adjustments conducive to fluid and electrolyte conservation are generally rapid and consistent. Surprisingly, Candas et al. (20) showed that marked hidromeiosis (reduction in sweat rate due to skin wettedness with prolonged sweating) during repeated exposures to hot, humid conditions did not elicit any changes in PA, PRA, or PVP. During active heat dissipation in the passive mode, visceral blood flow is attenuated and the peripheral share of cardiac output is increased to as much as 60% of the total (134). Despite the hormonal adjustments designed to conserve fluid and electrolytes, dehydration may occur and plasma volume may be noticeably reduced if fluid replenishment is inadequate or heat stress is intense and prolonged.

EXERCISE IN THE HEAT

When physical exercise is added to the stress of the hot environment, then the cascade of endocrinological and physiological adjustments necessary to meet metabolic and thermoregulatory demands is increased. When we exercised rats in the heat (35^oC) and removed a blood sample for analysis when T_{re} reached 40^oC, we observed significant elevations in PA in this sample which was taken just 8.25 min (mean) after the initiation of exercise (61). In humans increased cardiac output and blood flow to sustain the metabolic demands of the working muscles must be partially distributed also to the skin surface for sweat secretion and evaporation; the percentage of cardiac output to each may be determined by the work intensity and the ambient temperature. In any event, the surfeit of deep body heat, which can raise core temperatures to injurious levels, must be transferred to the periphery for radiative, convective, or evaporative dissipation. To meet the enormous demands placed upon the cardiovascular system during exercise in the heat (120) in man or animals, plasma volume must be protected and sustained. Fortunately, healthy humans ordinarily possess physiological and endocrinological mechanisms to defend plasma volume, reduce electrolyte loss, promote heat loss, and attenuate physiological strain during work in the heat.

Even at apparently moderate, but unspecified, environmental temperatures, Convertino et al. (30) observed that increasing the workload (bicycle-ergometer, 100, 175, 225 watt, W) among 15 healthy male test subjects elicited linear (with workload) increments in PRA which were significant at all three work intensities. Circulating AVP, however, manifested a more curvilinear increase which was markedly elevated at the highest work load. Decrements in plasma volume were also linearly (inversely) correlated with workload (-3.7% at 100 to -12.4% at 225 W). While changes in circulating Na^+ concentration and osmolality were closely correlated with changes in AVP, these variables were not correlated with PRA. These results indicate that PRA responds linearly to the reduction in renal blood flow due to the diversion of cardiac output to the exercising muscle mass. However, PVP release may be more closely correlated with elevated osmolality and plasma sodium levels. When the same group of investigators (31) later studied the effects of training on the responses of many of these same variables at an ambient temperature of 25°C, they reported that training increased resting PV by 12.3% although resting baseline levels of PRA and PVP were unaffected by training. Further, they demonstrated that the increments in PRA and AVP during exercise observed prior to training were attenuated by the training regimen. The effects of training on plasma protein concentrations and total circulating protein were not evaluated. It is noteworthy that, subsequent to training, the percentage decreases in plasma volume were reduced following 175 W and 225 W exercise (31) since total PV was increased by the training regimen. Also, because of the increased VO_2 max (11.2%), each workload represented a lowered relative intensity (% VO_2 max) and therefore a decreased physiological strain on the test subjects. This is certainly suggestive evidence that the magnitude of the response of the fluid regulatory hormones may be affected by the relative exercise intensity and the plasma volume itself.

Interestingly, when Finberg et al. (52) compared the responses of adult males to walking in the heat (level treadmill, 1.3 m/s, 90 min, 50°C) during the summer and winter months, they observed again an attenuated response of PRA during the summer trial which may be related to the increased plasma volume of natural acclimatization during the summer months. They also reported (52) that replacement of the estimated fluid loss during the 90 min walk with water and NaCl reduced the intensity of the PRA response pattern in 4 out of 5 subjects (Fig. 3), thus indicating that fluid replenishment probably helped to sustain renal blood flow, albeit at reduced levels. When Costill et al. (33,34) used exercise (60 min, 60% VO_2 max) at 30°C to study urinary sodium loss, they observed that levels of PRA and PA were elevated during and immediately following exercise in the heat, and returned to control levels usually by 6-12 h following exercise completion. Additionally, they reported that this scenario consisting of a single exercise interval was effective in reducing urinary Na^+ and Cl^- concentrations for up to 48h, presumably due to the effects of the single elevation in PA levels subsequent to exercise.

Similarly, when Orenstein et al. (122) exercised normal young adult test subjects at 50% VO_2 max at 37°C, also for 90 min, they observed significant elevations in PRA and PA immediately subsequent to exercise, and these increments contributed to marked reductions in urinary Na^+ loss with no effects on serum Na^+. Alternatively, in these studies (122) cystic fibrosis patients manifested normal hormonal responses to heat/exercise stress and similar reductions in urinary Na^+, but serum Na^+ levels were also reduced, probably due to excessive loss in sweat. Interestingly, the cystic fibrosis patients, who can and do manifest the physiological advantages of heat acclimation (123) yet respond to heat stress with an increased loss of sweat Na^+ and $C1^-$ (122), thus demonstrate normal responses to exercise in the heat with respect to PRA and PA.

Therefore, during exercise in the heat hormonal responses directed at fluid and electrolyte conservation are rapid and intense with probable persistent effects, and may be partially responsible for the defense of body water and extracellular fluid which help to maintain the efficiency of the cardiovascular

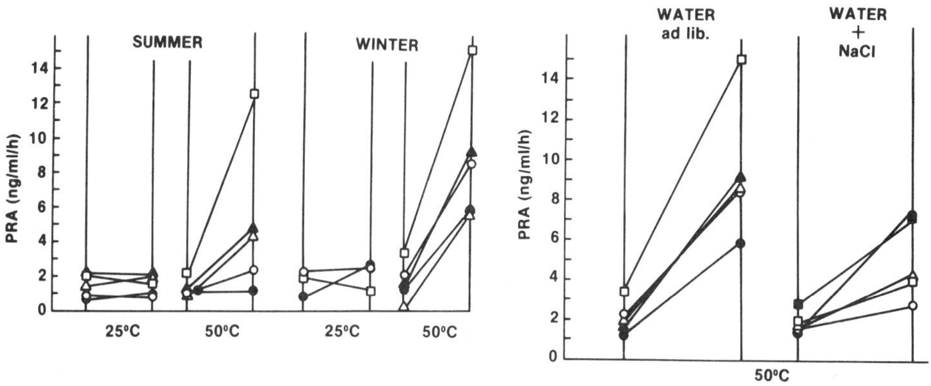

FIGURE 3. Effects of natural acclimatization and salt replacement on the responses of PRA to treadmill exercise at 25°C. and 50°C. in healthy, male volunteers. Individual data are depicted. In each section pre-values (on the left) are connected to post-values (on the right). Summer trials were conducted in September and October while winter tests were executed in December and January. Salt ingestion was based on the estimate that the NaCl content of sweat lost was 400 mg/100 ml, and replaced at 15 minute intervals during the 90 min walk at 4.7 km/hr. The increased intravascular volume of summer may blunt the PRA response in comparison to the winter trial as the NaCl ingestion relieves the demand to replace the NaCl lost in sweat. (Redrawn from: Finberg et al., J. Appl. Physiol., 36; 519, 1974 with permission of the publisher).

and thermoregulatory systems. In one of the very few studies which has quantitated fluid- and electrolyte-regulatory hormone levels after heat injury, Aarseth et al. (1) observed significant elevations in PRA and PVP at rest following incurrence of the injury in 6 athletes who suffered heatstroke with T_{re} in excess of 42.0°C.

When humans exercise in the heat even for relatively brief intervals, thermal sweating without fluid replacement is accompanied by general decrements in body weight with proportionately more intense reductions in plasma volume. Diaz et al. (38) investigated the effects of posture on plasma volume changes during rest (45 min) and exercise (45 min) in a hot environment. Subjects worked on a bicycle ergometer (30% and 45% VO_2 max, 49.5°C), in the upright, low-sit and supine postures without fluid replacement. During the total heat exposure, plasma volume was reduced by 20% in the upright, 16.1% in the low sit, and 13.3% in the supine positions with no differences noted between work loads. Body weight was reduced by only 1.3-1.4% in these experiments, thus eliciting substantial ratios in the percent decrease in PV versus percent decrease in body weight. No effects of posture were noted on either plasma protein levels or osmolality, suggesting an isooncotic and isosmotic fluid shift out of the plasma space, and, unfortunately, hormonal responses were not assessed.

When Harrison et al. (86) exercised adult unacclimated males for 50 min at 42°C and 3 months later at 30°C using the same experimental protocol without fluid replacement, they observed decrements in plasma volume of approximately 10-12% by the end of the exercise period in the fluid deprivation experiment. However, during a sedentary 50 min recovery period PV recovered to control or near control levels (depending on the method of calculation). These investigators (86) concluded that, as proposed by Senay (144, 145), the return of protein to the intravascular space via the lymphatic system during exercise and probably also during recovery contributed to an elevated oncotic pressure. This osmotic force in turn promotes water influx into the intravascular space at the expense of other fluid compartments. The same group (83) used radio-iodinated serum albumin to confirm that, following exercise, protein was transferred to the intravascular space more rapidly than it was lost through capillary permeability.

Senay and Fortney (149) compared the responses of untrained females to exercise (ergometer, 30% VO_2 max) at 16-20°C and 45°C and observed a PV decrement of nearly 13% in the thermoneutral environment and nearly 18% in the heat. While plasma protein increased markedly during the thermoneutral trial, no such increment was observed during the heat trial. This led Senay and Fortney (149) to conclude that the increased perfusion and, perhaps, permeability of the cutaneous capillaries, far more extensively perfused during exercise in the heat, counteract the retention or accumulation of intravascular protein during the heat/exercise regimen. When Greenleaf et al. (76) used 45% VO_2 max and 40°C Ta as an exercise/heat stress, they observed decrements in PV of approximately 11% after 60 min. Thus, it is clear that, despite the hormonal responses which favor fluid and electrolyte retention, plasma volume is nonetheless decreased during acute heat/cycle exercise stress. When such loss of body water results in frank hypohydration, then the physiological and endocrinological adaptations conserving fluid and electrolytes become even more crucial to the prevention of heat/exercise injury (1) and maintenance of physical performance (5).

The results indicate that passive heat exposure, exercise, and exercise in the heat are all rapidly and variably stimulatory to increased circulating levels of PRA, PA, and PVP. PRA may be stimulated most effectively by a reduction in renal blood flow secondary to increased muscle or skin blood flow. PA apparently may be initially elevated by generally increased adrenocorticotrophic activity secondary to exercise/heat stress while PVP, initially elevated by acute heat exposure or exercise heat stress, may be more severely affected by increased plasma Na^+, osmolality, or decreased plasma volume secondary to hypohydration.

HYPOHYDRATION

For those readers interested in the comparison among species, the apparent universality of the endocrinological responses to heat/hypohydration has been confirmed in a wide range of experimental animals. For example, Keil and Severs (98) observed in rats that 48 h of water deprivation was effective in eliciting marked elevations in plasma vasopressin levels, but these increments were attenuated with increasing weight of the experimental animals. Further, they reported (98) that the imposition of a non-thermal secondary stress (ether, acceleration) tended to reduce the elevations in PVP effected by hypohydration. Kenyon et al. (99) observed that when 1 ug/day of aldosterone was administered to adrenalectomized rats, the animals produced a small volume of more concentrated urine and plasma K^+ levels were increased. When rats were passively exposed to an ambient temperature of 40°C, PVP levels were increased and the increments were surprisingly exacerbated by propranolol treatment (77). Arad et al. (4) examined the hormonal, fluid, and electrolyte responses in domestic fowl and noted that hypohydration (13% bw, 48 h water deprivation) increased PA, PVP, Na^+, and osmolality, all of which were exaggerated when hypohydration was combined with heat exposure (final ambient = 42°C) and attenuated during a rehydration interval (30 min); however, heat exposure alone had no effects on these variables. During hypohydration and heat exposure, core temperature increased to 43.7°C from 42.8°C (heat alone); similarly, plasma osmolality increased from 319 to nearly 360 mOsm/kg H_2O, respectively.

Interestingly, Thrasher et al. (163) reported in dogs that 24 h of water deprivation (~5% body weight loss) caused significant elevations in Na^+, osmolality, PVP, and PRA which had returned to control levels after 1 day of rehydration. Alternatively, PA was not significantly affected during dehydration, but peaked at 24 h of recovery. They (163) attributed this 24 h peak to a decrement in plasma Na^+ occurring upon rehydration which was countermanded by this PA response, and hypothesized that a natriuresis during hypohydration helped to reduce the magnitude of the increments in plasma osmolality. However, using hyperhydrated goats Augustinsson et al. (8) reported no increments in excretion of AVP and a decrease in PA during acute

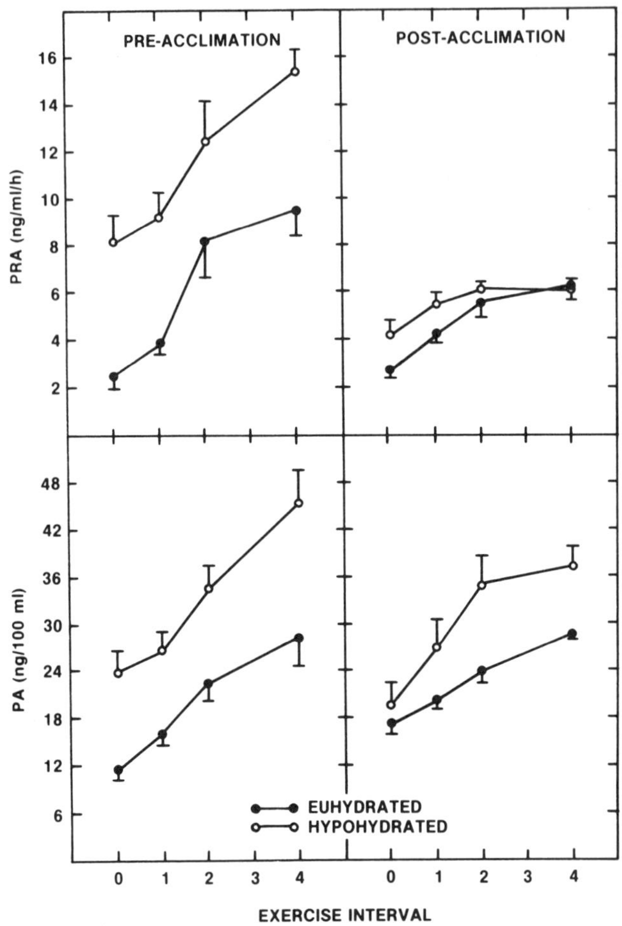

FIGURE 4. Effects of hypohydration (5% bw) and acclimation on plasma renin activity and aldosterone levels during exercise (four 25 min/10 min work/rest cycles, level treadmill, 1.34 m/sec) in the heat (49°C., 20% rh). Mean levels (±SEM) are depicted for 8 young adult male and 8 young adult female test subjects. Blood was taken prior to and approximately 15-20 min into the 1st, 2nd, and 4th exercise intervals. The increased plasma volume of acclimation may help to maintain renal blood flow and repress the PRA response. The effects of hypohydration are most notable pre-acclimation (time 0). Redrawn from: Francesconi et al., J. Appl. Physiol., 55; 1790, 1983 with permission of the publisher).

heat exposure (45°C); they attributed these observations to the significant respiratory alkalosis which developed by 60 min in this species.

Finally, even in animals as large as domestic cattle, El-Nouty et al. (45) reported that acute (8 h) heat stress (35°C) elicited a mean elevation in T_{re} of 2°C and a significant elevation in PVP which was further increased when water was withheld for 30 h. During 24 h of heat exposure PA levels were significantly depressed in these experiments (45), and recovered toward control levels during dehydration. Again, they attributed the decrement in PA to the increased plasma Na^+ observed during heat stress. Thus, although the responsiveness of the plasma hormones to hypohydration has been validated in a wide range of experimental species, the vast majority of this research has been accomplished using human test subjects.

In humans the effects of hypohydration during heat exposure and exercise in the heat have been extensively documented. Even in well heat-acclimated subjects, Strydom and Holdsworth (159) observed that during work in the heat increasing severity of hypohydration (3-5% and 5-8% body weight decrements) caused exaggerated increases in T_{re} and heart rates while sweat rates were reduced. In these studies optimal performance (i.e. minimal physiological strain) was observed when test subjects were compelled to rehydrate at 15 min intervals; it is generally believed that complete rehydration, even when palatable and potable fluids are conveniently available and drinking is encouraged, is

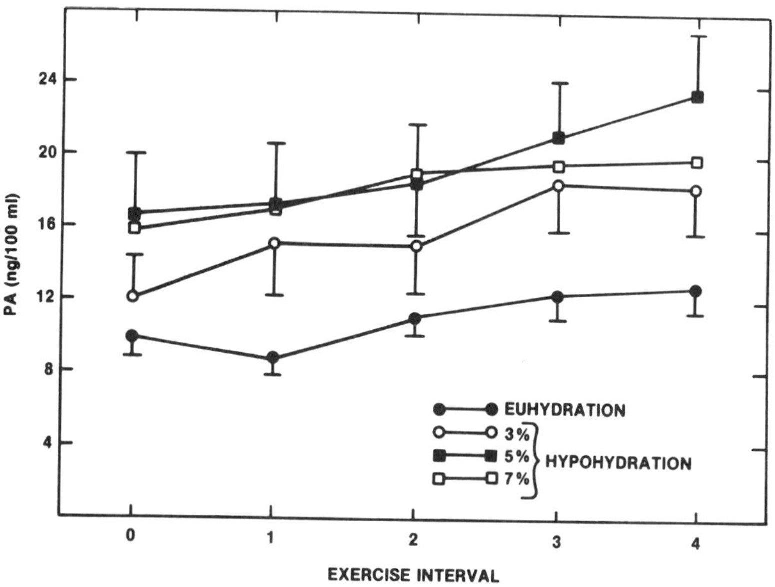

FIGURE 5. Effects of graded hypohydration levels (0-7%) on PA during exercise in the heat in 6 highly acclimated young adult male test subjects. Mean values ±SEM are depicted. Hypohydration to the appropriate level was accomplished by fluid denial during exercise in the heat during the afternoon prior to the morning of the test. The exercise intervals correspond to 4 consecutive exercise periods (25 min, level treadmill, 1.34 m/sec, 49°C.) interspersed by 10 min rest periods. Time 0 blood samples were taken after subjects remained upright in an antechamber (20°C.) for at least 20 min. Five and 7% hypohydration elicit similar elevations in resting PA levels; it is noteworthy that PV were reduced to similar degrees by 5 and 7% hypohydration indicating the role of volume receptors in controlling the endocrine responses. (Redrawn from: Francesconi et al., J. Appl. Physiol., 59;1855, 1985 with permission of the publisher).

ordinarily delayed during and immediately after exercise in the heat - a phenomenon termed voluntary dehydration (74).

The increased physiological strain of hypohydration partially results from the significant decrements in PV and increases in osmolality which usually occur concomitantly with hypohydration, resulting in decreased sweat rates and reduced skin blood flow (138). For example, Saltin (138) observed that hypohydration, elicited by thermal exposure to a 5.2% reduction in body weight, may be accompanied by reductions in PV by as much as 25%. He (138) further noted that the decrements in PV were accompanied by significantly reduced endurance capacities and maximal blood lactate while cardiac output may be maintained by increased heart rate. Costill and Fink (36) compared the effects of thermal- and exercise-induced hypohydration, and reported that at 4% body weight loss PV was reduced by 16-18% subsequent to either form of dehydration. In our own experiments induction of hypohydration (3-7% body weight) is ordinarily followed by a period (12-16 h) of inactivity before experimentation during which fluid is redistributed to the plasma, yet PV's consistently decrease by 5-15% (139-141).

When we dehydrated men by 5% body weight, we observed significant elevations in PRA and PA in blood samples taken prior to exercise; subsequent exercise in the heat reduced PV even further and PRA and PA were enhanced during hypohydration trials while the increases in PRA were modulated by acclimation (64) (Fig. 4). In a more recent study (65) in which we reported the effects of 3, 5, and 7% hypohydration on circulating hormone responses, we observed that increasing the intensity of hypohydration from 3% to 5% was usually accompanied by an increased elevation in PRA and PA; however, between 5 and 7% hypohydration, where no further decrements in PV were observed (141), we likewise noted no additional increments in either PRA or PA (Fig. 5). Consistent with these results Von Ameln et al. (165) demonstrated that, following thermal dehydration, PVP increased from 2.1 to 8.1 pg/ml, but this elevation was attenuated to 4.7 pg/ml by head-out water immersion. They attributed this attenuation of PVP response to "central hypervolemia" effected by water immersion.

When the same group (101) examined the effects of hypohydration induced by prolonged exercise (27-32 km) on PRA, they reported that four-fold increases in PRA levels 50-60 min after the completion of exercise were reduced to nearly control levels about 1 h later and following food and fluid consumption. In a separate experiment (16) subjects were exercised in the heat (34°C, 85 W, 4 h) with no fluid replacement, with water replacement, and with NaCl-sucrose consumption (Fig. 6). During the exercise interval levels of PA, PRA, and PVP were progressively increased during the "no fluid" trial; however, with either water or NaCl-sucrose replacement, increments in PRA and PVP were abolished. While water consumption attenuated the increment in PA elicited by no fluid replacement, NaCl-sucrose blunted this response even further, and after 4 h of exercise in the heat, levels were not different from controls.

Thus, the evidence seems to strongly favor a rapid and marked elevation in circulating levels of fluid and electrolyte regulatory hormones when

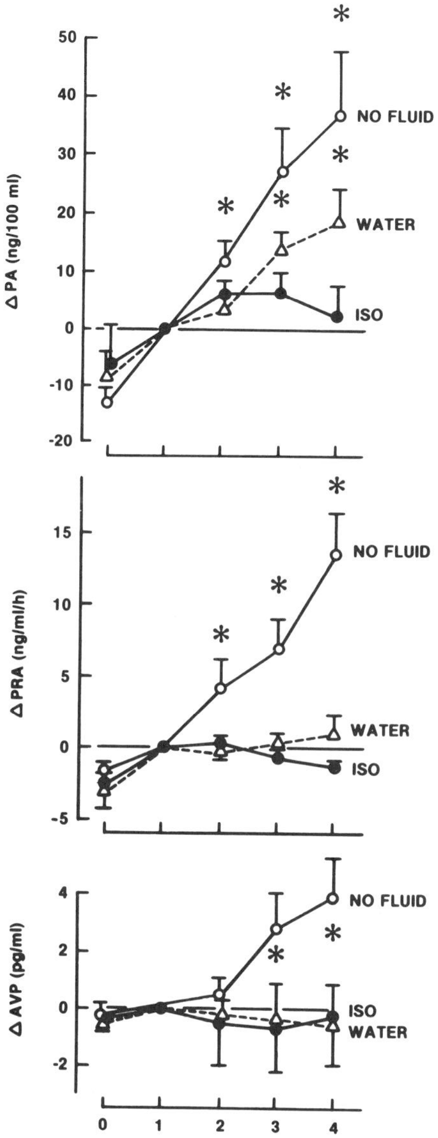

FIGURE 6. Effects of intermittent exercise in the heat (34°C.) on plasma renin activity, aldosterone, and vasopressin. Exercise consisted of four 25 min/5 min work/rest cycles followed by four 20 min/10 min work/rest cycles at approximately 85W. Three separate trials were evaluated: NO FLUID, exercise was accomplished with no fluid intake during the trial; WATER, 80% of the weight loss was replaced with spring water; ISO, 80% of the weight loss was replaced with an isotonic solution of sodium, chloride, potassium, and sucrose. Mean values (±SEM) are depicted for a group of 5 unacclimated young men. Asterisks indicate significant difference from the 1 hr value ($P < 0.05$). (Redrawn from: Brandenberger et al., Eur. J. Appl. Physiol., 55; 123, 1986 with permission of the publisher).

heat/exercise exposure induces progressive dehydration or a targeted level of hypohydration precedes the heat/exercise exposure. These responses may be related to increased osmolality, decreased plasma volume, or perhaps decreased blood pressure. While the responses of PVP and PRA have been consistent and unidirectional, there is some evidence that the control of aldosterone secretion may be superseded by the increasing Na^+ concentration which also may accompany hypohydration. In fact, reports on the influence of electrolyte supplements during heat exposure and exercise in the heat, the effects of prior high or low dietary consumption of electrolytes, and the experimental depletion of electrolytes provide a framework to investigate further the mechanisms and control of hormonal responses to heat/exercise stress.

ELECTROLYTES

In his review on fluid and electrolyte balance during exercise in hot environments, Halim (80) concluded that 3 g of salt should ordinarily be ingested for each liter of sweat loss. If the exercise intensity and the ambient temperature are sufficiently high, then it is not unusual that 6-12 L of sweat/day may be secreted requiring, accordingly, 300-600 mEq NaCl for replacement. However, in their more recent review, Epstein and Sohar (46) surveyed a variety of reports in the literature which suggested that well-acclimated individuals can tolerate work in the heat with NaCl intakes of even less than 100 mEq/day. Of course, several early reports had confirmed that the acquisition of acclimation is accompanied by a striking ability to secrete increased quantities of a more dilute sweat (39,130,131,162). The requirement for salt replacement during repeated or prolonged exercise in hot environments is dependent upon the individual's acclimation status as well as the normal amount of dietary salt to which the test subject or population may be accustomed.

When Smiles and Robinson (157) examined the effects of recurrent exercise in the heat (100 min, 1.58 m/s, 45°C) on young adult males in negative salt balance induced by dietary manipulation, they reported 3-6 fold increments in 24 h output of urinary tetrahydroaldosterone; this was accompanied by apparent 10-20-fold reductions in urinary Na^+. When the same experiments were repeated with the subjects in positive salt balance, both urinary tetrahydroaldosterone and Na^+ were at control levels, suggesting that the magnitude of the sodium conservation response during acclimation is dependent upon exogenous Na^+ availability. Shortly thereafter, Bailey and co-workers (10) placed 12 young adults males on high (>300 mEq/d), normal (182 mEq), and low (12 mEq) Na^+ diets during 3 consecutive weeks. Following the normal and low dietary intervals, heat stress was induced by sedentary exposure to 46-51°C ambient conditions and PA and PRA were assessed before and after the heat stress. The low-Na^+ diet elicited significant increments in both PA and PRA in the pre-heat samples, and the heat exposure increased the levels of both hormones following either dietary regimen though the elevations were more notable during the low salt trial. Interestingly, they noted that packed cell volumes were unaffected by thermal stress, and concluded that high thermal stress, *per se*, is a potent stimulator of renin and aldosterone secretion. In fact, these workers suggested that the level of heat stress elicited by sedentary exposure to approximately 50°C might be utilized as a marker of the normal response of these endocrine systems (10).

Recent results have generally indicated that exogenous salt loading does not markedly enhance the acquisition of acclimation or reduce the physiological strain of work in the heat. Although Armstrong et al. (6) observed several sporadic advantages to consuming a high sodium diet during acclimation to heat, Konikoff et al. (107) reported that salt supplementation in fully acclimated subjects provided no benefits during work in the heat while PA levels were repressed and PRA was unaffected. Earlier, Follenius et al. (54) had demonstrated that consumption of a low salt diet induced significant increments in basal levels of both PA and PRA; when these subjects were acutely exposed (90 min) to sedentary heat stress, the percent increases in PA and PRA were similar in subjects consuming either a high salt (200 mEq Na/d) or low salt (20-30 mEq Na/d) diet. The same group (17) used propranolol to illustrate a dissociation between the responses of PA and PRA to heat stress in that propranolol reduced the PRA response to heat exposure while PA was actually increased during the propranolol trial. We have observed dissociations in PRA and PA responses previously in both rats (57) and, under certain conditions, humans (65).

Likewise, when studying rehydration with a glucose-electrolyte solution or water, Costill et al. (35) concluded that, following dehydration to 3% body weight on 5 successive days, the glucose-electrolyte drink did not provide any physiological benefits to the test subjects. The authors cautioned, however, that electrolyte balance was being maintained by adequate dietary consumption. In fact, they hypothesized (35) that the supplementary Na^+ intake may have repressed PA secretion causing more Na^+ and fluid loss during the glucose-electrolyte trial. In addition, Nielsen et al. (119) recently reported no significant effects of rehydration with a control, high potassium, high sodium, or high sugar beverage; interestingly, they concluded that the high Na^+ drink specifically benefitted the extracellular fluid compartment while the high K^+ and high sugar drinks augmented intracellular fluid volume. Ikawa et al. (96) had previously exposed volunteers to a sauna (65-70°C) for 30 min and during a recovery period provided either no fluids, 500 ml of an isotonic sports supplement containing Na^+, or 500 ml of water. Circulating PA levels were significantly increased by the heat exposure, and were maintained at higher concentrations during the water or no-fluid experiment. The various drinks did not provide any advantages in reducing physiological strain with respect to either T_{re} or heart rate.

The evidence is weighted heavily toward the conclusion that in the presence of consistent dietary intake of salt, excessive salt consumption or the ingestion of salt-containing beverages does not have ergogenic effects during exercise in the heat or reduce the physiological cost of heat exposure. Harrison et al. (84) noted that when 1% NaCl was ingested to prevent dehydration, core temperatures were higher than when water was consumed. In fact, there is increasing evidence to suggest that consumption of modest or even low levels of salt (<100 mEq/d) is adequate to maintain electrolyte balance when the reduced dietary intake is followed by acute or prolonged heat exposure or exercise in the heat. Further, the maintenance of electrolyte balance under these conditions is dependent upon the effects of increased endocrinological activity as manifested in consistently elevated PA concentrations when dietary NaCl intake is low, and reduced circulating PA when NaCl intake is above normal.

Several of the world's population groups are able to withstand chronic heat exposure on low salt diets (20-50 mEq/d) without apparent increased rates of heat injury; this is probably testimony to the exquisite mechanisms for extremely efficient salt conservation by which humans adapt endocrinologically. From this it may be reasonable to conclude that individuals who are at most serious risk of developing salt depletion-induced heat cramps (14) are those who abruptly change from a high or average salt intake to a low consumption concomitant with sustained heat exposure and profuse sweating. In our experience we have observed this situation when large numbers of garrison quartered troops are abruptly transferred to desert environments in the southwestern US for field training exercises.

The effects of potassium deficiency upon the ability to work in the heat and the endocrinological responses to acute or chronic heat exposure have been less extensively studied. Malhotra et al. (113) reported that K deficiency can accrue even in well-acclimated individuals when exposed sedentarily to $40^{o}C$ for 4 consecutive days, and, further, that this K deficiency may contribute significantly to the development of heat injury. In fact, during acclimation to heat it is conceivable that the loss of K in sweat as well as the conservation of sodium by the kidney with attendant K loss could contribute to cellular potassium depletion and the development of heat illness (142).

Knochel and his co-workers (103,104) have demonstrated that recurrent work in hot environments may result in substantial negative K balance despite mean daily intakes of approximately 100 mEq; these investigators also observed that both PA and PRA, as well as urinary aldosterone were "unsuppressed" for the quantities of Na that their test subjects were ingesting although no explanation for the lack of suppression was offered. Alternatively, when Coburn et al. (21) acutely exposed unacclimated, K-deficient test subjects to heat stress, they observed repressed urinary aldosterone excretion which they attributed to a failure of plasma K to increase during heat exposure as a result of the K depletion. Interestingly, their regimen of K depletion (producing deficits of 230-465 mEq K) failed to induce consistent thermoregulatory decrements in their test subjects. When Francis and coworkers (66,67) used either water or a potassium supplemented electrolyte solution for rehydration during exercise (50% VO_2 max, 120 min, $32^{o}C$), they observed no marked beneficial effects of the electrolyte solution; PRA and PA were significantly reduced during the electrolyte supplement experiment. Generally, the consensus has been that carbohydrate/electrolyte supplements are unnecessary if balanced food consumption has not been curtailed (110).

When Hubbard et al. (95) used their rat model of human heatstroke (93,94) to investigate the effects of prolonged feeding (32 d) of a K deficient diet, they reported that exercise endurance was reduced by 37%, work done was decremented by 49%, and muscle K was depleted by 26%. At approximately the same time Haldy and Muller (79) had reported, also in rats, that consumption of a K-deficient diet (2 weeks, 0.8 mmole K/kg) markedly reduced the ability of excised and incubated adrenal glands to convert tritiated corticosterone to aldosterone. Since the biosynthesis of aldosterone in K-deficient rat adrenal glands could be stimulated by sodium deficiency, water deprivation, and furosemide treatment, these authors concluded (79) that enzymes regulating the final steps in the biosynthesis of aldosterone may be instrumental in the control of PA levels and inhibited by potassium deficiency.

In his review Knochel (102) concluded that K deficits may be associated with postural hypotension and syncope, reduced muscle membrane integrity, and the development of rhabdomyolysis. While frank intracellular hypokalemia will clearly predispose an individual to increased risk of heat injury, other potential sequelae of acute or chronic negative K balance have not been assessed in carefully controlled human studies. Interestingly, in our studies on heatstroke in rats we have demonstrated that the intensity of circulatory hyperkalemia subsequent to exercise in the heat was inversely correlated to survival time (60); conversely, rats which were able to run for prolonged periods with the achievement of a steady-state, moderate T_{re} (<40^oC) manifested reduced circulating K levels (59). Clearly, the relationships between K deficits and surfeits and plasma volume, sweat secretion, hormonal responses, Na balance, and the acquisition of acclimation in humans should be more extensively described (7).

HEAT ACCLIMATION

The effects of heat acclimation on the endocrinological responses to heat exposure/exercise in the heat are somewhat inconsistent and variable. When considering the number and range of experimental variables which could conceivably affect such responses, this is perhaps not surprising. For example, hydration level, acclimation status, aerobic fitness level, exercise intensity and type, ambient conditions, electrolyte balance, sampling time, subject posture and a variety of other experimental variables (19) could, singly or in combination, affect test results and conclusions. Of these, the acclimation state may especially provide significant variability due to the range of increments in resting plasma volume which has been consistently reported subsequent to heat acclimation.

When Greenleaf et al. (73, 75) exercised (45% VO_2 max) 2 groups of men at 23.8^oC and 39.8^oC for 8 d, they reported that during exercise in the heat, PRA and PVP levels were increased without effects of acclimation on the resting levels prior to or increments during exercise in the heat (Fig. 7). Likewise, when Finberg et al. (51) measured PRA and PA following exercise (ergometer, 40-50% VO_2 max, 30 min) in the heat (50^oC) for 7 consecutive days, they reported similar PRA (9.5 ± 4.4 and 8.0 ± 4.7, day 1 vs. day 7) and PA (22.6 ± 8.5 and 25.5 ± 8, day 1 vs. day 7) levels prior and subsequent to the acclimation regimen. Bonner et al. (15) had earlier reported similar elevations in PA prior and subsequent to acclimation and following both a sedentary and exercise interval in the heat. Davies and co-workers (22,37) concluded that an 11 day acclimation program did not attenuate the increments in PRA and PA observed during exercise in the heat, but prior saline ingestion did modulate these increments suggesting the more subtle effects of acclimation vs saline consumption on endocrinological responses. When Convertino and Kirby (32) observed a significant reduction in 24 h Na clearance following acclimation with no changes in resting PA levels, they concluded that renal sensitivity to PA may be increased during acclimation.

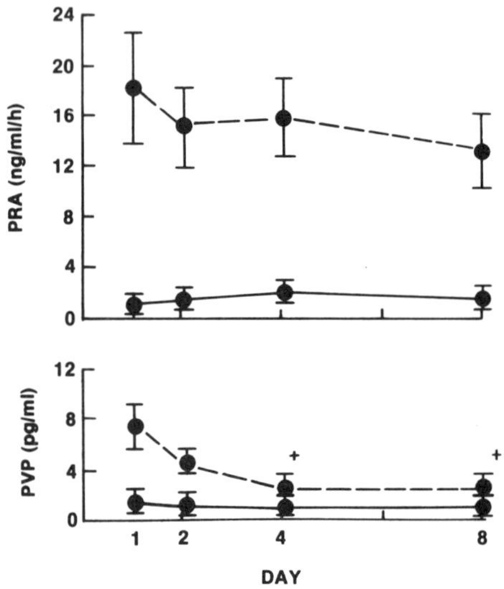

FIGURE 7. Effects of heat acclimation (39.8°C., 2 hr/d, 8 d, ergometer, 75W) on plasma renin activity and vasopressin levels immediately prior (solid line) and subsequent (dashed line) to exercise in the heat. Venous blood samples were taken on d 1,2,4, and 8 and the data represent mean levels for 5 healthy young males. The trend toward reduced PRA over the 8 d acclimation regimen did not achieve statistical significance although the data for PVP can be interpreted in terms of an increase in PV developing during acclimation. The continuous 2 hr exercise period may have contributed to the persistently high PRA even after acclimation. (+ = significantly different from day 1). (Redrawn from: Greenleaf et al., J. Appl. Physiol., 54; 414, 1983 with permission of the publisher).

A short time later the same workers (100) demonstrated reductions in sweat sodium loss concomitant with reductions in PA during exercise in the heat (45% VO_2 max, 40°C) on day 10 vs day 1 of heat acclimation. Again, they hypothesized that the reduced PA is compensated by an elevated eccrine sweat gland responsiveness to PA after acclimation. The pioneering work in this area had been accomplished much earlier by Conn who reported that acclimation can reduce the salt lost in sweat by as much as 95% (27). Finberg and Berlyne (50) had used both natural acclimatization (exposure to summer heat) and experimentally induced heat acclimation (90 min exercise, 50°C, 7 d) to demonstrate generally attenuated responses of PRA and PA to light exercise in the heat when compared to the responses elicited in winter or without acclimation. They (52) had earlier reported that not only natural acclimatization to summer heat, but also prehydration with a NaCl solution suppressed exercise/heat-induced increments in PRA.

Some of our own work (64,65) had also demonstrated attenuated responses of the fluid/electrolyte-regulatory hormones to exercise in the heat following heat acclimation. When Shvartz et al. (156) administered tilt-table tests prior and subsequent to heat acclimation and observed 50 and 75% decrements, respectively, in responses of PRA and PVP following acclimation, they ascribed these decreases to the increased resting plasma volume. Alternatively, when we acutely expanded PV by intravenous administration of hyperoncotic albumin, we reported that during exercise (63) or at rest (58) in the heat, PA levels were suppressed. Thus, the augmented cardiovascular stability (137,167) and plasma volume (151,166) of heat acclimation may combine to lessen the requirement and stimulus for the usual elevations in levels of fluid and electrolyte regulatory hormones during heat exposure or work in the heat.

Knochel and Vertel (105) hypothesized that the development of the acclimated condition is characterized by increased aldosterone secretion and excretion. Earlier, Fletcher et al. (53) had compared aldosterone excretion rates in residents of the United Kingdom (15-17°C) and British expatriates living in Kuwait (38°C) and reported mean 24 h urinary aldosterone levels of 8.7 and 13.4 ug, respectively. Knochel and Vertel (105) reasoned that the increased aldosterone secretion and excretion of heat acclimation could effect excessive urinary K loss and suggested that less vigorous NaCl replacement (especially in the form of salt tablets) may be appropriate in reducing electrolyte disorders, polyuria, and circulatory hypokalemia.

However, since these earlier suggestions that increased aldosterone secretion and activity may be necessary for the acquisition of heat acclimation (53,68,105), more recent evidence indicates that acclimation and aerobic exercise training (117) are accompanied by an increased sensitivity and responsiveness to endocrinological effects at the sites of both central control (118,129) and peripheral effectors (32,100,151). The majority of the data suggests that subjects who are fully heat acclimated respond to heat exposure/exercise in the heat with similar or attenuated levels of PVP, PA, and PRA when compared to their non-acclimated counterparts. Such responses appear to be consistent with the increased plasma volume, decreased physiological strain, increased perfusion of viscera, and electrolyte balance associated with heat acclimation.

PLASMA VOLUME

The thermoregulatory and cardiovascular advantages of increased plasma volume and total body water in reducing the physiological strain of exercise in the heat have been investigated and recognized for decades. Moroff and Bass (115) used the same test subjects in two experimental trials (90 min treadmill exercise, 49°C, 1.58 m/s), once after preingestion of 2000 ml water and once without preingestion. They reported (115) that hyperhydration resulted in lower

T_{re}, heart rate, and increased sweat secretion during exercise in the heat. Much later, Fortney et al. (56) studied the effects of hypovolemia (diuretic-induced) and hypervolemia (albumin infusion) on blood volume and sweating responses. They observed that hypovolemia (8.7% decrease in blood volume) and hypervolemia (7.9% elevation in blood volume) effected 20 min sweat rates of 270 ml and 541 ml, respectively (56), and hypothesized that the exacerbated release of PVP during hypovolemia may have contributed to this decrement. Earlier, Horstman and Horvath (91) reported that whole body, thigh, and abdomen sweat rates were significantly greater during euhydration than 3.6% hypohydration. Alternatively, Myhre and Robinson (116) used passive heat exposure (50°C) to reduce PV by 7.8% (no fluid replacement) or 2.9% (NaCl replacement) and demonstrated no effects on sweat rates; in these experiments the PV differential may have been insufficient to elicit observable differences (87). In a related experiment Shannon et al. (154) exercised men in a cool (15°C) environment, once after a subcutaneous administration of AVP and a second time when subjects ingested 2% of their body weight in water after AVP injection. Thirty through 60 min after the initiation of exercise, PV loss was reduced in the hyperhydrated group indicating the important effects of hydration level even when exogenous AVP is administered (154).

The mechanisms responsible for the increased PV of heat acclimation have been extensively investigated in recent years. Thus, Senay and co-investigators (152) exercised trained individuals (4 h/d, 40-50% VO_2 max, 3 d at 25°C and 10d at 45°C), and reported that between day 1 and day 2 of exercise in the heat total plasma protein was elevated by 11.6% and PV increased by 9%. Further, during acclimation more protein and fluid were retained within the circulatory system (152). Earlier, Senay (145) had compared the effects of stair-stepping in a cool environment (20°C) with the same exercise in the heat (40°C), and reported that following acclimation, exercise in the heat was accompanied by hemodilution and maintenance or increments in plasma protein. Conversely, before heat acclimation exercise at 40°C was characterized by hemoconcentration and net protein losses (145) while exercise in the cool environment even before heat acclimation was accompanied by hemodilution. These results led Senay (145, 147) to hypothesize that permeability changes in cutaneous capillaries and availability of translocatable protein were partially responsible for the increased PV of heat acclimation.

When Senay later (146) compared the effects of heat acclimation on block-stepping at 34°C, he again found that with acclimation, hemodilution was maintained for 2 h. He further hypothesized (146) that hemodilution or hemoconcentration responses may be dependent upon initial plasma osmolalities and circulating AVP levels with the degree of hemodilution inversely correlated with initial osmolality and AVP concentration. Interestingly, the same group (150) asserted that heat intolerant individuals (n=15) failed to hemodilute to the same extent as a group of heat tolerant men (n=19) when matched for VO_2 max, under similar ambient and work conditions. Moreover, reduced aerobic exercise in the heat or deacclimation was accompanied by a decrement in plasma volume mostly accounted for by significant reductions in total plasma protein (126). Even in rats, Horowitz and Samueloff (90) reported that dehydration following acclimation to 34°C ambient was characterized by decreased efflux of albumin while colloid osmotic pressure and total protein mass increased. Studying desert-originated mice, they demonstrated (89) that dehydration elicited no changes in plasma volume and a significant decrement in efflux of albumin from the circulatory system.

FUTURE STUDIES

It is noteworthy that in most of these studies addressing intercompartmental fluid shifts in acclimated, non-acclimated, heat tolerant and heat intolerant test subjects, potential endocrinological effectors have not been investigated. In fact, while a wide variety of physiological, pharmacological, and physical factors have been identified as predisposing an individual to heat/exercise injury (155), we are unaware of any studies which have evaluated the association between these factors and endocrinological adaptations to exercise in the heat.

For example, we have recently compared the physiological and hematological responses of older and younger men during 10 d of heat acclimation (124). While endocrinological responses are still being evaluated, the results of this study indicated no impairment of thermoregulatory responses when test subjects were separated by 25 years in age, but matched for VO_2 max and selected morphological factors. Alternatively, when Paolone et al. (125) compared the responses of young (26 y) and older (58 y) men to exercise in the heat, they observed that PRA was generally more markedly increased in the younger group. They further concluded (125) that increased PRA in the younger population may have contributed to their increased ability to protect PV during the first 60 min of exercise in the heat.

Additional studies on the role of endocrinological responses in the fluid shifts of heat acclimation, heat intolerance, and factors which predispose to heat injury may be useful in the design of pharmacological interventions to reduce the physiological strain of exercise in the heat. For example, although atrial hormone has been shown to counteract the vasoconstrictive effects of PRA and the anti-natriuretic effects of PA (111), to our knowledge no studies have been conducted assessing its response during heat exposure or exercise in the heat. We have demonstrated in a small animal model that during moderate (10%) hypohydration PV is protected by an influx of water from the interstitial fluid compartment, and at 15% hypohydration, both the interstitial and the intracellular compartment contribute to the maintenance of PV (42). However, no studies of hormonal control, if existent, of these intercompartmental shifts have been reported. In a much earlier study Giec (72) estimated the source of the water content of sweat during 2 h of sedentary heat (50°C) exposure and concluded that 66% originated in the interstitial fluid, 18% in the PV, and 16% in the erythrocytes and other cells.

Yet another understudied area is the complex series of endocrinological responses occurring in females during exercise in the heat with respect to circadian periodicity and phase of the menstrual cycle (88,158); for example, Horvath and Drinkwater (92) have reported a greater decrement in PV following exercise in the heat during the luteal phase of the cycle. Grucza et al. (78) have observed several significant differences in sweating responses to heat exposure between men and women yet to our knowledge no studies have been executed to investigate the endocrine correlates, if extant, of these differences with respect to either the monthly cycle or aging.

CONCLUSION

In this review we have attempted to address comprehensively the hormonal adaptations and responses which function in the maintenance of fluid and electrolyte homeostasis during heat/exercise stress (see also Table 1). Inconsistencies are apparent, but even more obvious are the myriad of experimental parameters which can affect experimental results. The exercise or, indeed, the heat may range from mild to severe, the time of exposure from acute to chronic, the fitness status of the subjects from poor to elite - clearly, all these can affect qualitatively and quantitatively adaptational profiles and response patterns. Add to these the variables that can be more subtle or difficult to assess - hydration status, acclimation level, prior dietary history, and it is not difficult to envision persistent inconsistencies or even apparent contradictions. However, frequently, a close reading of the methodology will reveal logical and valid reasons for what at first glance appear to be contradictory reports. In fact, in reviewing the literature over the past 40 years, one of the several striking differences to be noted is the more comprehensive and complete descriptions of the test scenarios, experimental conditions, test subjects, and methodologies that are currently provided. It is incumbent upon all investigators to maintain and expand this careful attention to experimental and methodological details so that data can be properly evaluated.

It would have been useful, if it were possible, to correlate plasma hormonal response patterns and intensities to fundamental physiological variables relevant to exercise/heat stress. Information on indices related to physiological strain (e.g. rectal temperature, heart rate, osmolality, sodium levels, plasma volume as estimated from hematocrit-hemoglobin changes) may have permitted comparisons of the endocrine response patterns with these physiological variables across experiments. For example, the endocrinological responses to sedentary (e.g. 1 h, 60°C, euhydrated) heat exposure or exercise (e.g. 15 min, 30°C, 3% hypohydrated, 50% VO_2 max) in the heat provide useful, but independent, information on human adaptations to exercise/heat stress. If in these two experiments, however, the response patterns could be related to common physiological criteria as indicated above, then much more comprehensive and useful interpretations could be made. For example, the intensity of the hormonal responses could be related to the physiological criteria affecting this intensity in both experiments. Conclusions might be drawn as to hormonal responses which contribute to the successful completion of either exercise or the heat stress in both experiments, and the role of baroreceptors, osmoreceptors, volume receptors and thermoreceptors could be assessed. The degree of stress would be related to a physiological rather than an environmental/exercise criterion, and the diversity of environmental/exercise criteria could be more comparable.

In closing, we would like to reemphasize that despite progress in understanding the role of hormonal action in regulating fluid and electrolyte balance during heat exposure/exercise in the heat, much remains unknown. A recent brief review by McDougall (114) underscores this. In this succinct report McDougall (114) discusses the factors which are instrumental to the control of aldosterone secretion. He notes that this hormone is secreted only by cells of the zona glomerulosa of the adrenal cortex. Further, he reports that angiotensin II, adrenocorticotropic hormone, potassium loading, and sodium deprivation are all stimulatory to aldosterone secretion while atrial natriuretic peptide is inhibitory. Despite these well-established regulatory factors, McDougall (114) asserts that several hypotheses and observations regarding the control of aldosterone biosynthesis remain unconfirmed and sometimes confusing: the role of monoamines and other hormones, alterations in adrenal sensitivity, occasional dissociation of the responses of angiotensin II and aldosterone, central stimulation of aldosterone secretion. McDougall concludes that much further in vitro and in vivo work is necessary "for full understanding of the physiological control of aldosterone secretion". More generally, we also conclude that much further work is necessary for a complete understanding of the role of the endocrine system in maintaining fluid and electrolyte homeostasis during the challenge of heat exposure/exercise in the heat.

The authors express their sincere appreciation to Mrs. Susan E.P. Henry and Mrs. Diane Danielski for their outstanding word processing support.

The views of the authors do not purport to reflect the positions of the Department of the Army or the Department of Defense.

Citations of commercial organizations and trade names in this report do not constitute an official Department of the Army endorsement or approval of the products or services of these organizations.

Table 1. Compendium of data from representative reports. Note that in some cases quantitative estimates were from interpretations of figure-depicted data.

LIST OF ABBREVIATIONS

PRA = PLASMA RENIN ACTIVITY; VO2 MAX = MAXIMAL OXYGEN CONSUMPTION; PADH = PLASMA ANTIDIURETIC HORMONE; NA = SODIUM; uU = MICROUNITS; PRE-EX = PRE-EXERCISE; POST-EX = POST-EXERCISE; H = HOURS; D = DAYS; M = METERS; ACCL = ACCLIMATIZED; PA = PLASMA ALDOSTERONE; HYPO = HYPOHYDRATED; ng = NANOGRAM; pg = PICOGRAM; PVP = PLASMA VASOPRESSIN; DEP = DEPRIVED; REHY = REHYDRATION; TRE = RECTAL TEMPERATURE; RT = (NORMAL) ROOM TEMPERATURE; W = WATTS; RH = RELATIVE HUMIDITY, KPM = KILOPOND METERS

CITATION	SPECIES	ACTIVITY	CONDITIONS AND RESULTS
GROZA ET AL., PHYSIOLOGIE, 14, 71, 1977	RAT	SEDENTARY	22°C, PADH = 3 uU/ml; 2H, 40°C, PADH = 6.75 uU/ml; 2H, 40°C, 5MG/KG PROPRANOLOL PADH = 10.5 uU/ml
FRANCESCONI ET AL., J. APPL. PHYSIOL. 58, 152, 1985	RAT	SEDENTARY	21°C, PA = 0.5 ng/ml; 35°C PA = 0.5 - 1.1 ng/ml; 71D, LOW NA DIET, 21°C PA = 3.9 ng/ml; 71D, LOW NA DIET, 6-168H 30°C, PA = 6 - 17 ng/ml
FRANCESCONI ET AL., J.APPL.PHYSIOL. 55, 870, 1983	RAT	EXERCISE, TREADMILL 9.14M/MIN	22°C PRE-EX, PA = 0.4 ng/ml; POST-EX, 35°C, PA = 0.9 ng/ml; 22°C, PRE-EX, LOW NA DIET 57D, PA = 1.37 ng/ml; POST-EX, 35°C, 57D LOW NA DIET, PA = 1.69 ng/ml
ARAD ET AL., J.COMP.PHYSIOL 155, 227, 1985	FOWL	SEDENTARY	25°C, PADH = 9.5 pg/ml, PA = 6.0 pg/ml; 42°C, ACCL, PADH = 10 pg/ml, PA = 11 pg/ml; 25°C, 13.4% HYPO, PADH = 17 pg/ml, PA = 11 pg/ml; 42°C ACCL, 13.4% HYPO, PADH = 21 pg/ml, PA = 34 pg/ml
THRASHER ET AL., AM.J.PHYSIOL. 247, R76, 1984	DOG	SEDENTARY	22°C, PVP = 2.5 pg/ml, PA = 5.0 ng/100ml; 22°C, 24H WATER DEP, PVP = 8 pg/ml; 22°C, 24H WATER DEP, 24H REHY, PA = 8ng/100ml
SZCZEPANSKA- SADOWSKA ET AL., AM.J.PHYSIOL. 226, 155, 1974	DOG	SEDENTARY	20-25°C, PADH = 2.4 uU/ml; HEAT BRAIN 1.5°C, PADH = 24 uU/ml HEAT HYPOTHALAMUS 2°C, PADH = 200 uU/ml

EL-NOUTY ET AL., J.APPL.PHYSIOL. 48, 249, 1980	CATTLE	SEDENTARY	20°C, PADH = 1.0–1.5 pg/ml; 35°C, PADH = 1.7–2.8 pg/ml; 35°C, WATER DEP 30H, PADH = 2.5–9.0 pg/ml
EISMAN ET AL., J.APPL.PHYSIOL. 43, 739, 1977	BABOONS	SEDENTARY (RESTRAINT)	25°C–30°C, NO CHANGE PRA; 42.5^{O}C–49°C, PRA UP 97.5%/^{O}C INCREASE Tre; PROPRANOLOL PREVENTED INCREASED PRA
GIBINSKI ET AL., EUR.J.APPL.PHYSIOL 42, 1, 1979	HUMAN	SEDENTARY	RT, PADH = 3.9 uU/ml; 1H, 43°C PADH= 17.7 uU/ml; 2H, 43°C PADH = 16.2 uU/ml
BAILEY ET AL., EXPERIENTIA, 28, 159, 1972	HUMAN	SEDENTARY	RT, NORMAL NA INTAKE PA = 13 ng/100ml, PRA = 2.3 ng/ml/h; RT, LOW NA INTAKE PA = 24.3 ng/100ml, PRA = 10.5 ng/ml/h; 46–51°C, NORMAL NA INTAKE PA = 22.8 ng/100ml, PRA = 6.3 ng/ml/h; 46–51°C, LOW NA INTAKE PA = 44.8 ng/100ml, PRA = 18.5 ng/ml/h
FOLLENIUS ET AL. EUR.J.APPL.PHYSIOL. 41, 41, 1979	HUMAN	SEDENTARY	28°C, LOW NA INTAKE PA = 11–20 ng/100ml, PRA = 3–3.5 ng/ml/h; 28°C, HIGH NA INTAKE PA = 5–7 ng/100ml, PRA = 2–2.5 ng/ml/h; 46°C, LOW NA INTAKE PA = 10–35 ng/100 ml, PRA = 3.5–6.5 ng/ml/h; 46°C, HIGH NA INTAKE PA = 5–12 ng/100 ml, PRA = 2.5–3.5 ng/ml/h
FOLLENIUS ET AL., HORM.METAB.RES. 11, 180, 1979	HUMAN	SEDENTARY	28°C, PA = 10–19 ng/100 ml; 46°C, PA = 10–30 ng/100 ml
ESCOURROU ET AL., J.APPL.PHYSIOL 52, 1438, 1982	HUMAN	SEDENTARY	RT, PRA = 102 ng/100ml/3h; TRE INCREASE 1^{O}C WATER-PERFUSED SUIT, PRA = 239 ng/100 ml/3h; PROPRANOLOL = INCONSISTENT EFFECTS ON PRA

(continued)

Table 1. (continued)

BRANDENBERGER ET AL., J.ENDOCRINOL.INVEST. 4, 395, 1980	HUMAN	SEDENTARY	28°C, LOW NA INTAKE, PA = 15-22 ng/100 ml, PRA = 4-5 ng/ml/h; 46°C, LOW NA INTAKE, PA = 15-37 ng/100 ml, PRA = 4.5-15 ng/ml/h; 28°C, PROPRANOLOL, LOW NA INTAKE, PA = 15-35 ng/100ml, PRA = 2-3 ng/ml/h; 46°C, PROPRANOLOL, LOW NA INTAKE, PA = 15-63 ng/100 ml, PRA = 2-7 ng/ml/h
ROCKER ET AL., EUR.J.APPL.PHYSIOL. 49, 59, 1982	HUMAN	SEDENTARY	19-21°C, PADH = 3.5 pg/ml; 70-75°C, PADH = 9.0 pg/ml; 90 MIN AFTER 70-75°C, PADH = 6.5 pg/ml
DUMOULIN ET AL., COMPTES RENDUS 174, 146, 1980	HUMAN	SEDENTARY	RT, PA = 143 pg/ml, PRA = 2.1 ng/ml/h; 80°C, PA = 207 pg/ml, PRA = 6.8 ng/ml/h
KOSUNEN ET AL., J.APPL.PHYSIOL. 41, 323, 1976	HUMAN	SEDENTARY	RT, PA = 140 pmole/l, PRA = 1.9 ug/l/h; 85°C-90°C PA = 750 pmole/l, PRA = 3.85 ug/l/h
BONNER ET AL., J.APPL.PHYSIOL. 41, 708, 1976	HUMAN	SEDENTARY, 155 MIN, EXERCISE, 50W, 30MIN ERGOMETER	28°C, PRE-ACCL, PA = 10.6ng/100ml, POST-ACCL, PA = 8.9 ng/100 ml; 48°C, PRE-ACCL, AFTER 155 MIN HEAT PA = 12.8 ng/100 ml POST-ACCL, PA = 11.1 ng/100ml; 48°C, PRE-ACCL, 30 MIN POST-EX, PA = 26.7 ng/100 ml, POST-ACCL PA = 24.8 ng/100 ml
KIRBY ET AL., J.APPL.PHYSIOL. 61, 967, 1986	HUMAN	EXERCISE, 45% VO2 MAX, ERGOMETER	40°C, DAY 1, 1H EX, PA = 75 ng/100ml, 2H EX, PA = 135 ng/100 ml; 40°C, D10, 1H EX, PA = 50ng/100ml, 2H EX, PA = 90ng/100ml

GREENLEAF ET AL., J.APPL.PHYSIOL. 54, 414, 1983	HUMAN	EXERCISE 75W ERGOMETER	24°C, DAY 1, POST-EX PRA = 6ng/ml/h, PVP = 2 pg/ml; 40°C, DAY 1, POST-EX, PRA = 18 ng/ml/h, PVP = 8 pg/ml; 24°C, DAY 8, POST-EX, PRA = 2.5 ng/ml/h, PVP = 2 pg/ml; 40°C, DAY 8, POST-EX, PRA = 14 ng/ml/h, PVP = 3 pg/ml
FINBERG ET AL., ISRAEL J.MED.SCI. 12, 844, 1976	HUMAN	EXERCISE ERGOMETER, 450kpm/min	PRE/EX PRA = 1.6 ng/ml/h, PA = 5.4 ng/100ml; 25°C POST-EX, PRA = 1.2 ng/ml/h, PA = 10.2 ng/100ml; 50°C, POST-EX, PRA = 5.7 ng/ml/h, PA = 22.6 ng/100ml
FINBERG ET AL., ISRAEL J.MED.SCI. 12, 1530, 1986	HUMAN	EXERCISE, ERGOMETER 40% VO2MAX	POST-EX, D1, PRA = 9.5 ng/ml/h, PA = 22.6 ng/100ml; POST-EX, D7, PRA = 8.0 ng/ml/h, PA = 25.5 ng/100ml
PAOLONE ET AL., MED.SCI.SPORTS.EXER. 15, 97, 1983	HUMAN	EXERCISE, ERGOMETER, 54% VO2MAX	25°C, YOUNG MEN PRE-EX, PRA = 1.48 pmole/ml/h, POST-EX, PRA = 3.05 pmole/ml/h; 35°C OLDER MEN, PRE-EX, PRA = 1.36 pmole/ml/h, POST-EX, PRA = 2.59 pmole/ml/h; 35°C, YOUNG MEN, PRA = 3.93 pmole/ml/h, 60 MIN EX, PRA = 5.91 pmole/ml/h 20 MIN EX
CONVERTINO ET AL., J.APPL.PHYSIOL 50, 123, 1981	HUMAN	EXERCISE, ERGOMETER, 100,175, AND 225W	RT, PRE-EX PRA = 2 ng/ml/h, PVP = 1 pg/ml; RT, POST-EX, 100W PRA = 3.5 ng/ml/h, PVP = 2 pg/ml; RT, POST-EX, 175W PRA = 5.5 ng/ml/h, PVP = 7 pg/ml; RT, POST-EX, 225W PRA = 7.5 ng/ml/h, PVP = 21 pg/ml
CONVERTINO ET AL., J.APPL.PHYSIOL 54, 508, 1983	HUMAN	EXERCISE, ERGOMETER, 100,175, AND 225W	PRE-TRAINING, POST-EX, 175 W, PRA = 6.8 ng/ml/h, PVP = 3.7 pg/ml; POST-TRAINING, POST-EX, 175W, PRA = 4.4 ng/ml/h, PVP = 1.5 pg/ml; PRE-TRAINING, POST-EX, 225W, PRA = 15.3 ng/ml/h, PVP = 8.3 pg/ml; POST-TRAINING, POST-EX, 225W, PRA = 8 ng/ml/h, PVP = 8 pg/ml

(continued)

Table 1. (continued)

BRANDENBERGER ET AL. EUR.J.APPL.PHYSIOL. 55, 123, 1986	HUMAN	EXERCISE ERGOMETER 85W	4H WORK, NO FLUID PRA UP 14 ng/ml/h, PA UP 37 ng/100ml, PVP UP 4 pg/ml; 4H WORK REPLACE FLUID LOSS WITH WATER, PRA UNAFFECTED, PA UP 19 ng/100ml, PVP UNAFFECTED; 4H WORK, REPLACE FLUID LOSS WITH NUTRIENT SOLN, PRA UNAFFECTED, PA UNAFFECTED, PVP UNAFFECTED
GREENLEAF ET AL., J.APPL.PHYSIOL. 51, 298, 1981	HUMAN	EXERCISE ERGOMETER 44% VO2max	24°C, D1, PVP = 2.0 pg/ml, PRA = 1.8 ng/ml/h; 24°C, D9, PVP = 2.0 pg/ml, PRA = 1.0 ng/ml/h; 40°C, D1, PVP = 7.5 pg/ml, PRA = 18.0 ng/ml/h; 40°C, D8, PVP = 2.8 pg/ml, PRA = 15.8 ng/ml/h
FINBERG ET AL., J. APPL. PHYSIOL. 42, 554, 1977	HUMAN	EXERCISE, ERGOMETER, 1.2L/min	NO ACCL, 50°C PRA = 6.0 ng/ml/h, PA = 18 ng/100ml; NATURAL ACCL, 50°C PRA = 3.75 ng/ml/h, PA = 9.5 ng/100ml; D1, 50°C PRA = 22 ng/ml/h, PA = 34.0 ng/100ml; D7, 50°C PRA = 11.1 ng/ml/h, PA = 24 ng/100ml
ORENSTEIN ET AL. PEDIATR. RES. 17, 167, 1983	HUMAN	EXERCISE, ERGOMETER 20W INCRE- MENTS TO EXHAUSTION	38°C, CONTROL, PRE-EX, PRA = 7.6 ng/ml/h, PA = 18.4 ng/100ml; 38°C, CONTROL, POST-EX, PRA = 13.0 ng/ml/h, PA = 36.4 ng/100ml; 38°C, CYSTIC FIBROSIS PATIENTS, PRE-EX, PRA = 5.5 ng/ml/h, PA = 10.4 ng/100ml; 38°C, CYSTIC FIBROSIS PATIENTS, POST-EX, PRA = 16.4 ng/ml/h, PA = 39.7 ng/100ml
DAVIES ET AL., J.APPL.PHYSIOL 50, 605, 1981	HUMAN	EXERCISE, ERGOMETER, 75W	45°C, PRE-ACCL, 45MIN EX, PRA = 5.6 ng/ml/h, PA = 500 pg/ml; 45°C, POST-ACCL, 45MIN EX PRA = 7.2 ng/ml/h, PA = 670 pg/ml; 45°C, PRE-ACCL, 45MIN EX, SALT ADMINISTERED DURING ACCL PRA = 7.0 ng/ml/h, PA = 340 pg/ml; 45°C, POST ACCL, 45 MIN EX, SALT ADMINISTERED DURING ACCL PRA = 7.0 ng/ml/h, PA = 420 pg/ml
FINBERG ET AL. J.APPL.PHYSIOL. 36, 519, 1974	HUMAN	EXERCISE, TREADMILL, 4.7 km/h	50°C, SUMMER, POST-EX, PRA = 5.1 ng/ml/h; 50°C, WINTER, POST-EX, PRA = 9.0 ng/ml/h; 50°C, POST-EX, WATER AD LIB, PRA = 9.3 ng/ml/h; 50°C, POST-EX, NACL, PRA = 5.0 ng/ml/h

FRANCESCONI ET AL. J. APPL. PHYSIOL. 55, 1790, 1983	HUMAN	EXERCISE, TREADMILL, 4.8km/h	35°C, 79% RH, PRE-EX, CONTROL PRA = 3.5 ng/ml/h, PA = 8.0 ng/100 ml; 35°C, 79% RH, PRE-EX, 5% HYPO, PRA = 8 ng/ml/h, PA = 13.5 ng/100ml; 35°C, 79% RH, POST-EX, CONTROL PRA = 6.5 ng/ml/h, PA = 6.3 ng/100ml; 35°C, 79% RH, POST-EX 5% HYPO, PRA = 11.8 ng/ml/h, PA = 13.5 ng/100ml; ACCL REDUCED PRA RESPONSES
FRANCESCONI ET AL., J.APPL.PHYSIOL. 59, 1855, 1985	HUMAN	EXERCISE, TREADMILL, 4.8km/h ACCL	49°C, PRE-EX, HYPO: 0% PRA = 3.8 ng/ml/h, PA = 10 ng/100ml; 3% PRA = 6.1 ng/ml/h, PA = 12 ng/100ml; 5% PRA = 7.5 ng/ml/h, PA = 16.5 ng/100ml; 7% PRA = 7.7 ng/ml/h, PA = 16 ng/100ml; 49°C, POST-EX, HYPO: 0% PRA = 5.2 ng/ml/h, PA = 12.2 ng/100ml; 3% PRA = 7.4 ng/ml/h, PA = 18.2 ng/100ml; 5% PRA = 9.2 ng/ml/h, PA = 23.5 ng/100ml; 7% PRA = 9.2 ng/ml/h, PA = 20.0 ng/100ml;
KIRSCH, ET AL., EUR. J.APPL.PHYSIOL. 47, 191, 1981	HUMAN	ENDURANCE, 27-32KM	PRE-EX, PRA = 0.17 ng/ml/h; POST-EX, PRA = 0.6 ng/ml/h; 45MIN POST-EX, PRA = 0.33 ng/ml/h
FRANCESCONI ET AL., EUR.J.APPL.PHYSIOL. 51, 121, 1983	HUMAN	EXERCISE TREADMILL, 5.6km/h	CONTROL, PRE-EX PA=10.5 ng/100ml; 45°C, POST EX PA = 23 ng/100ml; 45°C, POST EX, ALBUM INFUSION PA = 16 ng/100ml

REFERENCES

1. Aarseth, H.P., I. Eide, B. Skeie, and E. Thaulow. Heat stroke in endurance exercise. Acta Med. Scand. 220:279-283, 1986.
2. Adlerkreutz, H., K. Kosunen, K. Kuoppasalmi, A. Pakarinen, and S-L. Karonen. Plasma hormones during exposure to intense heat. In: Proc. 13th Cong. Internal Med., A. Louhija and V. Valtonen, eds., Karger, Basel, 1977, pp 346-355.
3. Allan, J.R., and G.G. Wilson. Influence of acclimatization on sweat sodium concentration. J. Appl. Physiol. 30:708-712, 1971.
4. Arad, Z., S.S. Arnason, A. Chadwick, and E. Skadhauge. Osmotic and hormonal responses to heat and dehydration in the fowl. J. Comp. Physiol. B 155:227-234, 1985.
5. Armstrong, L.E., D.L. Costill, and W.J. Fink. Influence of diuretic-induced dehydration on competitive running performance. Med. Sci. Sports Exerc. 17:456-461, 1985.
6. Armstrong, L.E., D.L. Costill, and W.J. Fink. Changes in body water and electrolytes during heat acclimation: effects of dietary sodium. Aviat. Space Environ. Med. 58:143-148, 1987.
7. Armstrong, L.E., R.W. Hubbard, P.C. Szlyk, W.T. Matthew, and I.V. Sils. Voluntary dehydration and electrolyte losses during prolonged exercise in the heat. Aviat. Space Environ. Med. 56:765-770, 1985.
8. Augustinsson, O., H. Holst, M. Forsgren, H. Andersson, and B. Andersson. Influence of heat exposure on acid/base and fluid balance in hyperhydrated goats. Acta. Physiol. Scand. 126:499-503, 1986.
9. Baer, P.G. Hormonal systems and renal hemodynamics. Ann. Rev. Physiol. 42:589-601, 1980.
10. Bailey, R.E., D. Bartos, F. Bartos, A. Castro, R.L. Dobson, D.P. Grettie, R. Kramer, D. Macfarlane, and K. Sato. Activation of aldosterone and renin secretion by thermal stress. Experientia 28:159-160, 1972.
11. Bakharev, V.D., A.T. Maryanovich, I.B. Slyusar, L.A. Levkin, O.S. Pansuevich, and G.I. Chipens. Effect of arginine-vasopressin neuropeptide on human tolerance of a hot dry environment. Fiziol. Chel. 9:819-827, 1983.
12. Bass, D.E., C.R. Kleeman, M. Quinn, A. Henschel, and A.H. Hegnauer. Mechanisms of acclimatization to heat in man. Medicine 34:325-380, 1955.
13. Bie, P. Osmoreceptors, vasopressin, and control of renal water excretion. Physiol. Revs. 60:961-1048, 1980.
14. Bligh, J., and K.G. Johnson. Glossary of terms for thermal physiology. J. Appl. Physiol. 35:941-961, 1973.
15. Bonner, R.M., M.H. Harrison, C.J. Hall, and R.J. Edwards. Effect of heat acclimatization on intravascular responses to acute heat stress in man. J. Appl. Physiol. 41:708-713, 1976.
16. Brandenberger, G., V. Candas, M. Follenius, J.P. Libert, and J.M. Kahn. Vascular fluid shifts and endocrine responses to exercise in the heat. Eur. J. Appl. Physiol. 55:123-129, 1986.
17. Brandenberger, G., M. Follenius, and S. Oyono. Effect of propranolol on aldosterone response to heat exposure in sodium-restricted men. J. Endocrinol. Invest. 4:395-400, 1980.

18. Braun, W.E., J.T. Maher, and R.F. Byrom. Effect of exogenous d-aldosterone on heat acclimatization in man. J. Appl. Physiol. 23:341-346, 1967.
19. Bunt, J.C. Hormonal alterations due to exercise. Sports Med. 3:331-345, 1986.
20. Candas, V., G. Brandenberger, B. Lutz-Bucher, M. Follenius, and J.P. Libert. Endocrine concomitants of sweating and sweat depression. Eur. J. Appl. Physiol. 52:225-229, 1984.
21. Coburn, J.W., R.C. Reba, and F.N. Craig. Effect of potassium depletion on response to acute heat exposure in unacclimatized man. Am. J. Physiol. 211:117-124, 1966.
22. Cochrane, L.A., J.A. Davies, R.J. Edwards, and M.H. Harrison. Some adreno-cortical responses to heat acclimatization. J. Physiol. 301:32P-33P, 1979.
23. Collins, K.J. Endocrine control of salt and water in hot conditions. Fed. Proc. 22:716-720, 1963.
24. Collins, K.J. The action of exogenous aldosterone on the secretion and composition of drug-induced sweat. Clin. Sci. 30:207-221, 1966.
25. Collins, K.J. The endocrine component of human adaptation to cold and heat. In: Environmental Endocrinology, I. Assenmacher and D.S. Farner, eds., pp.294-301, Springer-Verlag, New York, 1978.
26. Collins, K.J., J.D. Few, and J.P.M. Finberg. Metabolic clearance rate of cortisol and aldosterone during controlled hyperthermia in man. J. Physiol. 268:7P-8P, 1977.
27. Conn, J.W. Some clinical and climatological aspects of aldosteronism in man. Trans. Amer. Clin. Climatol. Assoc. 74:61-91, 1962.
28. Conn, J.W. Aldosteronism in man. J. Am. Med. Assoc. 183:775-781, 1963.
29. Conn, J.W., M.W. Johnston, and H.L. Louis. Acclimatization to humid heat. a function of adrenal cortical activity. J. Clin. Invest. 25:912-913, 1946.
30. Convertino, V.A., L.C. Keil, E.M. Bernauer, and J.E. Greenleaf. Plasma volume, osmolality, vasopressin and renin activity during graded exercise in man. J. Appl. Physiol. 50:123-128, 1981.
31. Convertino, V.A., L.C. Keil, and J.E. Greenleaf. Plasma volume, renin, and vasopressin responses to graded exercise after training. J. Appl. Physiol. 54:508-514, 1983.
32. Convertino, V.A., and C.R. Kirby. Expansion of total body water following heat acclimation. Physiologist 27:230, 1984.
33. Costill, D.L. Sweating: its composition and effects on body fluids. Ann. N.Y. Acad. Sci. 30:160-174, 1977.
34. Costill, D.L., G. Branam, W. Fink, and R. Nelson. Exercise induced sodium conservation: changes in plasma renin and aldosterone. Med. Sci. Sports 8:209-213, 1976.
35. Costill, D.L., R. Cote, E. Miller, T. Miller, and S. Wynder. Water and electrolyte replacement during repeated days of work in the heat. Aviat. Space Environ. Med. 46:795-800, 1975.
36. Costill, D.L. and W.J. Fink. Plasma volume changes following exercise and thermal dehydration. J. Appl. Physiol. 37:521-525, 1974.

37. Davies, J.A., M.H. Harrison, L.A. Cochrane, R.J. Edwards, and T.M. Gibson. Effect of saline loading during heat acclimatization on adrenocortical hormone levels. J. Appl. Physiol. 50:605-612, 1981.
38. Diaz, F.J., D.R. Bransford, K. Kobayashi, S.M. Horvath, and R.G. McMurray. Plasma volume changes during rest and exercise in different postures in a hot humid environment. J. Appl. Physiol. 47:798-803, 1979.
39. Dill, D.B., B.F. Jones, H.T. Edwards, and S.A. Obers. Salt economy in extreme dry heat. J. Biol. Chem. 100:755-767, 1933.
40. Doucet, A. Multiple hormonal control of kidney tubular functions. News Physiol. Sci. 2:141-146, 1987.
41. Dumoulin, G., N.U. Nguyen, M.T. Henriet, J. Bopp, and S. Berthelay. Variations des electrolytes plasmatiques et de leurs hormones de regulation, lors d'une exposition aigue a la chaleur. Etude au cours du sauna finlandais chez l'Homme. Compt. rend. 174:146-150, 1980.
42. Durkot, M.J., O. Martinez, D. Brooks-McQuade, and R. Francesconi. Simultaneous determination of fluid shifts during thermal stress in a small animal model. J. Appl. Physiol. 61:1031-1034, 1986.
43. Eisman, M.M., and L.B. Rowell. Renal vascular response to heat stress in baboons - role of renin-angiotensin. J. Appl. Physiol. 43:739-746, 1977.
44. Elizondo, R., M. Banerjee, and R.W. Bullard. Effect of local heating and arterial occlusion on sweat electrolyte content. J. Appl. Physiol. 32:1-6, 1972.
45. El-Nouty, F.D., I.M. Elbanna, T.P. Davis, and H.D. Johnson. Aldosterone and ADH response to heat and dehydration in cattle. J. Appl. Physiol. 48:249-255, 1980.
46. Epstein, Y., and E. Sohar. Fluid balance in hot climates: Sweating, water intake, and prevention of dehdyration. Public Health Rev. 13:115-137, 1985.
47. Escourrou, P., P.R. Freund, L. B. Rowell, and D.G. Johnson. Splanchnic vasoconstriction in heat-stressed men: role of renin-angiotensin system. J. Appl. Physiol. 52:1438-1443, 1982.
48. Fasciolo, J.C., G.L. Totel, and R.E. Johnson. Antidiuretic hormone and human eccrine sweating. J. Appl. Physiol. 27:303-307, 1969.
49. Finberg, J.P.M., and G.M. Berlyne. Renin and aldosterone secretion following acute environmental heat exposure. Israel J. Med. Sci. 12:844-847, 1976.
50. Finberg, J.P.M., and G.M. Berlyne. Modification of renin and aldosterone response to heat by acclimatization in man. J. Appl. Physiol. 42:554-558, 1977.
51. Finberg, J.P.M., Y. Kaplanski, and G.M. Berlyne. Renin and aldosterone secretion following heat exposure in man - relationship to VO_2 max and artificial acclimatization. Israel J. Med. Sci. 12:1530, 1976.
52. Finberg, J.P.M., M. Katz, H. Gazit, and G.M. Berlyne. Plasma renin activity after acute heat exposure in nonacclimatized and naturally acclimatized men. J. Appl. Physiol. 36:519-523, 1974.
53. Fletcher, K.A., C.S. Leithead, T. Deegan, M.A. Pallister, A.R. Lind, and B.G. Maegraith. Aldosterone excretion in acclimatization to heat. Ann. Trop. Med. Parasit. 55:498-504, 1962.

54. Follenius, M., G. Brandenberger, B. Reinhardt, and M. Simeoni. Plasma aldosterone, renin activity, and cortisol responses in sodium depleted and repleted subjects. Eur. J. Appl. Physiol. 41:41-50, 1979.
55. Follenius, M., G. Brandenberger, M. Simeoni, and B. Reinhardt. Plasma aldosterone, prolactin and ACTH: Relationships in man during heat exposure. Horm. Metab. Res. 11:180-181, 1979.
56. Fortney, S.M., E.R. Nadel, C.B. Wenger, and J.R. Bove. Effect of blood volume and sweating rate on body fluids in exercising humans. J. Appl. Physiol. 51:1594-1600, 1981.
57. Francesconi, R.P., and R.W. Hubbard. Chronic low sodium diet in rats: responses to severe heat exposure. J. Appl. Physiol. 58:152-156, 1985.
58. Francesconi, R.P., R.W. Hubbard, M.N. Sawka, W.T. Matthew, and M. Mager. Acute albumin-induced plasma volume expansion and heat exposure: effects on hormonal periodicity in men. J. Interdiscipl. Cycle Res. 15:23-32, 1984.
59. Francesconi, R., N. Leva, R. Hubbard, C. Matthew, M. Durkot, and M. Bosselaers. Exercise in the heat: effects of dinitrophenol. Fed. Proc. 46:1442, 1987.
60. Francesconi, R., and M. Mager. Heat-injured rats: pathochemical indices and survival time. J. Appl. Physiol. 45:1-6, 1978.
61. Francesconi, R., and M. Mager. Heat exposure and exercise: effects on plasma levels of renin, aldosterone, and vasopressin. Physiologist 24:13, 1981.
62. Francesconi, R.P., J. Maher, G. Bynum, and J. Mason. Recurrent heat exposure: effects on plasma and urinary sodium and potassium in resting and exercising men. Aviat. Space Environ. Med. 48:399-404, 1977.
63. Francesconi, R.P., M.N. Sawka, R.W. Hubbard, and M. Mager. Acute albumin-induced plasma volume expansion and exercise in the heat: effects on hormonal responses in men. Eur. J. Appl. Physiol. 51:121-128, 1983.
64. Francesconi, R.P., M.N. Sawka, and K.B. Pandolf. Hypohydration and heat acclimation: plasma renin and aldosterone during exercise. J. Appl. Physiol. 55:1790-1794, 1983.
65. Francesconi, R.P., M.N. Sawka, K.B. Pandolf, R.W. Hubbard, A.J. Young, and S. Muza. Plasma hormonal responses at graded hypohydration levels during exercise - heat stress. J. Appl. Physiol. 59:1855-1860, 1985.
66. Francis, K.T. Effect of water and electrolyte replacement during exercise in the heat on biochemical indices of stress and performance. Aviat. Space Environ. Med. 50:115-119, 1979.
67. Francis, K.T., and R. MacGregor. Effect of exercise in the heat on plasma renin and aldosterone with either water or a potassium-rich electrolyte solution. Aviat. Space Environ. Med. 49:461-465, 1978.
68. Furman, K.I., and G. Beer. Dynamic changes in sweat electrolyte composition induced by heat stress as an indication of acclimatization and aldosterone activity. Clin. Sci. 24:7-12, 1963.
69. Gibinski K., F. Kokot, S. Nowak, and L. Giec. Aldosterone and sweat gland function. Acta Med. Pol. 4:313-320, 1963.
70. Gibinski, K., F. Nowak, S. Nowak, and L. Giec. Aldosterone in the maintenance of the water-electrolyte balance. Acta Med. Pol. 4:321-328, 1963.

71. Gibinski, K., S. Kozlowski, J. Chwalbinska-Moneta, L. Giec, J. Zmudzinski, and A. Markiewicz. ADH and thermal sweating. Eur. J. Appl. Physiol. 42:1-13, 1979.
72. Giec, L. The effect of humid heat on the electrolyte-water balance in man. Acta Med. Pol. 2:345-351, 1961.
73. Greenleaf, J.E., P.J. Brock, L.C. Keil, and J.T. Morse. Drinking and water balance during exercise and heat acclimation. J. Appl. Physiol. 54:414-419, 1983.
74. Greenleaf, J.E., and F. Sargent II. Voluntary dehydration in man. J. Appl. Physiol. 20:719-724, 1965.
75. Greenleaf, J.E., D. Sciaraffa, E. Shvartz, L.C. Keil, and P.J. Brock. Exercise training hypotension: implications for plasma volume, renin and vasopressin. J. Appl. Physiol. 51:298-305, 1981.
76. Greenleaf, J.E., W. van Beaumont, P.J. Brock, L.D. Montgomery, J.T. Morse, E. Shvartz, and S. Kravik. Fluid-electrolyte shifts and thermoregulation: Rest and work in heat with head cooling. Aviat. Space Environ. Med. 51:747-753, 1980.
77. Groza, P., R. Carmaciu, and E. Daneliuc. Les effets de l'hyperthermie exogene et du propranolol sur la secretion de l'hormone antidiuretique chez le rat. Physiologie 14:71-78, 1977.
78. Grucza, R., J.L. Lecroart, J.J. Hauser, and Y. Houdas. Dynamics of sweating in men and women during passive heating. Eur. J. Appl. Physiol. 54:309-314, 1985.
79. Haldy, P., and J. Muller. Stimulation of the conversion of corticosterone to aldosterone by sodium and water depletion of potassium-deficient rats. Comparison of different experimental procedures. Acta Endocrinol. 96:519-526, 1981.
80. Halim, A. Fluid and electrolyte balance and physical training in hot climate. J. Sports Med. 20:347-350, 1980.
81. Handler, J.S., and J. Orloff. Antidiuretic hormone. Ann. Rev. Physiol. 43:611-624, 1981.
82. Harrison, M.H. Plasma volume changes during acute exposure to a high environmental temperature. J. Appl. Physiol. 37:38-42, 1974.
83. Harrison, M.H., and R.J. Edwards. Measurement of change in plasma volume during heat exposure and exercise. Aviat. Space Environ. Med. 47:1038-1045, 1976.
84. Harrison, M.H., R.J. Edwards, and P.A. Fennessy. Intravascular volume and tonicity as factors in the regulation of body temperature. J. Appl. Physiol. 44:69-75, 1978.
85. Harrison, M.H., R.J. Edwards, M.J. Graveney, L.A. Cochrane, and J.A. Davies. Blood volume and plasma protein responses to heat acclimatization in humans. J. Appl. Physiol. 50:597-604, 1981.
86. Harrison, M.H., R.J. Edwards, and D.R. Leitch. Effect of exercise and thermal stress on plasma volume. J. Appl. Physiol. 39:925-931, 1975.
87. Henschel, A. Water balance: A problem in occupational health. Occupat. Hlth. Revs. 17:11-13, 1965.
88. Hessemer, V., and K. Brueck. Influence of menstrual cycle on thermoregulatory, metabolic and heart rate responses to exercise at night. J. Appl. Physiol. 59:1911-1917, 1985.

89. Horowitz, M., and A. Borut. Plasma volume regulation in rodents: comparison of heat and dehydration effects. Israel J. Med. Sci. 12:864-867, 1976.
90. Horowitz, M., and S. Samueloff. Plasma water shifts during thermal dehydration. J. Appl. Physiol. 47:738-744, 1979.
91. Horstman, D.H., and S.M. Horvath. Cardiovascular and temperature regulatory changes during progressive dehydration and euhydration. J. Appl. Physiol. 33:446-450, 1972.
92. Horvath, S.M., and B.L. Drinkwater. Thermoregulation and the menstrual cycle. Aviat. Space Environ. Med. 53:790-794, 1982.
93. Hubbard, R.W., W.D. Bowers, and M. Mager. A study of physiological, pathological, and biochemical changes in rats with heat- and/or work-induced disorders. Israel J. Med. Sci. 12:884-886, 1976.
94. Hubbard, R.W., W.D. Bowers, W.T. Matthew, F.C. Curtis, R.E.L. Criss, G. Sheldon, and J.W. Ratteree. Rat model of acute heatstroke mortality. J. Appl. Physiol. 42:809-816, 1977.
95. Hubbard, R.W., M. Mager, W.D. Bowers, I. Leav, G. Angoff, W.T. Matthew, and I.V. Sils. Effect of low potassium diet on rat exercise hyperthermia and heatstroke mortality. J. Appl. Physiol. 51:8-13, 1981.
96. Ikawa, S., M. Suzuki, and M. Shiota. Effect of sports beverage intake after a sauna bath on water-electrolyte balance. Jpn. J. Phys. Fitness Sports Med. 34:1-10, 1985.
97. Katz, A.I., and M.D. Lindheimer. Actions of hormones on the kidney. Ann. Rev. Physiol. 39:97-134, 1977.
98. Keil, L.C., and W.B. Severs. Reduction in plasma vasopressin levels of dehydrated rats following acute stress. Endocrinol. 100:30-38, 1977.
99. Kenyon, C.J., N.A. Saccoccio, and D.J. Morris. Aldosterone effects on water and electrolyte metabolism. J. Endocrinol. 100:93-100, 1984.
100. Kirby, C.R., and V.A. Convertino. Plasma aldosterone and sweat sodium concentrations after exercise and heat acclimation. J. Appl. Physiol. 61:967-970, 1986.
101. Kirsch, K.A., H. Von Ameln, and H.J. Wicke. Fluid control mechanisms after exercise dehydration. Eur. J. Appl. Physiol. 47:191-196, 1981.
102. Knochel, J.P. Environmental heat illness. Arch. Int. Med. 133:841-864, 1974.
103. Knochel, J.P. Potassium deficiency during training in the heat. Ann. N.Y. Acad. Sci 30:175-182, 1977.
104. Knochel, J.P., L.N. Dotin, and R.J. Hamburger. Pathophysiology of intense physical conditioning in a hot climate. I. Mechanisms of potassium depletion. J. Clin. Invest. 51:242-255, 1972.
105. Knochel, J.P., and R.M. Vertel. Salt loading as a possible factor in the production of potassium depletion, rhabdomyolysis, and heat injury. Lancet I: 659-661, 1967.
106. Knox, F.G., and J.P. Granger. Control of sodium excretion: the kidney produces under pressure. News Physiol. Sci. 2:26-29, 1987.
107. Konikoff, F., Y. Shoenfeld, A. Magazanik, J. Epstein, and Y. Shapiro. Effects of salt loading during exercise in a hot dry climate. Biomed. Pharmacother. 40:296-300, 1986.

108. Kosunen, K.J., A.J. Pakarinen, K. Kuoppasalmi, and H. Adlerkreutz. Plasma renin activity, angiotensin II, and aldosterone during intense heat stress. J. Appl. Physiol. 41:323-327, 1976.
109. Ladell, W.S.S. The effect of desoxycorticosterone acetate on the chloride content of the sweat. J. Physiol. 104:13P-14P, 1945.
110. Lamb, D.R., and G.R. Brodowicz. Optimal use of fluids of varying formulations to minimize exercise induced disturbances in homeostasis. Sports Med. 3:247-274, 1986.
111. Laragh, J.H. The endocrine control of blood volume, blood pressure and sodium balance: atrial hormone and renin system interactions. J. Hypertens. 4:143-156, 1986.
112. Leithead, C.S. Water and electrolyte metabolism in the heat. Fed. Proc. 22:901-908, 1963.
113. Malhotra, M.S., S.K., Sridharan, and Y. Venkataswamy. Potassium losses in sweat under heat stress. Aviat. Space Environ. Med. 47:503-504, 1976.
114. McDougall, J.G. The physiology of aldosterone secretion. News Physiol. Sci. 2:126-128, 1987.
115. Moroff, S.V., and D.E. Bass. Effects of overhydration on man's physiological responses to work in the heat. J. Appl. Physiol. 20:267-270, 1965.
116. Myhre, L.G., and S. Robinson. Fluid shifts during thermal stress with and without fluid replacement. J. Appl. Physiol. 42:252-256, 1977
117. Nadel, E.R. Control of sweating rate while exercising in the heat. Med. Sci. Sports. 11:31-35, 1979.
118. Nadel, E.R., K.B. Pandolf, M.F. Roberts, and J.A.J. Stolwijk. Mechanisms of thermal acclimation to exercise and heat. J. Appl. Physiol. 37:515-520, 1974.
119. Nielson, B., G. Sjogaard, J. Ugelveg, B. Knudsen, and B. Dohlmann. Fluid balance in exercise dehydration and rehydration with different glucose-electrolyte drinks. Eur. J. Appl. Physiol. 55:318-325, 1986.
120. O'Donnell, T.F., and G.H.A. Clowes. The circulatory abnormalities of heat stroke. New Engl. J. Med. 287:734-737, 1972.
121. Ogawa, T., M. Asayama, and T. Miyagawa. Effects of sweat gland training by repeated local heating. Jpn. J. Physiol. 32:971-981, 1982.
122. Orenstein, D.M., K.G. Henke, D.L. Costill, C.F. Doershuk, P.J. Lemon, and R.C. Stern. Exercise and heat stress in cystic fibrosis patients. Pediatr. Res. 17:267-269, 1983.
123. Orenstein, D.M., K.G. Henke, and C.G. Green. Heat acclimation in cystic fibrosis. J. Appl. Physiol. 57:408-412, 1984.
124. Pandolf, K.B., B.S. Cadarette, M.N. Sawka, A.J. Young, R.P. Francesconi, and R.R. Gonzalez. Thermoregulatory responses of middle-aged and young men during dry-heat acclimation. J. Appl. Physiol. 65:65-71, 1988.
125. Paolone, A.M. A.O. Ajiduah, J.T. Troup, C.W. Stevens, and Z.V. Kendrick. The effects of age and heat stress on plasma renin activity and plasma volume during exercise. Med. Sci. Sports Exerc. 15:97-98, 1983.
126. Pivarnik, J.M., and L.C. Senay. Effects of exercise detraining and deacclimation to the heat on plasma volume dynamics. Eur. J. Appl. Physiol. 55:222-228, 1986.

127. Ratner, A.C., and R.L. Dobsen. The effect of antidiuretic hormone on sweating. J. Invest. Dermat. 43:379-381, 1964.
128. Reid, I.A., B.J. Morris, and W.F. Ganong. The renin-angiotensin system. Ann. Rev. Physiol. 40:377-410, 1978.
129. Roberts, M.F., C. B. Wenger, J.A.J. Stolwijk, and E.R. Nadel. Skin blood flow and sweating changes following exercise training and heat acclimation. J. Appl. Physiol. 43:133-137, 1977.
130. Robinson, S., R.K. Kincaid, and R.K. Rhamy. Effect of salt deficiency on the salt concentration in sweat. J. Appl. Physiol. 3:55-62, 1950.
131. Robinson, S. and A.H. Robinson. Chemical composition of sweat. Physiol. Revs. 34:202-220, 1954.
132. Rocker, L., K. Kirsch, and B. Agrawal. Long-term observations on plasma anti-diuretic hormone levels during and after heat stress. Eur. J. Appl. Physiol. 49:59-62, 1982.
133. Rocker, L., K. Kirsch, and H. Stoboy. The influence of heat stress on plasma volume and intravascular proteins in sedentary females. Eur. J. Appl. Physiol. 36:187-192, 1977.
134. Rowell, L.B. Human Circulation: Regulation During Physical Stress. Oxford University Press, New York, 1987, pp 174-212.
135. Rowell, L.B., J.R. Blackmon, R.H. Martin, J.A. Mazzarella, and R.A. Bruce. Hepatic clearance of indocyanine green in man under thermal and exercise stress. J. Appl. Physiol. 20:384-394, 1965.
136. Rowell, L.B., G.L. Brengelmann, J.R. Blackmon, R.D. Twiss, and F. Kusumi. Splanchnic blood flow and metabolism in heat-stressed man. J. Appl. Physiol. 24:475-484, 1968.
137. Rowell, L.B., K.R. Kraning, J.W. Kennedy, and T.O. Evans. Central circulating responses to work in dry heat before and after acclimatization. J. Appl. Physiol. 22:509-518, 1967.
138. Saltin, B. Circulatory response to submaximal and maximal exercise after thermal dehydration. J. Appl. Physiol. 19:1125-1132, 1964.
139. Sawka, M.N., R.P. Francesconi, A.J. Young, and K.B. Pandolf. Influence of hydration level and body fluids on exercise performance in the heat. J. Am. Med. Assoc. 252:1165-1169, 1984.
140. Sawka, M.N., M.M. Toner, R.P. Francesconi, and K.B. Pandolf. Hypohydration and exercise: effects of heat acclimation, gender, and environment. J. Appl. Physiol. 55:1147-1153, 1983.
141. Sawka, M.N., A.J. Young, R.P. Francesconi, S.R. Muza, and K.B. Pandolf. Thermoregulatory and blood responses during exercise at graded hypohydration levels. J. Appl. Physiol. 59:1394-1401, 1985.
142. Schamadan, J.L., and W.D. Snively, Jr. The role of potassium in heat stress disease. Indust. Med. Surg. 36:785-788, 1967.
143. Schrier, R.W., J. Hano, H.I. Keller, R.M. Finkel, P.F. Gilliland, W.J. Cirksena, and P.E. Teschan. Renal, metabolic, and circulatory responses to heat and exercise. Ann. Int. Med. 73:213-223, 1970.
144. Senay, L.C., Jr. Movement of water, protein, and crystalloids between vascular and extra-vascular compartments in heat exposed men during dehydration, and following limited relief of dehydration. J. Physiol. 210:617-635, 1970.

145. Senay, L.C., Jr. Changes in plasma volume and protein content during exposures of working men to various temperatures before and after acclimatization to heat; separation of the roles of cutaneous and skeletal muscle circulation. J. Physiol. 224:61-81, 1972.
146. Senay, L.C., Jr. Early response of plasma contents on exposure of working men to heat. J. Appl. Physiol. 44:166-170, 1978.
147. Senay, L.C., Jr. Effects of exercise in the heat on body fluid distribution. Med. Sci. Sports 11:42-48, 1979.
148. Senay, L.C., Jr., M. Christensen, and A.B. Hertzman. Cutaneous Vasodilatation elicited by body heating in calf, forearm, cheek and ear. J. Appl. Physiol. 16:655-659, 1961.
149. Senay, L.C., Jr., and S. Fortney. Untrained females: effects of submaximal exercise and heat on body fluids. J. Appl. Physiol. 39:643-647, 1975.
150. Senay, L.C., Jr., and R. Kok. Body fluid responses of heat tolerant and intolerant men to work in a hot wet environment. J. Appl. Physiol. 40:55-59, 1976.
151. Senay, L.C., Jr., and R. Kok. Effects of training and heat acclimatization on blood plasma contents of exercising men. J. Appl. Physiol. 43:591-599, 1977.
152. Senay, L.C., Jr., D. Mitchell, and C.H. Wyndham. Acclimatization in a hot, humid environment: body fluid adjustments. J. Appl. Physiol. 40:786-796, 1976.
153. Senay, L.C., Jr., and W. van Beaumont. Antidiuretic hormone and evaporative weight loss during heat stress. Pfluger's Arch. 312:82-90, 1969.
154. Shannon, T., J. Pivarnik, and L.C. Senay, Jr. Influence of hyperhydration on body fluid dynamics during rhythmic exercise. Fed. Proc. 43:627, 1984.
155. Shibolet, S., M.C. Lancaster, and Y. Danon. Heatstroke: a review. Aviat. Space Environ. Med. 47:280-301, 1976.
156. Shvartz, E., V.A. Convertino, L.C. Keil, and R.F. Haines. Orthostatic fluid electrolyte and endocrine responses in fainters and nonfainters. J. Appl. Physiol. 51:1404-1410, 1981.
157. Smiles, K.A., and S. Robinson. Sodium ion conservation during acclimatization of men to work in the heat. J. Appl. Physiol. 31:63-69, 1971.
158. Stephenson, L.A., and M.A. Kolka. Menstrual cycle phase and time of day alter reference signal controlling arm blood flow and sweating. Am. J. Physiol. 249:R186-R191, 1985.
159. Strydom, N.B., and L.D. Holdsworth. The effects of different levels of water deficit on physiological responses during heat stress. Int. Z. angew. Physiol. 26:95-102, 1968.
160. Strydom, N.B., C.H. Wyndham, C.G. Williams, J.F. Morrison, G.A.G. Bredell, A.J.S. Benade, and M. von Rahden. Acclimatization to humid heat and the role of physical conditioning. J. Appl. Physiol. 21:636-642, 1966.
161. Szczepanska-Sadowska, E. Plasma ADH increase and thirst suppression elicited by preoptic heating in the dog. Am. J. Physiol. 226:155-161, 1974.

162. Taylor, H.L., A. Henschel, O. Mickelsen, and A. Keys. The effects of the sodium chloride intake on the work performance of man during exposure to dry heat and experimental heat exhaustion. Am. J. Physiol. 140:439-451, 1944.
163. Thrasher, T.N., C.E. Wade, L.C. Keil, and D.J. Ramsay. Sodium balance and aldosterone during dehydration and rehydration in the dog. Am. J. Physiol. 247:R76-R83, 1984.
164. van Beaumont, W., H.L. Young, and J.E. Greenleaf. Plasma fluid and blood constituent shifts during heat exposure in resting men. Aerospace Med. 45:176-181, 1974.
165. Von Ameln, H., M. Lanido, L. Rocker, and K.A. Kirsch. Effects of dehydration on the vasopressin response to immersion. J. Appl. Physiol. 58:114-120, 1985.
166. Wyndham, C.H. The physiology of exercise under heat stress. Ann. Rev. Physiol. 35:193-220, 1973.
167. Wyndham, C.H., A.J.H. Benade, C.G. Williams, N.B. Strydom, A. Goldin, and A.J.A. Heyns. Changes in central circulation and body fluid spaces during acclimatization to heat. J. Appl. Physiol. 25:586-593, 1968.
168. Zgoda, N.V., V.D. Bakharev, V.I. Yunkerov, N.E. Domal'chuk, and Y.P. Osipov. Effect of 8-arginine-vasopressin during adaptation to hyperthermia. Fiziol. Chel. 9:828-836, 1983.

3

EFFECT OF EXPOSURE TO COLD ON FLUID AND ELECTROLYTE EXCHANGE

Melvin J. Fregly

Department of Physiology
University of Florida College of Medicine
Gainesville, FL 32610

INTRODUCTION

Experimental evidence has been accumulating during the past twenty years to suggest that exposure of mammals to cold air is accompanied by a voluntary dehydration (21). In this regard, the rat has received a considerable amount of attention.

My interest in this subject stems from my days as a graduate student studying the physiological changes accompanying acclimation of rats to cold. I noted that each time I brought rats from the cold into a warm (26°C) room, they began to drink immediately, and consumed water for at least half an hour Some years passed before I actually quantitated this post-cold exposure, or thermogenic, drinking response of rats.

EFFECTS OF EXPOSURE TO COLD ON WATER INTAKE

Effects of Acute Exposure to Cold in Rats

Twenty-nine male Sprague Dawley rats were kept in individual cages in air at 5°C for 10 days (27). Twenty-one controls were kept at 26°C. All rats received tap water and Rockland Rat Diet ad libitum during the two weeks prior to beginning the study. At this time, water bottles were removed from the cages of all rats. The cold-treated rats were then transferred from cold to warm air, and preweighed beakers containing water (26°C) were placed in the cage of each control and cold-treated rat. Water intakes were measured gravimetrically at 0.5, 1.0, and 2.0 hr thereafter (Figure 1). Water intake of the cold-treated group was significantly ($P<0.01$) greater than that of the control group at all times measurements were made. The change in water intake of the cold-treated group was also greater than that of controls at each

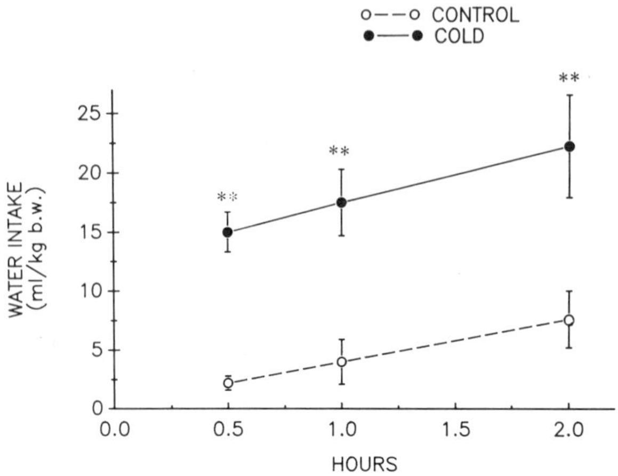

*FIGURE 1. Cumulative water intake of 21 control and 29 cold-treated rats at graded intervals after removal from cold (5°C) air. One standard error is set off at each mean. ** = $P<0.01$ compared to control.*

time measurements were made. The volume of water ingested within one hr after removal from cold was approximately 10% of the total daily water intake of these rats.

<u>Duration of Exposure to Cold Required to Induce Thermogenic Drinking in Rats</u>

Different groups of male rats were exposed to 5°C for periods of time varying from 1 to 22 hr. Appropriate controls were maintained at 26°C. Food and water were freely available during these times. At the end of each period, the water and food containers were removed from each cage and all rats were transferred in their cages to a room at 26°C. Preweighed bottles of water (26°C) were placed on each cage. Water intakes of both control and cold-treated groups were measured gravimetrically during the first 15, 30, and 60 min following removal from cold. Additional details of this experiment have been described elsewhere (44). A previous study showed that transfer per se at the same room temperature did not affect water intake (43).

The results of this study showed that exposure to cold for either 1 or 3 hr failed to induce thermogenic drinking at 30 min after removal from the cold (Figure 2). However, thermogenic drinking occurred after 6 or more hours of exposure to cold air.

Although thermogenic drinking can be initiated after as little as 6 hr of exposure to cold, additional studies showed that it persists during at least 120 days of exposure to cold (Figure 3) (22).

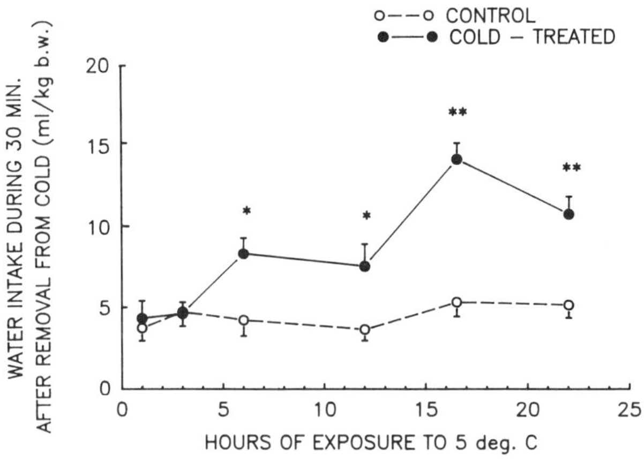

*FIGURE 2. Water intake during 30 min. after removal from cold is expressed as a function of hours of exposure to 5°C. One standard error is set off at each mean. * = P<0.05; ** = P<0.01 compared to control.*

Effects of Food Intake on Water Intake in the Cold

The thermogenic drinking response following removal from cold prompted studies to characterize food and water intakes, as well as urine output, accompanying exposure to cold. Male rats were maintained individually in metabolic cages and their food and water intakes and urine outputs were measured daily for 7 days at 26°C. At the end of this time, air temperature

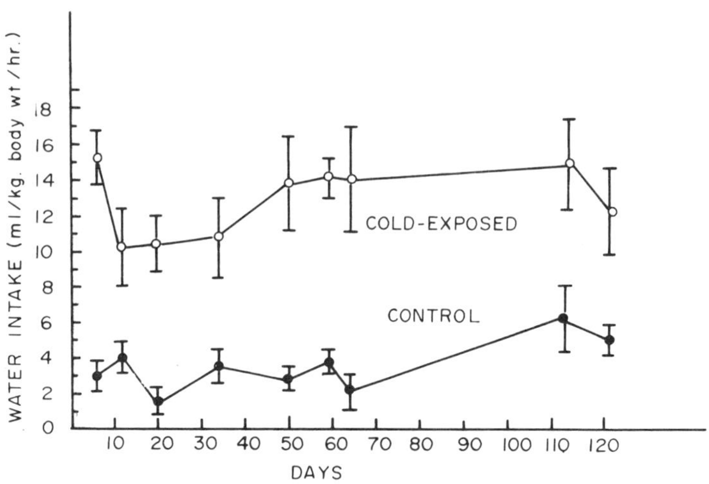

FIGURE 3. Water intakes of cold-treated and control groups measured during the first hr the cold-treated group was removed from cold. Measurements were made after 5 through 120 days of cold exposure. One standard error is set off at each mean. (Reproduced with permission, Ref 22).

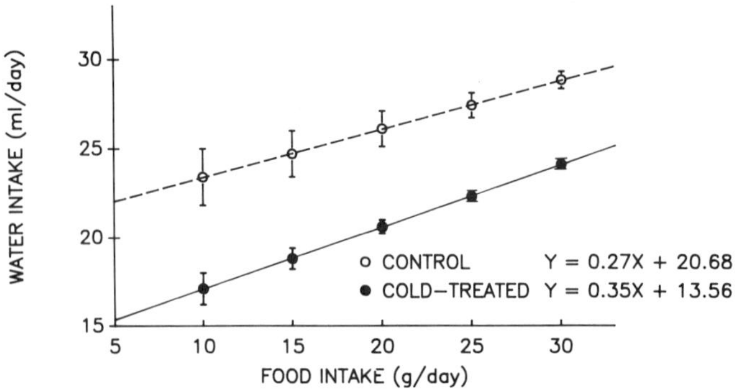

FIGURE 4. Regressions of water intake at a given food intake are shown for control and cold-treated groups. One standard error is set off at each mean. Regression equations for each group are given in the figure.

was reduced to 6°C for the next 10 days, and the same measurements continued. The cold-treated rats were returned to air at 26°C during the last 7 days of the study. Details of this experiment have been described elsewhere (27). A regression analysis of water intake on food intake revealed that the intercepts, but not the slopes of the two lines differed significantly ($P<0.01$). Thus, water intake for a given food intake was less during than before cold exposure (Figure 4). This occurred in spite of the increase in food intake initiated by exposure to cold and the well-known, direct relationship between food and water intakes in the rat (13,24-27). This suggests that the cold-treated rats may be dehydrating themselves voluntarily. Indeed, a regression analysis of urine output on water intake for these same animals indicated that both the slopes ($P<0.05$) and the intercepts ($P<0.01$) of the two lines differed significantly. Thus, more

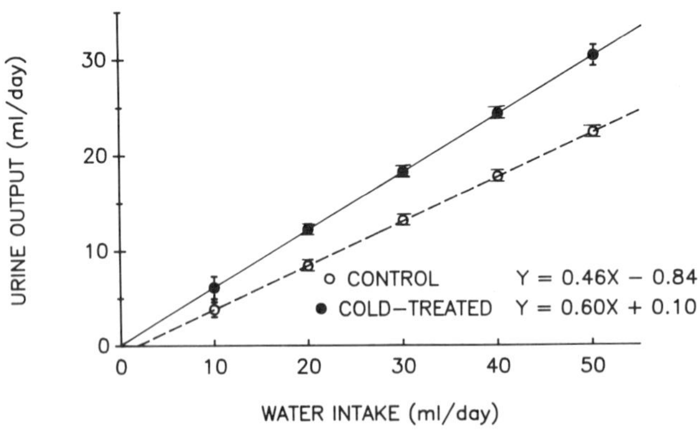

FIGURE 5. Regressions of water intake at a given urine output are shown for control and cold-treated groups. One standard error is set off at each mean. Regression equations for each group are given in the figure.

urine was excreted at a given water intake by cold-treated rats than by controls (Figure 5). This also suggests that exposure to cold induces a relative dehydration in rats.

Additional studies with a sensitive electronic balance revealed that the evaporative water loss of rats exposed to cold was more than twice that of warm-acclimated controls (0.298 ± 0.060 versus 0.124 ± 0.016 g/100 g body weight per hr, respectively) (17).

EFFECTS OF COLD ON URINE PRODUCTION: ROLE OF ANTIDIURETIC HORMONE

A possibility existed that the kidneys of cold-treated rats compensated for the reduced water intake and increased evaporative water loss by concentrating urine to a greater extent than controls. To test this possibility, male rats were exposed to cold for 10 days and urine osmolality of individual rats measured daily. At the end of this time, the rats were dehydrated without food for 24 hr. Four days later each rat was injected with 500 mU Pitressin Tannate in oil, s.c. Their urine outputs and osmolalities were compared with controls maintained at 26°C. Cold-treated rats increased urine output during the 10 days of exposure to cold, but urine osmolality was unchanged (Figure 6). Cold-treated rats failed to decrease urine volume and increase urine osmolality to the levels of controls after either dehydration or administration of Pitressin (26). The extra solute load resulting from the increased food intake by cold-treated rats appeared to be excreted in urine of similar osmolal concentration to that of control rats. The extra solutes thus appeared to be eliminated in a greater volume of urine rather than by concentration of urine to a greater extent.

Itoh (32) showed that the concentration of antidiuretic substance in the plasma of acutely (2 hr) cold-exposed rats was reduced below that of controls. Itoh et al. (33) also showed that the urine output of acutely cold-exposed rats administered Pitressin was reduced to a lesser extent than that of control rats. Further, Bray (9) reported that the urinary volume and osmolal response to daily injection of 500 mU Pitressin were negated when the rats were exposed to air at 3°C. These results suggest that exposure to cold may reduce both production of, and response to, endogenous antidiuretic hormone in rats. Other mechanisms may also play a role. Thus, it is known that the renal tubular response to administered Pitressin is blunted when either glucocorticoid hormones (28) or catecholamines (35) are administered simultaneously. Both of these hormones are elevated in the rat exposed to cold chronically (38,42,53) and could also account for the results observed.

Inasmuch as the cold-treated rat does not appear to make up for its reduced water intake by concentrating its urine to a greater extent than controls, a problem of continuing dehydration with no apparent stimulation of thirst appeared to exist during the 10-day exposure to cold. It is possible that a portion of the deficit may be made up by the preferential metabolism of lipids that would yield more water of oxidation per g than carbohydrates or proteins. Metabolism of body fat stores accounts, in part at least, for the reduction in

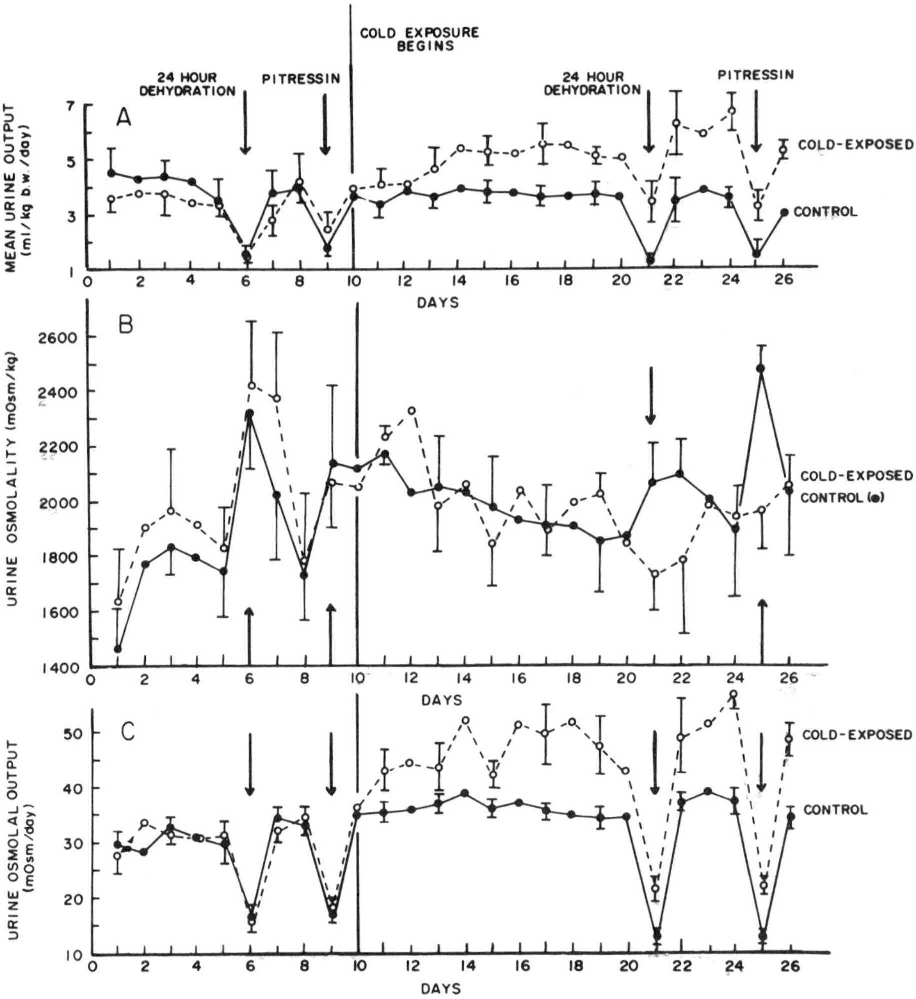

FIGURE 6. Mean urine output (A), urine osmolality (B) and urine osmolal output (C) are shown for control and cold-exposed groups throughout the experiment. All rats were dehydrated for 24 hr during the 6th and 21st days and were administered 500 mU Pitressin on the 9th and 25th days. One standard error is set off at the means.

body weight accompanying exposure to cold. This aspect merits additional study.

It also seems clear that dehydration occurs in cold-treated rats as judged by serum osmolality (20,23-25). Within 1 day of exposure to cold (either 7.5 or 5.0°C), serum osmolality increased significantly (Table 1). Increasing the time of exposure to either temperature did not appear to increase serum osmolality further (20).

TABLE 1. Effect of exposure to cold air for various periods of time on serum osmolality of rats.

Experimental group	No. of rats	Serum osmolality, mOsm/kg
Control	22	290 ± 2[a]
Exposure to 7.5°C air		
1 day	9	301 ± 5[b]
6 days	5	308 ± 1[c]
9 days	8	302 ± 2[c]
Exposure to 5°C air		
1 day	5	302 ± 5[b]
6 days	4	299 ± 2[c]
9 days	6	303 ± 2[c]

[a]Values are given ± 1 SEM.
[b]Significantly different from control group ($P<0.05$).
[c]Significantly different from control group ($P<0.01$).

MECHANISM OF THERMOGENIC DRINKING

Thermogenic drinking was not thwarted by preventing access to water for either 1 or 2 hr after transfer from 5 to 26°C (44). These results are similar to those reported by Adolph et al. (2) and Barker et al. (4) for thirst induced in rats and dogs, respectively, by a hypertonic saline load.

The similarities between thermogenic drinking and postdehydration drinking suggest that the effect of exposure to cold is to induce a dehydration in rats. The increased serum osmolality of rats exposed to air at 5°C supports this suggestion (20,23-25). In addition, cold-induced or thermogenic drinking is similar to thirsts induced by either dehydration or hypertonic saline loading in that delayed access to water did not modify the urge to drink whereas intragastric administration of a water load before removal from cold inhibited drinking (44).

These results raise the question of the mechanism by which the thermogenic drinking response may arise: i.e., absolute dehydration, extracellular dehydration, or involvement of the renin-angiotensin system (31,45). The results of studies described above favor dehydration and activation of osmoreceptors as the mechanism in view of the following: (a) a greater urine output compared to water intake; (b) a smaller water intake at a given food intake; (c) increased serum osmolality; (d) abolition of thermogenic drinking by prior administration of a water load, and (e) persistent thirst when cold-treated rats are allowed to have water only after 2 hr in air at 26°C.

Role of the Renin-Angiotensin System in Thermogenic Drinking

Additional studies were carried out to determine whether the renin-angiotensin system might play a role in thermogenic drinking. A possibility existed that at least one factor stimulating the secretion of angiotensin II and drinking might be the increased rate of secretion of catecholamines induced by either acute or chronic exposure of rats to cold (38). To assess this possibility, d,l-propranolol, a beta-adrenergic antagonist, was tested to determine its effect on thermogenic drinking (22). d,l-Propranolol, administered at 6, (but not at 3), mg/kg b.w. 0.5 hr prior to removal from cold, significantly inhibited thermogenic drinking in cold-treated rats. This dose of propranolol did not affect significantly the drinking response of control rats. Cold-treated rats, given propranolol, drank about one-third the amount of water ingested by control, cold-treated rats. However, this dose of propranolol failed to reduce water intake of the cold-treated rats to that of the untreated control group.

To determine whether the effect of d,l-propranolol might be related to its membrane-stabilizing and central nervous effects, d-propranolol (6 mg/kg) was also used. This isomer contains little beta-adrenergic antagonistic activity, but has the membrane-stabilizing and central nervous characteristics of the l-isomer. d-Propranolol failed to influence the thermogenic drink (22).

Since beta-adrenergic receptors can be subdivided into $beta_1$- and $beta_2$-subtypes, additional studies were carried out to characterize further the receptor type concerned with thermogenic drinking (22). Administration of practolol, a selective $beta_1$-adrenergic antagonist, at either 50 or 150 mg/kg b.w. 0.5 hr prior to removal from cold, had no significant effect on thermogenic drinking. However, administration of the selective $beta_2$-adrenergic antagonist, butoxamine, at 35 mg/kg 0.5 hr prior to removal from cold reduced significantly the thermogenic drink.

Thus, it appears that the thermogenic drinking response arises, in part at least, as a result of stimulation of $beta_2$-adrenergic receptors during transfer of rats from a cold to a warm environment. Whether $beta_2$-adrenergic receptors may also mediate the release of renin from the juxtaglomerular cells of the kidney is debatable at present (12,55). If it can be shown ultimately that they do, it will add another dimension to the role that the renin-angiotensin system plays in the thermogenic drinking response. To test whether the renin-angiotensin system became activated under these conditions, plasma renin activity (PRA) was measured in control rats maintained at 26°C, in cold-adapted rats maintained at 5°C, and in treated rats 15 min after removal from 5 to 26°C (20,34). The results of this study revealed that cold exposure per se did not affect PRA significantly. However, within 15 min after removal from cold, PRA increased four-fold. An additional study showed that administration of propranolol prior to removal from cold prevented the increase in PRA. Since a similar treatment blunted the thermogenic drinking response, the results suggest that removal from cold is associated with an increase in the formation of angiotensin II which could account, in part at least, for the thermogenic drink.

To test further this possibility, the angiotensin I converting enzyme inhibitor, captopril, was administered to rats 15 min prior to transfer from the cold to a neutral environment (34). These studies revealed a graded reduction in the thermogenic drinking response with graded increases in the dose of captopril administered prior to transfer from the cold to a thermoneutral environment.

These results suggest that thermogenic drinking may be mediated, in part at least, by activation of the beta-adrenergic system, which induces an increase in PRA and the formation of angiotensin II. The latter is the dipsogenic agent responsible, at least in part, for the induction of drinking. Support for a role of angiotensin II in thermogenic drinking is obtained from the elevated PRA of rats removed from the cold to a neutral environment. The time-course for the increase in PRA also coincides with the time-course for induction of a thermogenic drinking response. Additional evidence that angiotensin II may be important in the thermogenic drinking response is found in the dose-dependent blocking effect of captopril, which inhibits conversion of angiotensin I to angiotensin II (34).

Experimental results to date suggest that thermogenic drinking is mediated both by osmoreceptors and angiotensin II receptors. Present results do not show the extent to which each may contribute to the thermogenic drink. Thus, a possibility exists that the thermogenic drinking response of the cold-treated rat is of sufficient physiological importance to have redundancy in the mechanisms initiating it. While thermogenic drinking has been well studied in the rat, the studies of Conley and Nickerson (14) and Spealman et al. (52) indicate that cold-exposed man may have a similar response.

EFFECT OF A TEN-DAY COLD EXPOSURE ON ELECTROLYTE EXCHANGE

The results of the studies described above suggest an imbalance between intakes of food and water during exposure to cold. It is obvious that an imbalance could not continue indefinitely. If food, and therefore solute, intake increases by fifty percent, and there is at best only a slight increase in water intake, dehydration could be prevented by increasing the solute concentration of urine; by decreasing extra-renal water loss; by increasing fecal electrolyte excretion; by increased metabolism of fat with an accompanying gain of metabolic water, or all of these. The study described next was designed to address some of these points.Twelve male Sprague-Dawley rats were maintained in individual metabolic cages under the same conditions described above. During a 7-day control period in air at 26°C, intakes of distilled water and food (Rockland Diet) as well as urine and fecal outputs were measured daily (18). At the end of the control period, six of the rats, chosen at random, were exposed to air at 6°C while the remaining six were kept at 26°C. Intakes and outputs were measured daily for an additional 10 days, after which the cold-treated rats were returned to air at 26°C. Measurement of intakes and outputs continued for

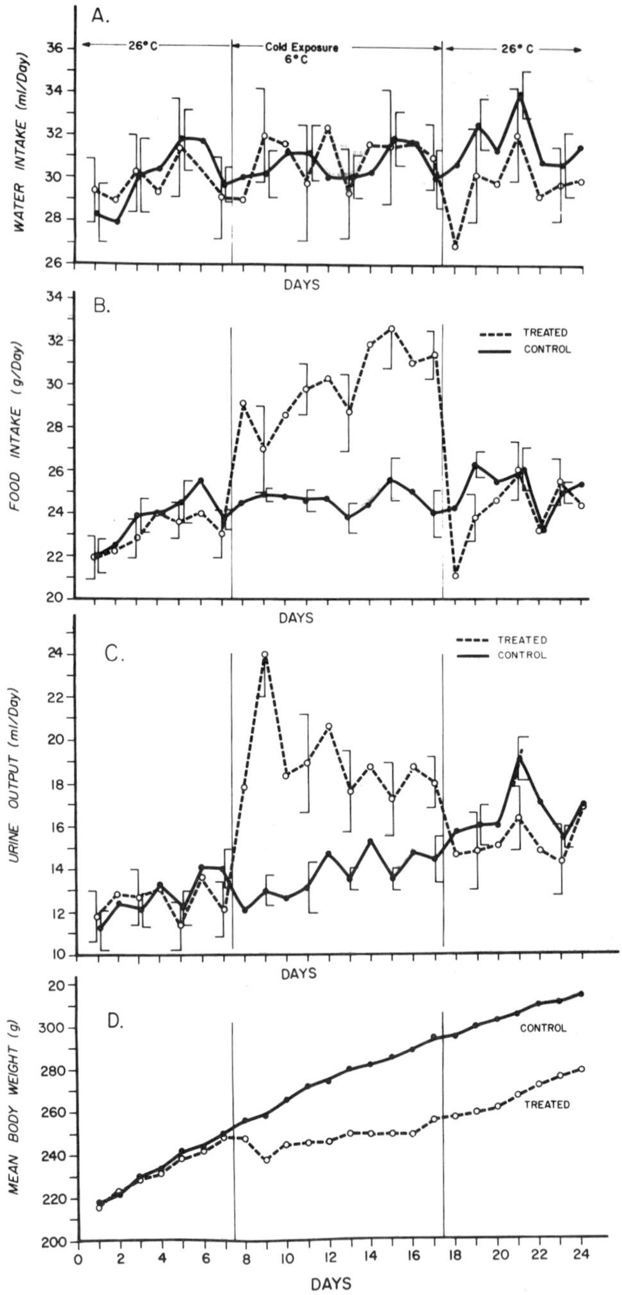

FIGURE 7. Effect of exposure to air at 6°C on water intake (A), food intake (B), urine output (C), and mean body weight (D) of rats. Control, cold, and post-cold periods are shown. The broken line represents cold-treated rats and the solid line represents control. One standard error is set off at each mean. (Reproduced with permission, Ref 18).

an additional 7 days. Urine was analyzed for sodium, potassium, and chloride concentrations. The daily fecal collection from each rat was wet-ashed in concentrated nitric acid and analyzed for sodium and potassium content.

Water intake again failed to increase during exposure to cold (Figure 7A) and decreased during the first day after removal from cold in spite of a robust thermogenic drinking response. Food intake increased within the first day of exposure to cold and reached a value about 35% above the average control level by the 10th day (Figure 7B). Food intake also decreased sharply during the first day after removal from cold. Urine output doubled during the first days of cold exposure but gradually diminished toward control levels by the 10th day (Figure 7C). The urine output of control rats tended to increase gradually throughout the experiment. Body weight of cold-treated rats failed to increase during exposure to cold but remained nearly constant (Figure 7D). Following removal from cold, the rate of body-weight gain was similar to that of controls.

The relationships between water intake and urinary output for control and cold-treated rats were similar to those shown earlier (Figure 5). The regression equations for the relationships in control and cold-treated rats are: $Y = 0.54X - 2.79$ (control) and $Y = 0.52X - 1.60$ (cold-exposed), where Y is urinary output (ml/day) and X is water intake (ml/day). Correlation coefficients for these relationships are 0.86 and 0.85 for control and cold-treated groups, respectively ($N = 144$ and 59; $P<0.01$ for each group). The results indicate that only the intercepts ($P<0.05$) of the lines differ significantly from each other. Thus, for a given water intake, urinary output of cold-exposed rats was greater than that of controls.

The relationships between water and food intakes for control and cold-treated rats were also similar to those shown in Figure 4. The regression equations for the relationships are the following: $Y = 0.60X + 15.83$ (control) and $Y = 0.70X + 10.69$ (cold-exposed group), where X is food intake (g/day) and Y is water intake (ml/day). Correlation coefficients for these relationships are 0.43 and 0.43 for control and cold-treated groups, respectively ($N = 144$ and 59; $P<0.01$ for each group). The intercepts, but not the slopes, of the lines differ significantly ($P<0.01$). The results indicate that for a given food intake, there is a smaller water intake in cold-treated rats than in controls.

Mean intakes of food, water, sodium, and potassium for the two groups of rats during control, cold, and post-cold periods are shown in Table 2. During exposure to cold, the experimental group ingested significantly ($P<0.01$) more food, sodium, and potassium than controls. Within 1 day after cold exposure ended, these increased intakes had returned to the level of the control group.

The effect of exposure to cold on mean urinary and fecal electrolyte excretion rates during control, cold, and post-cold periods is shown in Table 3.

Again, exposure to cold increased significantly ($P<0.01$) urinary osmolar, chloride, sodium, and potassium outputs. Fecal sodium and potassium outputs were also increased significantly. Excepting urinary potassium outputs, all

TABLE 2. Effect of exposure to cold air on intake of food, water, and electrolytes.

	Control period§	Cold period^t	First day after return to 26°C	Post cold period
Food (g/day)				
Control	24.5 ± 0.5+	24.9 ± 0.8	24.8 ± 0.6	24.6 ± 0.8
Treated	24.2 ± 1.0	29.4 ± 1.3**	21.1 ± 2.2	26.0 ± 0.8
Water (ml/day)				
Control	30.0 ± 0.6	30.6 ± 0.4	30.7 ± 1.7	31.8 ± 0.6
Treated	29.9 ± 0.8	30.9 ± 1.0	26.9 ± 1.2	30.2 ± 0.7
Sodium (meq/day)				
Control	4.52 ± 0.09	4.58 ± 0.11	4.47 ± 0.11	4.58 ± 0.14
Treated	4.45 ± 0.20	5.41 ± 0.23**	3.88 ± 0.41	4.49 ± 0.26
Potassium (meq/day)				
Control	6.21 ± 0.15	6.28 ± 0.19	6.15 ± 0.16	6.21 ± 0.60
Treated	6.27 ± 0.25	7.43 ± 0.32**	5.34 ± 0.57	6.16 ± 0.62

§Each period consisted of 3 days excepting column 3, which contains values for 1 day only.
^{t}Measurements were made during the last 3 days of control, cold, and post-cold periods.
+Mean ± standard error.
**Significantly different from control (P<0.01).

electrolyte outputs returned to the control level within 1 day after removal from cold.

The relationships between sodium intake and simultaneous total (urinary plus fecal) sodium output for each group were subjected to a regression analysis (Figure 8). The correlation coefficients for these relationships are 0.48 and 0.48 for control and cold-treated groups, respectively (N = 54 and 18; P<0.01, P<0.05). The results indicated that the slopes of the lines were not different whereas the intercepts differed significantly (P<0.01). When compared at the same sodium intake, cold-exposed rats excreted more sodium than did controls.

The relationships between potassium intake and simultaneous total potassium output are also shown in Figure 8 for the two groups of rats. The correlation coefficients for these relationships are 0.28 and 0.54 for control and cold-treated groups, respectively (N = 54 and 18; P<0.05, P<0.02). Both the slopes and intercepts of the two lines are significantly different (P<0.01). For potassium intakes above 5 mEq/day, as they were during both control and cold

Table 3. Effect of exposure to cold air on urinary and fecal electrolyte excretion.

	Control period[§]	Cold period[ƚ]	First day after return to 26°C	Post-cold period[ƚ]
Urinary osmolar output (mOsm/day)				
Control	29.8±0.7[+]	27.0±0.4	30.9±0.9	28.0±0.4
Treated	27.9±1.0	36.0±1.4**	25.6±1.1	28.9±1.1
Urinary chloride output (meq/day)				
Control	3.21±0.07	3.63±0.07	3.83±0.09	3.53±0.01
Treated	3.20±0.09	4.28±0.16**	3.17±0.01	3.53±0.17
Urinary sodium output (meq/day)				
Control	3.18±0.02	3.47±0.03	4.00±0.33	3.57±0.10
Treated	3.10±0.08	4.13±0.1**	3.28±0.17	3.53±0.12
Fecal sodium output (meq/day)				
Control	0.31±0.02	0.34±0.04	0.36±0.04	0.43±0.06
Treated	0.39±0.04	0.66±0.10**	0.47±0.08	0.40±0.04
Total sodium output (meq/day)				
Control	3.49±0.06	3.81±0.08	4.36±0.32	4.01±0.12
Treated	3.46±0.09	4.81±0.19**	3.76±0.17	3.98±0.14
Urinary potassium output (meq/day)				
Control	4.43±0.02	4.43±0.02	5.06±0.04	4.82±0.01
Treated	4.60±0.02	5.14±0.06**	3.96±0.02**	4.53±0.02
Fecal potassium output (meq/day)				
Control	0.55±0.03	0.55±0.06	0.59±0.04	0.61±0.06
Treated	0.68±0.06	1.01±0.10**	0.65±0.08	0.63±0.07
Total potassium output (meq/day)				
Control	4.95±0.26	4.99±0.13	5.69±0.31	5.41±0.08
Treated	5.28±0.48	6.12±0.27**	4.65±0.21	5.13±0.22

[§]Each period consisted of 3 days excepting column 3, which contains values for 1 day only.
[ƚ]Measurements were made during the last 3 days of control, cold, and post-cold periods.
[+]Mean ± standard error.
** Significantly different from control ($P < 0.01$).

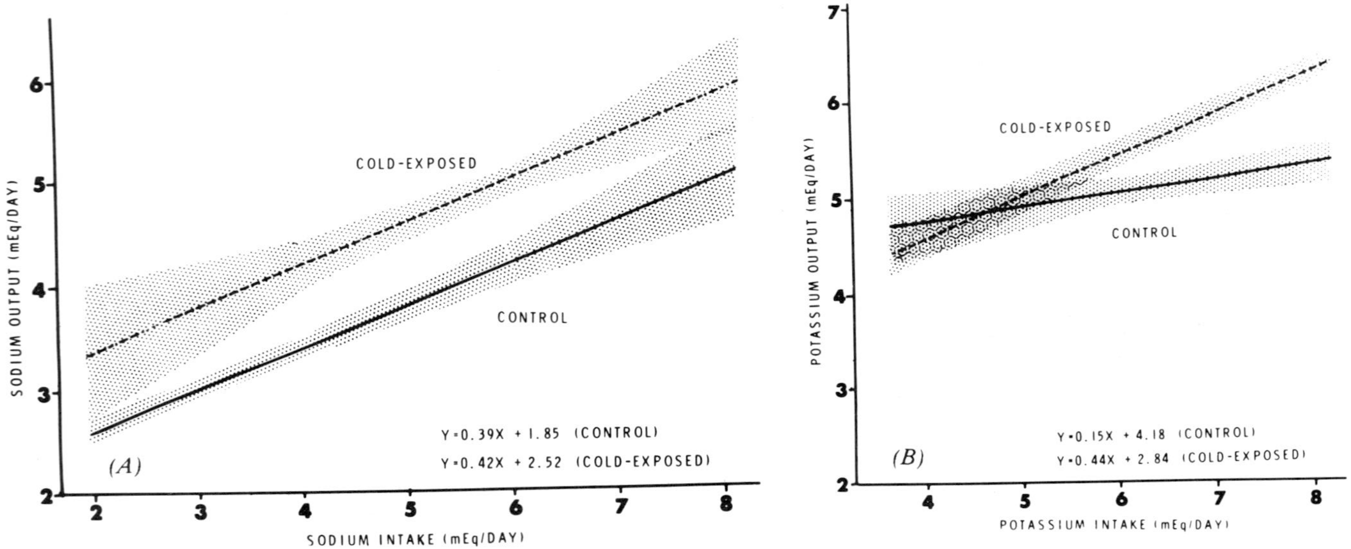

FIGURE 8. The relationship between sodium output and sodium intake for control and cold-treated groups is shown in (A). Similar relationships for potassium are shown in (B). The shaded area around each line represents the 95% confidence interval. (Reproduced with permission, Ref 18).

periods (Table 2), potassium output of cold-exposed rats was greater than that of controls.

To determine whether greater proportions of the total sodium and potassium outputs were excreted by the fecal route during exposure to cold than before it, the ratio of either fecal sodium or potassium to total sodium or potassium was calculated for control and cold periods and analyzed by an analysis of covariance. The results (Table 4) show that both the ratios of fecal sodium/total sodium and fecal potassium/total potassium increased significantly during exposure to cold. This suggests that the fecal route was used to a greater extent for electrolyte excretion during cold than before it. Figure 8 shows that about half of the difference between the two lines (i.e. about half the difference between intercepts) can be accounted for by the increased fecal sodium excretion induced by cold (Table 3).

The daily urinary osmolalities (mOsm/kg of water) of control and experimental groups during control and cold periods were compared by an analysis of covariance to determine whether exposure to cold was accompanied by a significant change in urinary total solute concentration. The results indicate that cold exposure failed to affect urinary osmolality significantly (Table 5). Thus, the greater solute output (mOsm/day) accompanying exposure to cold (Table 3) was accomplished by increasing urinary flow rather than by concentrating urine to a greater extent.

TABLE 4. Effect of exposure to cold on ratios of fecal Na/total Na and fecal K/ total K excretion.

Group	Control period		Cold period	
	Fecal Na / total Na (%)	Fecal K / total K (%)	Fecal Na / total Na (%)	Fecal K / total K (%)
Control	8.7	11.5	8.8	10.9
Experimental	10.9	12.8	13.7	16.4

Analysis of covariance:

Source	*df*	Fecal Na/total Na			Fecal K/total K		
		MSS	*F*	*P**	*MSS*	*F*	*P**
Treatment	1	144.92	10.4	<0.01	237.60	19.9	<0.01
Error	34	13.96			11.93		
Total	35						

*Probability value.

TABLE 5. Effect of exposure to cold on urine osmolality of rats.

Group	Milliosmoles/kg water Control period	Cold period
Control	2343	2337
Experimental	2150	2262

Analysis of covariance:

Source	*df*	*MSS*	*F*	*P**
Treatment	1	40991.75	1.89	>0.05
Error	9	21665.52		
Total	10			

*Probability value.

The results of this study reinforce earlier findings that cold-treated rats do not increase their urinary concentration of total solutes to conserve water. Since cold-treated rats cannot increase their renal concentrating ability to the level of controls when required to do so by either dehydration or following administration of Pitressin, the possibility exists that reduced renal concentrating ability is another factor contributing to the dehydrating effect of exposure to cold.

Cold-treated rats excreted more sodium in their urine and feces than controls when compared at the same intake of sodium (Figure 8, Table 4). Although the slope of the line relating sodium output to intake was unchanged by exposure to cold, the intercepts were significantly different. In large measure, the difference between intercepts is related to an increased fecal sodium excretion induced by exposure to cold (Table 4). The physiological significance of the increased fecal sodium excretion occurring during exposure to cold may be in its contribution to the conservation of body water. Thus, the average urinary sodium concentration both before and during exposure to cold was 160 mEq/l, or 6.25 ml urine was required for excretion of each mEq of sodium. On average, 0.32 mEq more sodium per day was excreted via feces by cold-exposed rats than by controls, resulting, on this basis alone, in a net saving of about 1.9 ml of water/day. This rough calculation suggests the extent of contribution of the increased fecal electrolyte excretion to water balance during exposure to cold. Although exposure to cold induces a relative dehydration in rats, an important factor limiting the extent of the dehydration may be the increased fecal electrolyte loss. However, the occurrence of dehydration in spite of this indicates that even this adjustment is not adequate. The increased fecal electrolyte excretion occurring during cold exposure may be an artifact of the increased fecal bulk accompanying increased food intake induced by exposure to cold. The possibility that the necessity to ingest more food of high bulk during exposure to cold contributed to the dehydrating effect of exposure to cold was considered next.

Effect of Dietary Bulk on Water and Electrolyte Exchange in the Cold

Twelve male Sprague-Dawley rats were kept in individual metabolic cages at 26°C. During a 7-day control period, daily intakes of distilled water and food (Sodium Deficient Test Diet, Nutritional Biochemicals Co., supplemented with 0.8 g of NaCl/100 g of food), as well as urinary and fecal outputs, were measured (19).

At the end of the control period, six of the rats, chosen at random, were exposed to air at 6°C while the remainder were kept at 26°C. The intakes and outputs listed above were measured for an additional 10 days, after which the cold-exposed rats were returned to air at 26°C. Measurements of intakes and outputs continued for an additional 5 days. Urine was analyzed for sodium and potassium concentrations by flame photometry using lithium as the internal standard. The daily fecal collection from each rat was pooled for each period. The pooled sample from each rat for each period was then analyzed for its sodium and potassium contents by flame photometry. Additional details of this experiment are given elsewhere (19).

At the end of the period of cold exposure and immediately upon return to air at 26°C all rats were given water at 6°C to drink. The fluid drunk was then measured at hourly intervals for 3 hr.

Water intake failed to increase during exposure to cold, and actually decreased somewhat below the pre-cold exposure control level (Figure 9A). Food intake increased within the third day of exposure to cold and reached a value about 35% above the average control level by the 8th day. Food intake decreased sharply during the 1st day after removal from cold (Figure 9B). Urinary output increased during the first days of cold exposure and reached maximal levels by the fourth day (Figure 9C). Mean body weight of the experimental group actually decreased during cold exposure. Following removal from cold, the rate of body weight gain was similar to that of controls (Figure 9D).

Upon return of the experimental group to air at 26°C, their accumulative water intake during the 1st, 2nd, and 3rd hr increased significantly ($P<0.01$) above that of controls that had been maintained in air at 26°C (19). Thus, ingestion of a diet low in bulk had no effect on thermogenic drinking.

The relationships between water intake and urinary output for control and cold-exposed rats were determined by linear regression analysis. During the control period, neither slopes nor intercepts of this relationship for either control or experimental groups differed. Hence, all data were combined and compared against the control group during the experimental period. Again, neither slopes nor intercepts differed significantly and these data were

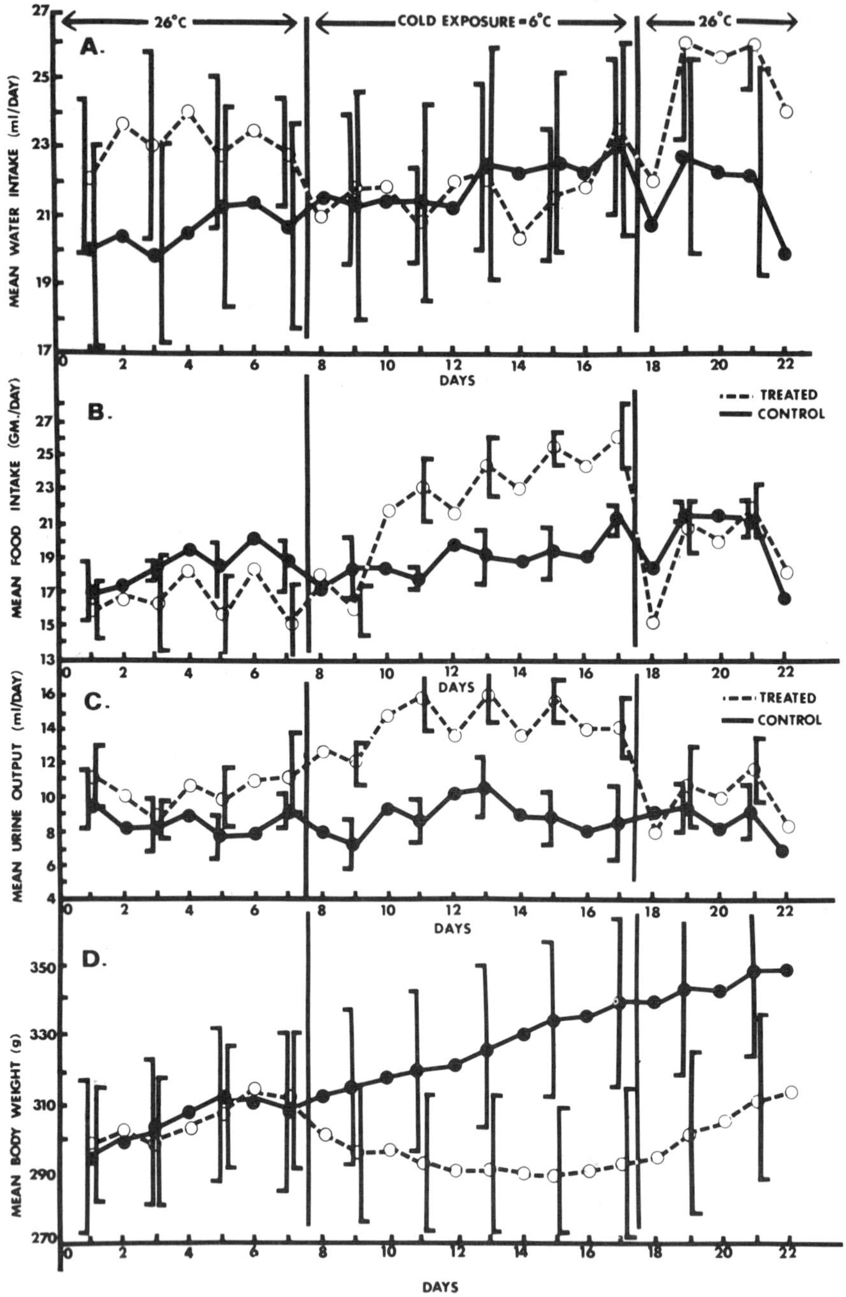

FIGURE 9. Effect of exposure to air at 6°C on water intake (A), food intake (B), urine output (C), and mean body weight (D) of rats. Control, cold, and post-cold periods are shown. The broken line represents the experimental group while the solid line represents controls. One standard error is set off at each mean. (Reproduced with permission, Ref 19).

TABLE 6. Effect of exposure to cold on intake of food, water, and electrolytes.

	Control period	Cold period	First day after return to 26°C	Post-cold period
Food (g/day)				
Control	18.0 ± 0.8[+]	18.7 ± 0.8	18.2 ± 1.3	18.7 ± 0.7
Treated	16.5 ± 2.1	22.3 ± 0.8**	15.1 ± 1.6	19.1 ± 1.4
Water (ml/day)				
Control	20.8 ± 2.8	21.9 ± 2.6	20.7 ± 3.1	21.6 ± 2.9
Treated	23.1 ± 1.9	21.7 ± 1.8	22.0 ± 2.4	24.7 ± 2.5
Sodium (mequiv/day)				
Control	4.66 ± 0.21	4.88 ± 0.20	4.80 ± 0.34	5.52 ± 0.40
Treated	4.35 ± 0.53	5.82 ± 0.35*	3.98 ± 0.42	5.86 ± 0.30
Potassium (mequiv/day)				
Control	5.77 ± 0.21	5.96 ± 0.32	5.66 ± 0.40	4.58 ± 0.20
Treated	5.29 ± 0.66	7.17 ± 0.44*	4.72 ± 0.50	5.16 ± 0.30

[+]Mean ± standard error.
*Significantly different from control ($P<0.05$).
**Significantly different from control ($P<0.01$).

combined into the previous groups. The combined control data were then compared with data from the experimental group during the period of cold exposure. The following relationships between water intake (X, ml/day) and urinary output (Y, ml/day) are given for the combined control and experimental groups: $Y = 0.493X - 1.725$; $r = 0.82$; $P<0.01$; $N = 124$ (combined control) and $Y = 0.412X + 5.991$; $r = 0.691$; $P<0.01$; $N = 59$ (cold-exposed group). Statistical comparison revealed that the slopes of the lines did not differ but the intercepts were significantly ($P<0.01$) different. Under these conditions, the urinary output for a given water intake was also greater in cold-treated than in control rats.

During exposure to cold, the experimental group, on average, ingested significantly more food ($P<0.01$), sodium ($P<0.05$), and potassium ($P<0.05$) than controls (Table 6). Within 1 day after cold exposure ended, these increased intakes had returned to the levels of the control group. The intakes of the treated group failed to differ from those of the control group during the remainder of the post-cold period.

The effect of exposure to cold on mean urinary and fecal electrolyte excretion rates during control, cold, and post-cold periods is shown in Table 7. Again exposure to cold increased significantly the urinary outputs of chloride,

Table 7. Effect of exposure to cold on urinary and fecal electrolyte excretion.

	Control period	Cold period	First day after return to 26°C	Post-cold period
Urinary chloride output (meq/day)				
Control	4.73±0.23 +	4.98±0.27	5.55±0.66	4.80±0.24
Treated	4.65±0.35	6.74±0.30**	3.95±0.67	5.25±0.24
Urinary sodium output (meq/day)				
Control	2.98±0.19	3.01±0.19	3.54±0.45	3.16±0.24
Treated	3.05±0.28	3.89±0.21**	2.52±0.42	3.19±0.24
Fecal sodium output (meq/day)				
Control	0.117±0.022	0.101±0.012	-	0.098±0.011
Treated	0.091±0.006	0.102±0.013	-	0.098±0.001
Total sodium output (meq/day)				
Control	3.11±0.17	3.11±0.19	-	3.26±0.24
Treated	3.14±0.41	3.99±0.27*	-	3.29±0.23
Urinary potassium output (meq/day)				
Control	3.47±0.24	3.56±0.22	4.46±0.49	3.87±0.19
Treated	3.45±0.29	4.66±0.16**	3.34±0.47	3.74±0.31
Fecal potassium output (meq/day)				
Control	0.107±0.022	0.099±0.012	-	0.113±0.019
Treated	0.076±0.005	0.126±0.011	-	0.098±0.011
Total potassium output (meq/day)				
Control	3.58±0.25	3.66±0.22	-	3.98±0.20
Treated	3.53±0.42	4.79±0.32*	-	3.84±0.30

+Mean ± standard error

*Significantly different from control ($P<0.05$).

**Significantly different from control ($P<0.01$).

sodium, and potassium. However, fecal outputs of sodium and potassium were not increased significantly by exposure to cold. During the 5-day post-cold period, all electrolyte outputs of cold-exposed rats returned to control values.

The relationship between sodium intake and simultaneous total (urinary plus fecal) sodium output for each group was subjected to a regression analysis. This relationship did not differ for control and cold-exposed animals and is shown in Figure 10A where each point represents the mean sodium intake and output of an individual rat during either the control or experimental periods. The equation describing the relationship between total sodium output (Y,

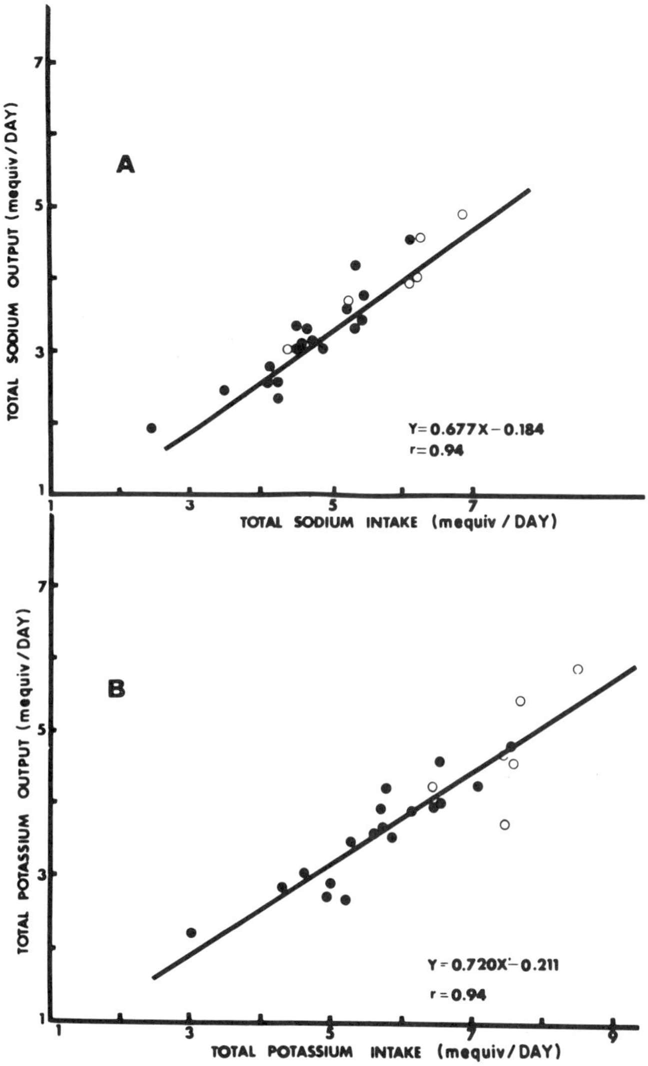

FIGURE 10. The relationship between sodium intake and sodium output (A) and potassium intake and output (B) for rats maintained either in air at 26°C or in air at 6°C. The equations of the lines and the correlation coefficients are given in each figure. (●) Control and experimental rats at 26°C, (○) experimental rats at 6°C. (Reproduced with permission, Ref 19).

mEq/day) and total (food) sodium intake (X, mEq/day) for all rats is the following: Y = 0.68X - 0.18; N = 24; r = 0.94; P<0.01. Thus, the low bulk diet used in this experiment apparently prevented the increased fecal sodium excretion by cold-exposed rats observed earlier with a high-bulk diet (18). The relationships between potassium intake and simultaneous potassium output are shown in Figure 10B. Again the relationship did not differ for control and cold-exposed animals. The relationship between total potassium output (Y, mEq/day) and food potassium intake (X, mEq/day) for all rats is described by the following equation: $Y = 0.72X - 0.21$; $N = 24$; $r = 0.94$; $P<0.01$. These results also suggest that the low-bulk diet used here prevented the increased fecal potassium excretion by cold-treated rats observed earlier with a high-bulk diet (18).

To determine whether greater proportions of the total sodium and potassium outputs were excreted by the fecal route during cold exposure than before it, the ratio of either fecal sodium or potassium to total sodium or potassium output was calculated for control and cold periods and analyzed by an analysis of covariance. The results are not shown but indicate that the same percentages of either total sodium or potassium output were excreted by the fecal route during cold exposure as during the control period. The results reveal that the increased fecal sodium and potassium outputs observed earlier with a high-bulk diet did not occur when a low-bulk diet was used. However, fluid exchange during exposure to cold was essentially unchanged by administration of a diet low in bulk, including the greater urinary output for a given fluid intake, the smaller water intake for a given food intake, and the thermogenic drinking response.

FLUID EXCHANGE DURING FOUR WEEKS OF EXPOSURE TO COLD

This experiment was carried out to assess the effect of a 4-week exposure to cold on fluid exchange of rats. This long-term exposure to cold seemed important to carry out since the results of the 10-day exposure to cold suggested that the rats were in negative fluid balance. Obviously, an increasingly negative fluid balance during exposure to cold is not compatible with life. Hence, the objective of the present experiment was to determine whether compensatory changes occurred during a longer term of exposure to cold that might reverse some of the effects of cold observed during the shorter-term exposure.

Six male Sprague-Dawley rats (250-290 g) served as controls while 6 others served as experimental subjects. The rats were caged individually. During a 5-day control period, daily measurements of food and water intakes, urine outputs, and body weights were made as described in the previous experiments. At the end of this time, the experimental group was transferred to air at $5^{o}C$. Measurements of intakes and outputs continued every second day for 4 weeks.

Water intake of the control group remained relatively constant throughout the experiment while that of the cold-treated group decreased slightly when placed initially into cold and gradually increased to reach control intake on the 13th day (Figure 11A). Intake then exceeded that of controls for the remainder of the study. Food intake of the control group also remained relatively constant throughout the experiment while that of the cold-treated group increased upon initial exposure to cold, but reached maximal level at 8 days after exposure to cold (Figure 11B). Again, urinary output of the control group remained relatively constant throughout the period of exposure to cold while urinary

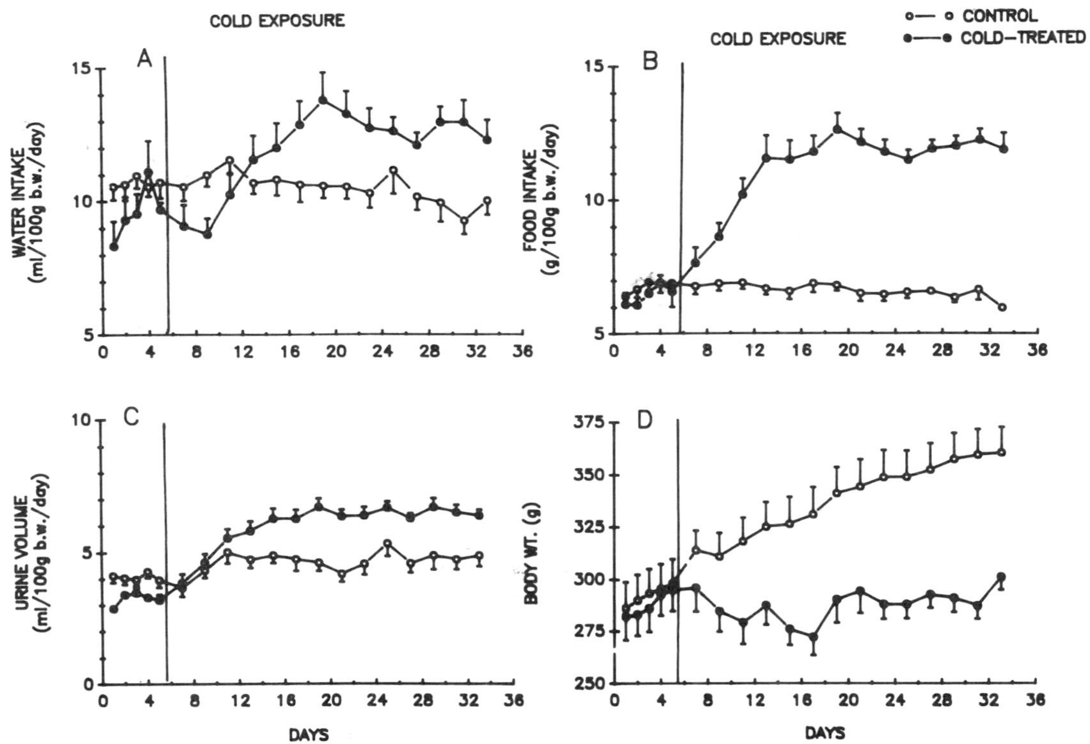

FIGURE 11. Effect of exposure to cold on mean water intake (A), food intake (B), urine output (C), and body weight (D) of control and cold-treated groups. One standard error is set off at each mean.

output of the cold-treated group increased on the 6th day of exposure to cold and reached maximal level on the 10th day of exposure to cold (Figure 11C). Mean body weight of the control group increased during the experiment while that of the cold-treated group decreased slightly initially, but remained relatively fixed throughout the experiment (Figure 11D).

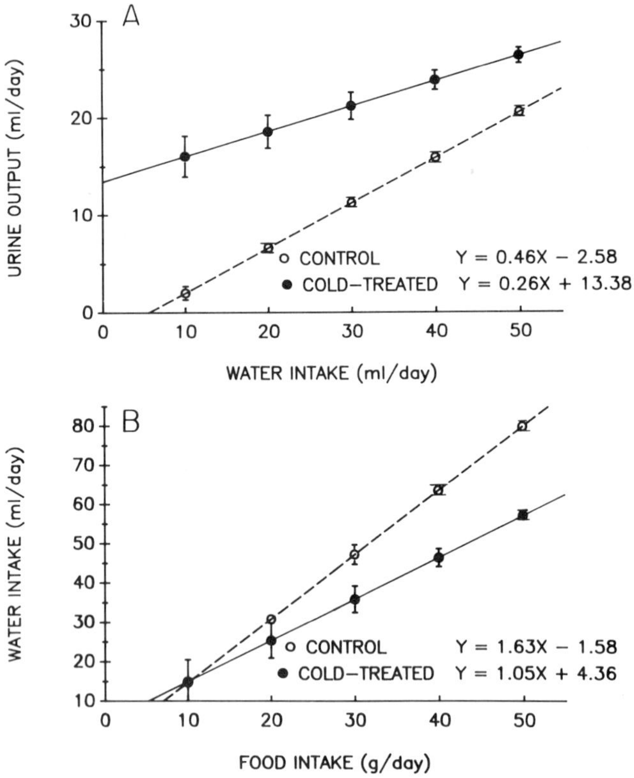

FIGURE 12. Regressions of water intake versus urine output (A) and food intake versus water intake (B) are shown. One standard error is set off at each mean. Equations of the lines are given in the figure.

The results suggested initially that longer-term exposure to cold can actually increase the water intake of rats. To assess whether the ratio of water intake / urinary output had been altered, these two variables were graphed against each other as had been done for the shorter-term exposure to cold (Figure 12A). The same relationship observed earlier was also present in this study; viz., urinary output of the cold-treated group was greater at a given water intake than it was for the control group. Further, water intake for a given food intake was less for the cold-treated than for the control group (Figure 12B). These results suggest that the cold-treated rats in this study were relatively dehydrated, a suggestion verified by a significant ($P<0.01$) increase in serum osmolality (314 ±4 S.E. mOsm/kg) in the cold-treated compared to the control (293 ± 2) group. These results suggest that a level of dehydration is maintained during exposure to cold, even of 4 weeks' duration. This suggests that voluntary dehydration may be an important aspect of acclimation and survival in the cold. It does, however, also present certain limitations to survival. Thus, the dehydrated, cold-treated rat should be more susceptible to circulatory shock following a given loss of blood than warm-adapted controls. This aspect deserves additional study.

WATER BALANCE IN MAN EXPOSED TO COLD

Acute exposure to cold is well known to induce a diuresis in man (1,3,5,7,8,29,39,50). It begins within the first half-hour, and differs from a water diuresis in that the rate of solute excretion is also increased (29,39,50). It may depend on the state of hydration prior to exposure to cold. Whether the diuresis is blockable by exogenous administration of antidiuretic hormone has been the subject of debate (3,39).

A large number of investigators have now reported an increase in both plasma protein concentration, hemoglobin concentration, and hematocrit ratio in men and women exposed acutely to cold (1,3,6,16,29,30,39,41,51,54). It is tempting to suggest that the physiological importance of cold-induced diuresis is to provide a mechanism for a rapid reduction in extracellular fluid volume to match the decreased vascular capacity resulting from cold-induced vasoconstriction.

Burton et al. (10) measured evaporative water loss, plasma volume, plasma colloid osmotic pressure, water intake, and urine output of six male subjects exposed for 1-6 days to a cool environment (21.0 to 23.7°C). They observed a reduction in evaporative water loss by more than 50% when the subjects were transferred from a warm to a cool environment. These subjects also had an increase in colloid osmotic pressure of the plasma; a reduction in plasma volume (between 65 and 1430 ml in five subjects); a reduction in water intake, and an increased urine output that occurred throughout 6 days of exposure to the cool environment.

Conley and Nickerson (14) also exposed men to mild cold (16-18 °C). In the case of the five subjects for whom complete data are available, all reduced water intake and increased urinary output on exposure to cold. The changes in urinary output and water intake were maintained during the 3-day cold exposure. Plasma volumes were measured prior to, and 3-5 days after, exposure to cold. Decreases of 3, 4, 7, and 8% were observed for the 4 subjects in whom the measurements were made. Extracellular fluid volume decreased by 0.8, 2.8, 6.1, and 13.8% in these same subjects. Further, Spealman et al. (51) observed negative water balances of from about 200 to 1000 ml in four humans exposed to an air temperature of 16 °C for 2-6 days. The reduction in water intake by humans exposed to cold may be related to a reduction in the sensation of thirst noted by Rogers et al. (49).

The studies cited above suggest that man exposed to cold for periods up to a week may be in negative fluid balance. It is clear, however, that additional studies in the area are needed. A recent in depth review (21) of this subject is recommended to the reader seeking additional information.

COMMENTS

Studies from this laboratory showed that dehydration accompanies exposure of rats to cold air for 1 to 120 days (22). This was manifested by an alteration in the relationship between water intake and urinary output such that more urine was excreted for a given water intake by cold-treated than by control rats (18). Further evidence that exposure to cold induced a relative dehydration was found in the increased serum osmolality and chloride concentration as well as in the striking thirst following removal from cold (20,24,25). These changes were also observed in rats given a low-bulk diet to eat.

A number of factors may contribute to the cold-induced dehydration. Evaporative water loss has been measured and is nearly doubled during exposure of rats to air at $5^{o}C$ (44). However, the increased evaporative water loss of cold-treated rats may be counterbalanced by their increased food intake since Radford (48) estimated that evaporative water loss approximated the water present in the food ingested by his rats. Proof that this is the case during exposure to cold would require additional study. The relationship between food intake and water intake is also changed such that less water is ingested at a given food intake by cold-exposed than by control rats (18). A possibility exists that this food-water imbalance results in an accumulation of solutes and thereby contributes to the increased serum osmolality and the dehydrating effect of cold. In addition, the altered relationship between urinary output and water intake induced by cold suggests changes in either the thirst mechanism or in the mechanisms influencing renal water loss. Mefford et al. (30) also observed a reduction in the relationship between water intake and urinary output in rats exposed to cold. Thus, the ability both to produce and to respond to endogenous antidiuretic hormone, or both, may be reduced in rats exposed to cold.

The phenomenon of a reduction in relationship of water intake to urinary output during exposure to cold was also observed by Mefford et al. (40) in rats. Under these conditions the cold-exposed rats might be expected to concentrate their urine to a greater extent than control rats. The results presented here also show that exposure to cold failed to affect urinary osmolality significantly (18). Thus, the greater solute output accompanying cold exposure was accomplished by increasing urinary flow rather than by concentrating urine to a greater extent. The mechanism responsible for the greater urinary flow in chronically cold-exposed rats is not completely understood. Itoh (32) showed that the concentration of antidiuretic substance in the plasma of acutely (2 hr) cold-exposed rats administered Pitressin was reduced to a lesser extent than that of control rats. Further, Bray (9) showed that the urinary volume and osmolal responses to daily injection of 500 mU Pitressin were negated when the rats were exposed to air at 3°C. These results, as well as those presented here, suggest that exposure to cold may reduce both production of, and response to, endogenous antidiuretic hormone in rats. Other mechanisms such as changes in renal blood flow and glomerular filtration rate may also contribute and await further study. It is of interest that the renal response of cold-exposed rats to exogenous Pitressin mentioned above is different from that of cold-exposed man. Bader et al. (3) reported complete inhibition of cold diuresis in humans administered Pitressin.

An important contribution to fluid balance under conditions of cold may also be made by the metabolism of body fat since both the utilization and turnover of lipids are increased by exposure to cold (36), and both body fat content (47,56) and respiratory quotient are reduced (46). The reduction in body weight accompanying exposure to cold can be attributed, in part at least, to the metabolism of body fat stores. Page and Babineau (46) reported that high-fat diets promote growth of cold-exposed rats. In addition, high-fat diets may enhance the ability of rats to maintain their body temperatures on exposure to cold (37), and to adapt to a cold environment (46). Dietary self-selection studies also suggest that an enhanced adaptive resistance to cold accompanies increased ingestion of fat (15). While the importance of fat in the maintenance of energy balance of animals exposed to cold has been well studied, its added importance and contribution to the maintenance of water balance require further study.

Exposure to cold air is well known to increase excretion of sodium and potassium in rats (11,18). Studies using a high-bulk diet revealed that cold-exposed rats excreted more sodium than controls when compared at the same sodium intake (18). In large measure, the difference between cold-exposed and control rats was related to an increased fecal sodium excretion. However, when the rats were given a low-bulk diet, cold-treated rats still excreted more sodium and potassium than controls. When these cold-treated rats were compared at the same sodium intakes, outputs of either sodium or potassium failed to differ from those of controls. Hence, increased fecal electrolyte excretion of cold-exposed rats given Rockland Diet to eat is most likely to be a consequence of the fecal bulk rather than the consequence of exposure to cold per se.

With respect to thermogenic drinking, the results are quite clear that abrupt removal of rats from a cold to a warm environment results in a striking thermogenic drinking response. However, little still is known about the failure to drink adequate amounts of water during exposure to cold, at least up to 12 days. A possibility exists that a blunting of the mechanisms for induction of thirst occurs during exposure to cold. This is not a function of the fact that only cold water was available to the rats to drink since studies in which the rats were supplied with warm water while in the cold failed to affect their daily fluid intake (43). At present, it is possible only to speculate why exposure to cold, with its consequent increase in food intake and solute load, fails to induce an increased water intake. The possibility must also be considered that dehydration is a facet of the process of adaptation to cold.
Supported by contract N00014-88-J-1221 with the U.S. Navy.

REFERENCES

1. Adolph, E.F. and G.W. Molnar. Exchanges of heat and tolerance to cold in men exposed to outdoor weather. Am. J. Physiol. 146:507-537, 1946.
2. Adolph, E.F., J.P. Barker and P.A. Hoy. Multiple factors in thirst. Am. J. Physiol. 178:538-562, 1954.
3. Bader, R.A., J.W. Eliot and D.E. Bass. Hormonal and renal mechanisms of cold diuresis. J. Appl. Physiol. 4:649-658, 1952.
4. Barker, J.P., E.F. Adolph and A.D. Keller. Thirst tests in dogs and modifications of thirst with experimental lesions of the neurohypophysis. Am. J. Physiol. 171:233-238, 1953.
5. Bass, D.E. and A. Henschel. Responses of body fluid compartments to heat and cold. Physiol. Rev. 36:128-144, 1956.
6. Bass, D.E., D.C. Fainer, R.K. Blaisdell and F. Daniels, Jr. Adrenal cortical activity and hematological changes in man during cold acclimatization. Fed. Proc. 10:10, 1951.
7. Bazett, H.C. Studies on the effects of baths on man. I. Relationship between the effects produced and the temperature of the bath. Am. J. Physiol. 70:412-429, 1924.
8. Bazett, H.C., S. Thurlow, C. Crowell and W. Stewart. Studies on the effects of baths on man. II. The diuresis caused by warm baths, together with some observations on urinary tides. Am. J. Physiol. 70:430-452, 1924.
9. Bray, G.A. Rhythmic changes in renal function in the rat. Am. J. Physiol. 209:1187-1192, 1965.
10. Burton, A.C., J.C. Scott, B. McGlone and H.C. Bazett. Slow adaptations in the heat exchanges of man to changed climatic conditions. Am. J. Physiol. 129:84-101, 1940.
11. Canguilhem, B. Influence du froid sur l' limination urinaire du sodium et du potassium chez le rat. C. R. Soc. Biol. 161:2048-2054, 1967.
12. Capponi, A.M., M. Gourjon and M.B. Vallotton. Effect of beta-blocking agents and angiotensin II on isoproterenol-stimulated renin release from rat kidney slices. Circ. Res. 40:89-93, 1977.
13. Cizek, L.J. and M.R. Nocenti. Relationship between water and food ingestion in the rat. Am. J. Physiol. 208:515-520, 1965.
14. Conley, C.L. and J.L. Nickerson. Effects of temperature change on the water balance in man. Am. J. Physiol. 143:373-384, 1943.
15. Dugal, L.P., C.P. LeBlond and M. Therien. Resistance to extreme temperatures in connection with different diets. Can. J. Res. 23:244-258, 1944-1945.
16. Eliot, J.W., R.A. Bader and D.E. Bass. Blood changes associated with cold diuresis. Fed. Proc. 8:41, 1949.
17. Fregly, M.J. Effect of exposure to cold on evaporative loss from rats. Am. J. Physiol. 213:1003-1008, 1967.
18. Fregly, M.J. Water and electrolyte exchange in rats exposed to cold. Can. J. Physiol. Pharmacol. 46:873-881, 1968.
19. Fregly, M.J. Effect of a low bulk diet on water and electrolyte exchange in rats exposed to cold. Can. J. Physiol. Pharmacol. 49:959-966, 1971.
20. Fregly, M.J. Thermogenic drinking: mediation by osmoreceptor and angiotensin II pathways. Federation Proc. 41:2515-2519, 1982.
21. Fregly, M.J. Water and electrolyte exchange during exposure to cold. Pharmacol. Therap. 18:199-231, 1982.
22. Fregly, M.J., M.J. Katovich, P.E. Tyler and R. Dasler. Inhibition of

thermogenic drinking by beta-adrenergic antagonists. Aviat. Space Environ. Med. 49:861-867, 1978.
23. Fregly, M.J., L.O. Lutherer and P.E. Tyler. Variation of both ambient temperature and duration of cold exposure on water intake following removal from cold. In: International Symposium On Environmental Physiology: Bioenergetics, edited by R.E. Smith, J.P. Hannon, J.L. Shields and B.A. Horwitz. Washington, DC: FASEB, 1972, p. 96-100.
24. Fregly, M.J., L.O. Lutherer and P.E. Tyler. The effect of exposure to cold, hypoxia and both combined on water exchange in rats. Aerospace Med. 45:1223-1231, 1974.
25. Fregly, M.J., E.L. Nelson, Jr. and P.E. Tyler. Water exchange in rats exposed to cold, hypoxia and both combined. Aviat. Space Environ. Med. 47:600-607, 1976.
26. Fregly, M.J. and P.E. Tyler. Renal response of cold-exposed rats to Pitressin and dehydration. Am. J. Physiol. 222:1065-1070, 1972.
27. Fregly, M.J. and I.W. Waters. Water intake of rats immediately after exposure to a cold environment. Can. J. Physiol. Pharmacol. 44:651-662, 1966.
28. Gaunt, R., C.W. Lloyd and J.J. Chart. The adrenal-neurohypophyseal interrelationship. In: The Neurohypophysis, edited by H. Heller. London: Butterworths, 1957, p. 233-250.
29. Gibson, A.G. On the diuresis of chill. Q. J. Med. 3:52-60,1909-1910.
30. Glaser, E.M. Acclimatization to heat and cold. J. Physiol. (Lond.) 110:330-337, 1949.
31. Greenleaf, J.E. and M.J. Fregly. Dehydration-induced drinking: peripheral and central aspects. Federation Proc. 41:2507-2508, 1982.
32. Itoh, S. The release of antidiuretic hormone from the posterior body on exposure to heat. Japan. J. Physiol. 4:185-190, 1954.
33. Itoh, S., Y. Toyomasu and T. Konno. Water diuresis in cold environment. Japan. J. Physiol. 9:438-443, 1959.
34. Katovich, M.J., C.C. Barney, M.J. Fregly, P.E. Tyler and R. Dasler. Relationship between thermogenic drinking and plasma renin activity in the rat. Aviat. Space Environ. Med. 50:721-724, 1979.
35. Klein, L.A., B. Liberman, M. Laks and C.R. Kleeman. Interrelated effects of antidiuretic hormone and adrenergic drugs on water metabolism. Am. J. Physiol. 221:1657-1665, 1971.
36. Kodama, A.M. and N. Pace. Effect of environmental temperature on hamster body fat composition. J. Appl. Physiol. 19:863-867, 1964.
37. LeBlanc, J. Prefeeding of high fat diet and resistance of rats to intense cold. Can. J. Biochem. Physiol. 35:25-30, 1957.
38. Leduc, J. Catecholamine production and release in exposure and acclimatization to cold. Acta Physiol. Scand. 53 (Suppl. 183):1-101, 1961.
39. Lennquist, S. Cold-induced diuresis. Scand. J. Urol. Nephrol. 6 (Suppl. 9): 1-46, 1972.
40. Mefford, R.B., Jr., H.B. Hale and H.H. Martens. Nitrogen and electrolyte excretion of rats chronically exposed to adverse environments. Am. J. Physiol. 192:209-218, 1958.
41. Miller, M.R. and A.J. Miller. Physiological effects of brief periods of exposure to low temperatures. J. Aviat. Med. 20:179-185, 1949.
42. Munday, K.A. and G.F. Blane. Changes in electrolytes and 17-oxysteroids in the rat subjected to a cold environment. J. Endocrinol. 20:266-275, 1960.
43. Nelson, E.L., Jr., M.J. Fregly and P.E. Tyler. Effects of water temperature

on post-cold exposure drinking response of rats. Am. J. Physiol. 227:977-980, 1974.

44. Nelson, E.L., Jr., M.J. Fregly and P.E. Tyler. Factors affecting thermogenic drinking in rats. Am. J. Physiol. 228:1875-1879, 1975.

45. Oatley, K. Stimulation and theory of thirst. In: The Neuropsychology Of Thirst: New Findings And Advances In Concepts, edited by A.N. Epstein, H.R. Kissileff and E. Stellar. Wash., DC: Winston, 1973, p. 199-223.

46. Page, E. and L.M. Babineau. The effects of diet and cold on body composition and fat distribution in the white rat. Can. J. Med. Sci. 31:22-40, 1953.

47. Page, E. and L. Chernier. Effects of diet and cold environment on respiratory quotient of the white rat. Rev. Can. Biol. 12:530-541, 1953.

48. Radford, E.P., Jr. Factors modifying water metabolism in rats fed dry diets. Am. J. Physiol. 196:1098-1108, 1959.

49. Rogers, T.A., J.A. Setliff and J.C. Klopping. Energy cost, fluid and electrolyte balance in subarctic survival situations. J. Appl. Physiol. 19:1-8, 1964.

50. Segar, W.E. and W.W. Moore. The regulation of antidiuretic hormone release in man. J. Clin. Invest. 47:2143-2150, 1968.

51. Spealman, C.R., M. Newton and R.L. Post. Influence of environmental temperature and posture on volume and composition of blood. Am. J. Physiol. 150:628-639, 1947.

52. Spealman, C.R., W. Yamamoto, E.W. Bixby and M. Newton. Observations on energy metabolism and water balance of men subjected to warm and cold environments. Am. J. Physiol. 152:233-241, 1948.

53. Straw, J.A. and M.J. Fregly. Evaluation of thyroid and adrenal-pituitary function during cold stimulation. J. Appl. Physiol. 23:825-830, 1967.

54. Walsh, R.J., I. Kaldor and H. Cotter. The effect of ambient temperature on haemoglobin concentration. Aust. J. Exp. Biol. 34:59-64, 1956.

55. Weber, M.A., F.S. Stokes and J.M. Gain. Comparison of the effects on renin release of beta adrenergic antagonists with differing properties. J. Clin. Invest. 54:1413-1419, 1974.

56. Young, D.R. and S.F. Cook. Body lipids in small mammals following prolonged exposures to high and low temperatures. Am. J. Physiol. 181:72-74, 1955.

4

HORMONAL AND RENAL RESPONSES TO HYPERBARIA

Suk Ki Hong[1] and John R. Claybaugh[2]

[1]Department of Physiology
State University of New York at Buffalo
Buffalo, New York 14214

[2]Department of Clinical Investigation
Tripler Army Medical Center
TAMC, HI 96859-5000

INTRODUCTION

With the advent of a new diving technique "the saturation dive" about three decades ago, human divers are now able to engage in a multi-day dive to a considerable depth. In a dry simulation (chamber) dive carried out at Duke University in 1981, several divers exposed themselves to a depth of 686 m (nearly 70 atmospheres absolute or ATA) for 24 h and then safely returned to sea level. Apparently, human divers seem to be able to cope with such high pressures and can maintain normal activities albeit on a somewhat limited basis.

During a typical deep saturation dive the divers breathe a normoxic gas mixture which is usually composed of O_2 (0.3 - 0.5 ATA), N_2 (0.8 ATA) and He (the balance). Helium is most widely used as a diluent gas because it has a lower density and narcotic potency as compared to N_2. However, at high ambient pressure, the density of He-O_2 mixture is still much higher than that of air at 1 ATA and, therefore, the divers exposed to a high pressure environment are subject to an increased resistance to breathing. In fact, the divers exposed to 47-66 ATA He-O_2 environment (the density 8-15 fold greater than that of 1 ATA air) have complained of an extreme dyspnea during moderate exercise (42). Another major problem associated with exposure to >20 ATA He-O_2 environment is the occurrence of the so-called "high pressure nervous syndrome" (HPNS) which often develops during the compression phase and can severely limit the performance of divers. Fortunately, one can attenuate HPNS by slow compression or by using a trimix (He-N_2-O_2) (2).

A significant increase in daily urine flow (50-100% increase in two subjects) associated with some indirect evidence for mild dehydration was first observed during a short (1-2 days on the bottom) He-O_2 dry saturation dive conducted at a simulated depth of 650 ft (20.6 ATA) by Hamilton et al. (14) more than 20 years ago. Since then, a similar hyperbaric diuresis has been observed in many dives to various depths (see below). If such a diuresis is sustained during a prolonged dive, a severe dehydration could develop which will not only affect divers' performance but also endanger their safety.

In this review, attempts will be made to characterize in detail the renal, endocrine and body fluid responses to hyperbaric exposure, with a view to elucidating the mechanism underlying the hyperbaric diuresis. This topic has been reviewed, though not extensively, previously by Hong (17), Hong et al. (19), Shiraki (44) and Shiraki et al. (47).

URINARY RESPONSES TO HYPERBARIC EXPOSURE

Urine flow has been determined before, during and after hyperbaric exposure in many saturation dives. However, many early saturation dives were

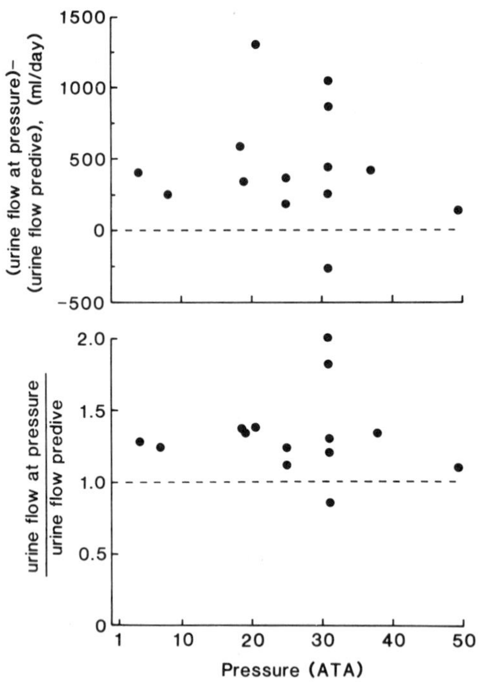

Figure 1. Daily urine flow responses to hyperbaric exposure. Both daily increments over and above the 1 ATA predive level (top panel) or relative urine flows (bottom panel) are shown as a function of the environmental pressure. All data points shown in this figure are from Table 1.

Table 1. Average daily urine flow before (pre) and during hyperbaric exposure as observed in 14 different saturation dives.

Chamber Pressure (ATA)	Bottom time (days)	No. of subjects	Urine flow (ml/day) Pre (V_c)	At pressure (V_p)	(V_p-V_c)	V_p/V_c	Reference
4*	14	6	1372	1768	396	1.29	Alexander et al. (1)
7	3	3	1079	1323	244	1.23	Matsuda et al. (29)
18.6	12	5	1864	2537	673	1.36	Hong et al. (18)
19-31	2	2	930	1260	330	1.35	Schaefer et al. (43)
20.6	2	2	1475	2775	1300	1.88	Hamilton et al. (14)
25-30	6	12	1604	1981	377	1.23	Neuman et al. (34)
25-37	5-6	4	1459	1640	181	1.12	Leach et al. (27)
31	3	3	1680	1413	-267	0.84	Buhlmann et al. (3)
31	14	4	1419	1864	445	1.31	Nakayama et al. (33)
31	3	4	1280	1540	260	1.20	Shiraki et al. (48)
31	7	4	1039	1891	852	1.82	Shiraki et al. (45)
31	7	3	1032	2100	1068	2.03	Unpublished data of Sagawa et al.
37-49.5	5-6	4	1224	1645	421	1.34	Leach et al. (27)
49.5	7	6	1540	1677	137	1.09	Raymond et al. (38)
		x	1357	1815	458	1.36	
		SE	73	115	107	0.09	

* represents the sole N_2-O_2 dive (all others are He-O_2 dives)

conducted in the presence of a significant cold stress and hence it is difficult to assess the pressure effect on urinary function. Although it was appreciated early on that the body heat loss would increase markedly in the hyperbaric helium environment, it took many years before investigators were able to determine the thermoneutral ambient temperature as a function of the environmental pressure.

Based on the level of thermoneutral temperature recommended for a given pressure, we were able to select 14 saturation dives in which the daily urine flow was determined in the absence of a significant cold stress. The results obtained from these dives are summarized in Table 1. It is evident that the daily urine flow increased during hyperbaric exposure in all dives with the sole exception of a dive reported by Buhlmann et al. (3). In the latter dive, the daily urine flow decreased by 16% during a 3-day exposure to 31 ATA. Why the subjects in this dive showed a mild antidiuresis in contrast to the diuretic response observed in all other dives is not at all clear. From what we can gather from the description of this dive, the overall experimental conditions are very similar to all other dives and hence we are unable to even speculate on the mechanism for this anomalous urine flow response. On the average, the magnitude of the increase in daily urine flow during the hyperbaric period was 458 ml, equivalent to a 36% increase as compared to the predive control period.

In order to examine the relationship between the diuretic response and the level of the environmental pressure, either the pressure-induced increase in daily flow (top panel) or the ratio of daily urine flow at high pressure to that at 1 ATA predive control period (bottom panel) is plotted as a function of the environmental pressure in Fig. 1. It is evident that there is no correlation between the degree of the hyperbaric diuresis and the pressure. However, Fig. 1 should not be interpreted to mean that the diuresis observed during a saturation dive is independent of pressure. As shown in the top of Fig. 2, the urine flow increases upon compression and this diuresis is sustained during the course of a 2 week exposure to high pressure (31 ATA in the dive shown in the figure); during the decompression period, the diuresis slowly disappears and the urine flow returns to the predive control level toward the end of decompression. In other words, the hyperbaric diuresis is clearly a pressure

Table 2. Average daily urine flow before (predive) and during early (week 1) and late (week 2) hyperbaric exposure periods in 3 long saturation dives.

Chamber Pressure (ATA)	Urine Flow (ml/day)			Reference
	Predive	At Pressure		
		week 1	week 2	
4	1372	1896	1653	Alexander et al. (1)
18.6	1864	2666	2407	Hong et al. (18)
31	1419	1848	1924	Nakayama et al. (33)

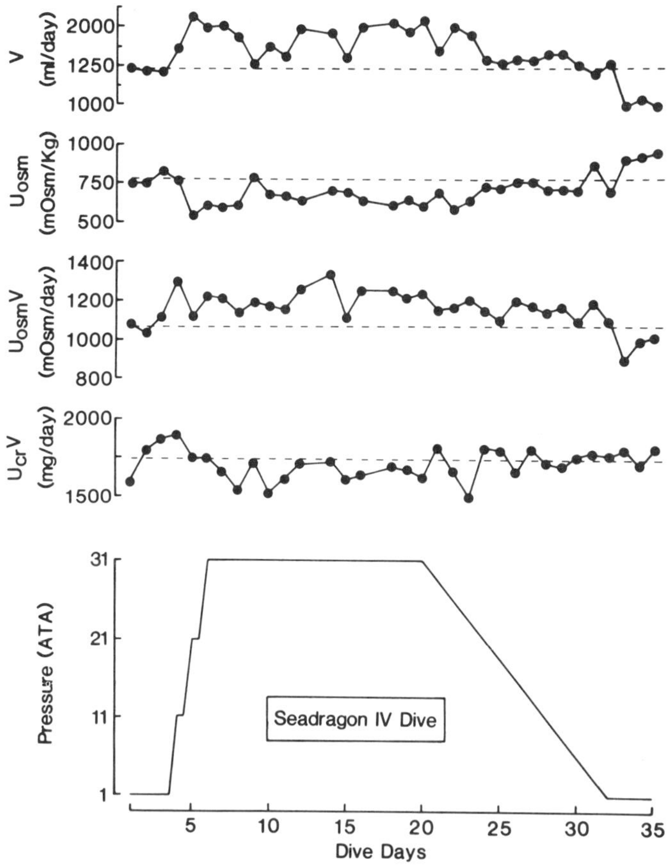

Figure 2. Daily urine flow (V), urine osmolality (U_{osm}), urinary excretion of total osmotic substances ($U_{osm}V$) and endogenous creatinine ($U_{cr}V$), and the dive profile during a 35-day, 31 ATA He-O_2 dry saturation dive (Seadragon IV). Broken lines indicate the respective predive average values.

dependent phenomenon. Apparent lack of the dependence of the degree of hyperbaric diuresis on the environmental pressure (Fig. 1) may be attributed to the subtle differences in the experimental conditions such as the history of hydration (or dehydration) of the subjects, the chamber environment (temperature and relative humidity), the degree of emotional/psychological stress, and the presence of subtle HPNS. It is possible that the combined effects of these factors may serve to counteract the effects of pressure per se, thus imposing a self-limiting step.

The hyperbaric diuresis is also time-dependent. In two out of three dives in which the duration of hyperbaric exposure (excluding the compression and decompression phases) was 12-14 days, the magnitude of hyperbaric diuresis was found to be considerably greater during the first week as compared to the second week of hyperbaric exposure (Table 2).

The hyperbaric diuresis is always accompanied by a significant reduction in urine osmolality as shown in Fig. 2 and Table 3. In 9 dives, urine osmolality decreased from the predive level of 794±61 (SE) to 633±38 mOsm/Kg H_2O during hyperbaric exposure. In no instance has urine osmolality at pressure been found to decrease to a level below the plasma osmolality. As urine flow

Table 3. Urine flow (V), urine osmolality (U_{osm}), and urinary excretion of antidiuretic hormone ($U_{ADH}V$) before (pre), during (press) and after (post) hyperbaric exposure.

Pressure (ATA)	V (ml/day)			U_{osm} (mOsm/kg)			$U_{ADH}V$ (mU/day)			Reference
	pre	press	post	pre	press	post	pre	press	post	
4	1372	1768	1118	781	742	877	39.6	28.9	21.1	Alexander et al. (1) Leach et al. (26)
7	1079	1323	980	1031	880	1000	2.4	4.3	6.2	Matsuda et al. (29)
18.6	1864	2537	2133	650	500	500	40.0	29.2	23.0	Hong et al. (18)
25-30	1604	1981	1434	693	618	666	20.7	22.4	22.1	Neuman et al. (34)
25-37	1459	1640	1279	695	605	659	55.7	40.7	32.0	Leach et al. (27)
31	1419	1864	1100	770	650	930	50.0	36.7	-	Nakayama et al. (33) Claybaugh et al. (4)
31	1039	1891	1205	954	553	917	66.3	30.3	47.0	Shiraki et al. (45) Claybaugh et al. (5)
37-49.5	1224	1645	1176	779	603	736	29.4	29.7	19.1	Leach et al. (27)
49.5	1540	1677	1900	800	550	680	8.0	10.0	5.0	Raymond et al. (38)
$\bar{x}$	1400	1814	1369	794	633	774	34.7	25.8	21.9	
SE	87	110	130	61	38	55	7.2	3.9	4.7	

slowly decreases to the predive level during decompression, urine osmolality increases to the predive level.

Despite this inverse relationship between urine flow and osmolality, the product of these two variables (i.e., the rate of the urinary excretion of total osmotic substances) increased in some dives during hyperbaric exposure, as shown in Fig. 2. According to data obtained from the literature on saturation dives conducted in the absence of cold stress, the daily excretion of total osmotic substances increased (by ~10%) in 4 dives while it remained unchanged in 6 dives (Table 4). It is also interesting to note that a greater increase in the urinary excretion of total osmotic substances is generally observed during the early phase of the hyperbaric exposure as compared to the later steady-state phase (18,33). The daily excretion of K and inorganic phosphate has been shown to increase while that of Ca tends to decrease in many dives (Table 4). On the other hand, the daily excretion of Na at pressure either increases, decreases or remains unchanged (Table 4). These changes in the excretion of osmotic solutes during hyperbaric exposure do not seem to be related to the corresponding changes in the glomerular filtration rate, as indicated by the pattern of endogenous creatinine excretion, which remains largely unchanged at pressure in the face of a constant plasma creatinine level (Table 4). Plasma concentrations of Na, K, and total osmotic substances also showed small changes during hyperbaric exposure in some dives but there is no consistent pattern (Table 4).

These findings strongly suggest that the small changes in daily excretion of osmotic substances (including Na and K) observed during hyperbaric exposure are not primarily due to the corresponding changes in the filtered load but to the effect of the hyperbaric environment on the tubular transport functions. In fact, the fractional excretion of these osmotic substances is increased in many saturation dives (Table 5), indicating that the tubular reabsorption of osmotic substances may be affected in the hyperbaric environment. This notion is clearly supported by the data shown in Fig. 2, which indicates a sustained increase in $U_{osm}V$ at 31 ATA in the face of a decreased level of creatinine excretion (indicative of decreased glomerular filtration rate). A consistent increase in the osmolal clearance (C_{osm}) is also noted in all 5 dives in which the data necessary for the calculation of C_{osm} are available (Table 5). This indicates that the hyperbaric diuresis is, at least in part, osmotic in nature. On the other hand, the negative free water clearance relative to C_{osm} ($T^c_{H_2O}/C_{osm}$) decreases consistently at pressure (Table 5), indicating that there is also a water diuresis component in the hyperbaric diuresis. In other words, the hyperbaric diuresis consists of both osmotic and water diuresis components.

BODY FLUID BALANCE DURING HYPERBARIC EXPOSURE

There is a tight coupling between the fluid intake and the urinary output of water, which is essential for body fluid balance. Therefore, it is most important to find out if the saturation divers maintain a higher fluid intake while they are confined to the hyperbaric chamber environment. The relationship between urine flow and fluid intake was investigated in 8 dives as

Table 4. Summary of changes in the hematocrit, plasma chemistry and urinary excretion of solutes observed during hyperbaric exposure.

Pressure (ATA)	Hematocrit	Plasma Conc.					Urinary Excretion						Reference
		Osm	Na	K	Creatinine	Protein	Osm.	Na	K	Ca	P	Creatinine	
4	+	+	+	+	0	+	+	+	+	+	+	+	Alexander et al. (1)
7		0	0	0	0	0	0	0	0			-	Matsuda et al. (29)
18.6	+	-	-	-	0	+	+	0	+	-	+	0	Hong et al. (18)
19-25	0		0	0				+	0	0	+		Schaefer et al. (43)
25-30		-	-			+		0	+				Neuman et al. (34)
25-37							0	-	+	-	+	0	Leach et al. (27)
31	-	0	-	-		-		-	+	-	+	0	Buhlman et al. (3)
31	+	+	0	0		+	+	+	+			-	Nakayama et al. (33) Claybaugh et al. (4)
31	0	0					0	0	-				Shiraki et al. (48)
31	+	-	-	0	0	+	0	0	+	0	+	0	Shiraki et al. (45)
31	+	0	+	0	0		+	+	+	+	+	0	Unpublished data of Sagawa et al.
37-49.5							0	0	0	0	0	0	Leach et al. (27)
46								+					Moon et al. (32)
49.5			+			+	0	-	+	-	0	0	Raymond et al. (38)
61								+					Moon et al. (32)

+ increase, - decrease, 0 no change

Table 5. Osmolal (C_{osm}) and negative free water clearances ($T^c_{H_2O}$), and fractional excretions of total osmotic substances (FE_{osm}), Na (FE_{Na}) and K (FE_K) during hyperbaric exposure.

Pressure (ATA)	C_{osm}	$T^c_{H_2O}$	$T^c_{H_2O}/C_{osm}$	FE_{osm}	FE_{Na}	FE_K	Reference
7					+	+	Matsuda et al. (29)
18.6	+			+	0	+	Hong et al. (18)
25-30	+	0	-	+	0	+	Neuman et al. (34)
31	+	-	-	+	+	+	Nakayama et al. (33) Claybaugh et al. (4)
31				0	0	0	Shiraki et al. (48)
31	+	-	-	0	0	+	Shiraki et al. (45)
31	+	0	-	+	+	+	Unpublished data of Sagawa et al.
46					+		Moon et al. (32)
61					+		Moon et al. (32)

+ increase
- decrease
0 no change

summarized in Table 6. In these dives, the daily urine flow increased by ~450 ml during the hyperbaric period as compared to the predive period. Despite this sustained diuresis, the daily fluid intake actually decreased from the predive level of 2,373 to 2,033 ml at pressure. Thus, the hyperbaric diuresis can not be accounted for by a corresponding increase in the daily fluid intake. In fact, the divers exposed to high pressure seem to subject themselves to a negative sensible fluid balance of nearly 800 ml per day. This would indicate a loss of body fluid amounting to nearly 11 liters during the 14 days of a saturation dive, which is equivalent to a body weight loss of 11 Kg (~24 lb). As shown in Tables 1 and 2, there are at least 3 dives with a duration of 2-14 days at depth (1,18,33). The magnitude of the decrease in body weight in

Table 6. Daily fluid intake and urine flow before (predive) and during hyperbaric exposure.

Pressure (ATA)	Fluid intake (ml/day)		Urine flow (ml/day)		Reference
	Predive	At Pressure	Predive	At Pressure	
7	2,495	2,000	1,079	1,323	Matsuda et al. (29)
18.6	2,770	2,625	1,864	2,537	Hong et al. (18)
19-31	1,840	1,580	930	1,260	Schaefer et al. (43)
25-37	1,887	1,730	1,604	1,981	Leach et al. (27)
31	2,673	2,400	1,419	1,864	Nakayama et al. (33)
31	2,100	1,750	1,280	1,540	Shiraki et al. (48)
31	2,893	2,802	1,039	1,891	Shiraki et al. (45)
37-49.5	2,330	1,382	1,224	1,645	Leach et al. (27)
$\bar{x}$	2,373	2,033	1,305	1,755	
SE	142	183	110	51	

these divers amounts to only 0.7 - 1.0 Kg, strongly suggesting that the body fluid balance seems to be maintained remarkably well despite the continuous diuresis with somewhat reduced fluid intake. In fact, actual measurements of the body fluid volume before, during and after a prolonged exposure to 4 ATA N_2-O_2 (22) or 18.6 ATA He-O_2 environments (18) clearly indicate that there is no net loss of the total body fluid volume during hyperbaric exposure, as shown in Fig. 3.

In one chamber dive conducted at 18.6 ATA He-O_2 environment, a careful body fluid balance study was conducted (18). In this analysis, it was assumed that the body fluid balance is maintained throughout the dive, based on the above mentioned fact that the total body water volume remained unchanged (Fig. 3) and the body weight remained virtually constant (see above). As shown

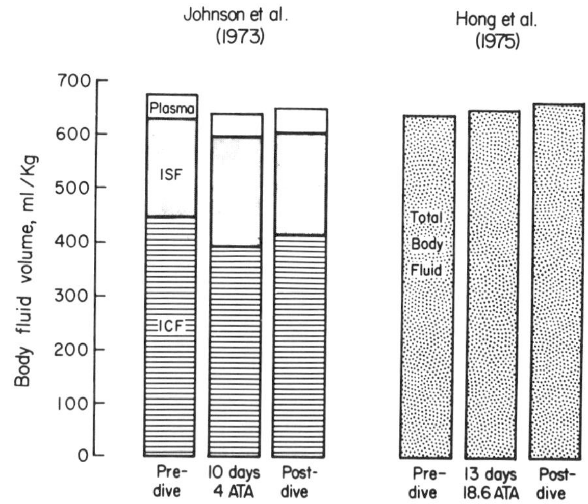

Figure 3. Body fluid volume before (predive), during and after (postdive) exposure to 4 ATA N_2-O_2 (left panel) or 18.6 ATA He-O_2 (right panel) dives. Data obtained from Johnson et al. (22) and Hong et al. (18).

in Fig. 4, the increased sensible (urinary and fecal) water loss in the face of a slightly reduced water intake at 18.6 ATA indicates a marked reduction in the sensible water balance which represents the insensible water loss. In other words, the increased urine flow observed at 18.6 ATA appears to be accompanied by a corresponding reduction in the insensible water loss, whereby an overall body water balance is maintained at high pressure. The notion that the insensible water loss indeed decreases at pressure has been verified by actual measurements in four dives. As shown in Fig. 5, the insensible water loss decreased significantly at pressure in all four dives; the magnitude of the reduction was 400-500 ml/day which is remarkably similar to the average magnitude of the increase in daily urine flow at pressure (Table 1). It is thus hypothesized that the hyperbaric diuresis is primarily due to the suppression of the insensible water loss at pressure.

There are at least two reasons for the decrease of the insensible water loss at pressure. The first factor is the high (pressure) chamber temperatures which would increase the water vapor pressure of the environment into which the water vapor would diffuse according to the water vapor pressure gradient. Since the mean skin temperature is maintained at the comparable level at all pressures, the higher thermoneutral chamber temperature at pressure (see above) would tend to decrease the skin-to-environment water vapor pressure gradient even if the relative humidity is kept at the same level at high pressure. The second factor is the reciprocal relationship between gas diffusivity and pressure given by the Chapman-Enskog equation (40). Based on this equation, Paganelli and Kurata (36) predicted the skin insensible water loss in subjects exposed to 18.6 ATA He-O_2 environment to be reduced to 1/6 of its value in air at 1 ATA. However, the data shown in Fig. 5 show a considerably smaller reduction, in

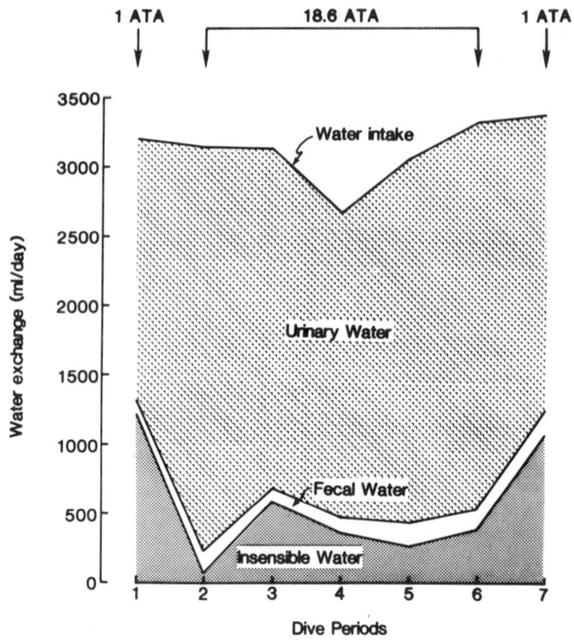

Figure 4. Pattern of daily water exchange before, during and after 17 days of exposure to the 18.6 ATA He-O_2 environment (Hana Kai II dive). Water intake and sensible water loss (urinary water loss) was attributed to the insensible water loss. Each dive period consisted of 3 days. Data obtained from Hong et al. (18).

addition to the lack of pressure dependence of insensible water loss. Reasons for the discrepancies between predicted and observed effects of high pressure on insensible water loss are not obvious and we may merely attribute them to unmeasured changes in other factors such as skin temperature, boundary layer thickness (as a result of altered convective air flow), ambient water vapor density, and the activity pattern of the subjects. In addition, systematic evaluation of skin resistance to gas diffusion under hyperbaric conditions is lacking.

Although the suppression of the insensible water loss appears to be primarily responsible for the hyperbaric diuresis observed during a prolonged, steady-state phase of exposure to high pressure, it may not account for the diuresis observed during the early phase of hyperbaric exposure. When urine was collected every other hour on the compression day to determine the time course of development of the hyperbaric diuresis in a dive to 18.6 ATA, it was found that the urine flow increased markedly 6 h after the start of compression (at about 10 ATA) (18). Thus, the diuresis seems to develop too soon to be accounted for by the suppression of the insensible water loss. Moreover, the urine flow during the first two days following compression exceeded 3,000 ml/day, after which it gradually decreased to approximately 2,500 ml/day. As

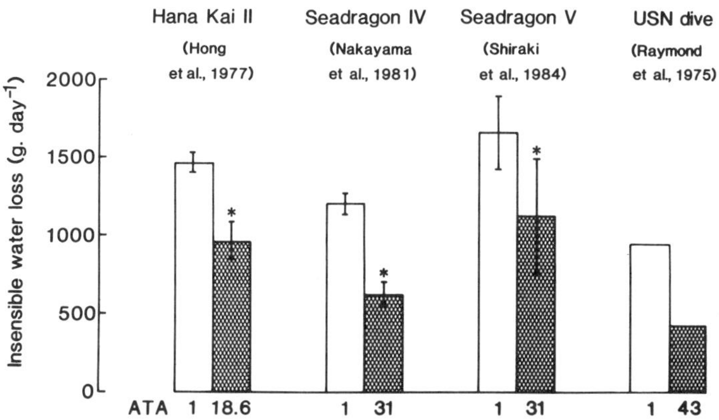

*Figure 5. Daily insensible water loss before (1 ATA) and during exposure to various environmental pressures. Vertical bars represent ±1 SE. * $P < 0.05$ as compared to the corresponding 1 ATA value. Data obtained from Hong et al. (18), Nakayama et al. (33), Shiraki et al. (48), and Raymond et al. (39).*

stated above, this early hyperbaric diuresis was accompanied by the increased excretion of osmotic substances as well as by indirect evidence of dehydration (e.g., increases in hematocrit and plasma protein concentration). In addition, the body weight also decreases during the first several days of hyperbaric exposure after which it either becomes stabilized or slowly returns to the predive level. The time course of changes in the body weight, plasma protein concentration, hematocrit and the plasma volume (calculated from changes in hematocrit values using Van Beaumont's formula (51)) is illustrated in Fig. 6. Similar results have been obtained from several other dives (18,38,48). These characteristics of the early hyperbaric diuresis are clearly different from those of the steady-state hyperbaric diuresis (see above), suggesting that another mechanism not related to the suppression of the insensible water loss may be involved in the development of the early hyperbaric diuresis.

There are two possible mechanisms, one involving fluid shifts associated with gas-induced osmosis (43) and the other involving blood redistribution associated with breathing a denser gas mixture (18), which may account for the early hyperbaric diuresis. Kylstra et al. (25) pointed out in 1968 that, when a diver is exposed to increased atmospheric pressures, the partial pressure of inert gas in his blood temporarily exceeds the partial pressure of inert gas in poorly perfused tissues. In other words, dissolved-gas concentration gradients, producing osmotic gradients, may cause water to flow from poorly perfused tissues to the vascular compartment, thus increasing the circulating plasma volume. However, later studies indicated that osmotic gradients caused by dissolved inert gas are not only very small but are also transient because of the extremely low Staverman reflection coefficient. If it is assumed that a membrane between the cardiovascular system and the other body fluids is permeable only to water, 35 ATA He would increase the blood osmolality by 13 mOsm/l (equivalent to a 4.2% increase) (13). In reality, however, the capillary

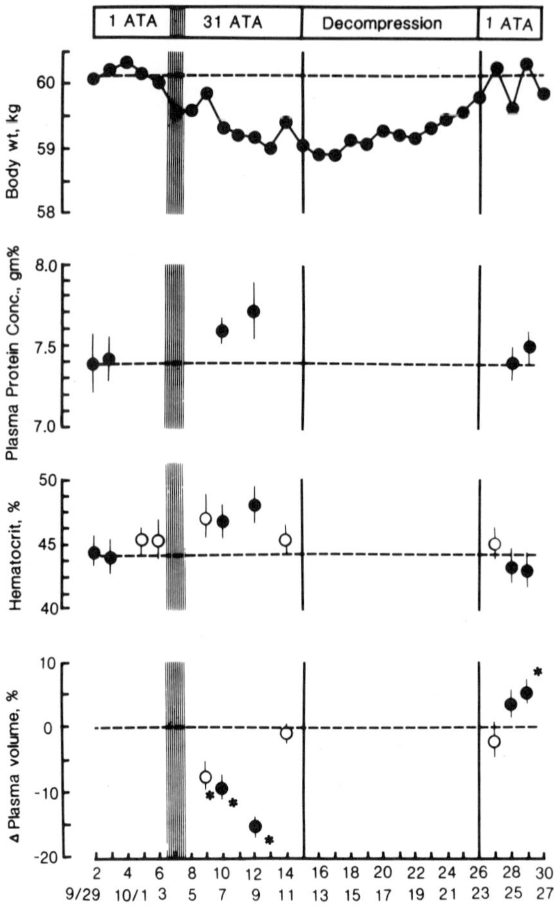

*Figure 6. Body weight, plasma protein concentration, hematocrit, and percent change in plasma volume during the course of a 30-day 31 ATA He-O_2 dry saturation dive (Seadragon VI). The "shaded area" indicates the compression phase. Vertical bars indicate ± 1 SE. * $P < 0.05$ as compared to the corresponding predive 1 ATA level. Adapted from Shiraki et al. (45) with permission.*

membrane is highly permeable to inert gases (e.g., a reflection coefficient of 0.04 for N_2O which is a much larger molecule than He), and hence the true transient fluid shift is probably at best an order of magnitude less than the calculated figure (13,16). Therefore, it is doubtful if gas-induced osmosis plays any important role during hyperbaric exposure.

During compression, the density of breathing gas increases progressively, thus altering the mechanics of respiration. One of the consequences of breathing a denser gas is an increase in the negative intrathoracic pressure as measured by the esophageal pressure (49), which would lead to increases in venous return and thoracic blood volume. In fact, Smith et al. (49) observed that thoracic impedance at a fixed lung volume decreased progressively during the course of compression to 18.6 ATA, strongly suggesting an increase in the thoracic blood volume. The calculated thoracic conductive volume tended to increase during compression to about 10.5 ATA and then fell. Interestingly, when thoracic conductive volume reached a peak (at 10.5 ATA) the urine flow began to increase (see above). In other words, an increased gas density at pressure and consequently more negative intrathoracic pressure (during inspiration) may be the cause of a redistribution of blood into the thorax. Such an increase in thoracic blood volume is known to affect cardiovascular and body fluid regulation via high and low pressure intravascular stretch receptors. Thus it is hypothesized that the increase in thoracic blood volume during compression may be the mechanism for the early hyperbaric diuresis which seems to produce a mild systemic dehydration (18).

ENDOCRINE RESPONSES

Antidiuretic Hormone (ADH)

Urinary excretion of ADH has been determined in nine saturation dives and the results are summarized in Table 3. Overall, a characteristic hyperbaric diuresis associated with decreased urine osmolality is observed in all dives during the steady state phase of the hyperbaric period. Urinary excretion of ADH showed a 30-50% decrease during hyperbaric exposure in five dives while it remained virtually unchanged at pressure in the remaining four dives. On the average, urinary excretion of ADH decreased by 25% at pressure as compared to the predive level. Plasma ADH level was determined in only one dive (5) and was also found to decrease by ~40% during exposure to 31 ATA. Taken together, these observations indicate that the ADH system is inhibited under high pressure, which would in turn induce a free water diuresis. As discussed above (also see Table 5), the negative free water clearance decreases in hyperbaria, indicating an increase in free water excretion (or a decrease in free water reabsorption). It thus appears that at least the free water component of the hyperbaric diuresis can be accounted for by hyperbaric inhibition of the ADH system.

However, a careful inspection of the time course of changes in ADH excretion during a prolonged exposure to high pressure suggests that there may be other factors modulating renal function during both the early phase and the postdive period. As shown in Fig. 7, urinary excretion of ADH increased significantly on the compression day despite the development of a marked diuresis (largely osmotic in nature) (18). Similar findings were reported by Raymond et al. (38). The data summarized in Table 3 also suggest a dissociation of the relationship between renal function and ADH during the postdive period. Both urine flow and urine osmolality returned virtually to the predive level during the postdive period while urinary excretion of ADH remained low; thus, renal function returned to normal during the postdive period even though the ADH system was still suppressed. This phenomenon suggests either that the sensitivity of the renal (collecting) tubule to ADH is

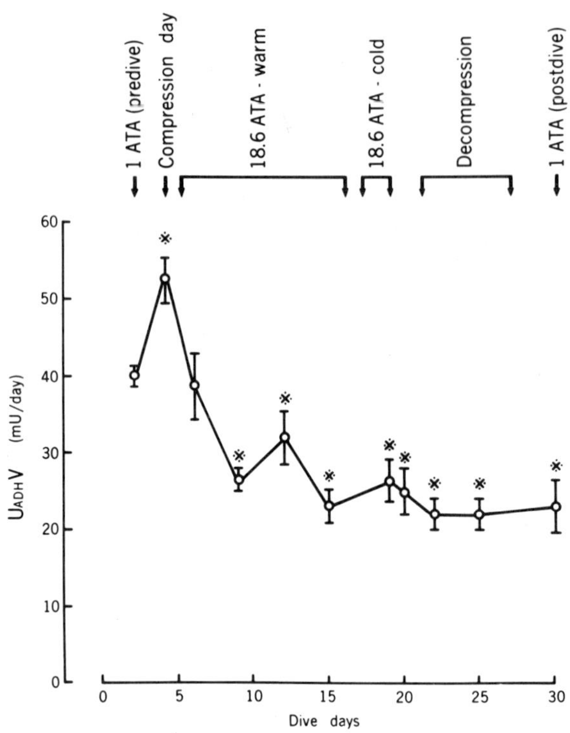

*Figure 7. Daily urinary excretion of antidiuretic hormone during various phases of a 30-day, 18.6 ATA He-O_2 dry saturation dive (Hana Kai II). Vertical bars indicate ± 1SE. * $P < 0.05$ as compared to the predive (1 ATA) value. Adapted from Hong et al. (18) with permission.*

increased after a prolonged hyperbaric exposure or that factors other than ADH control the water permeability of the renal tubule during the postdive period.

The suppression of the ADH system during the steady-state phase of hyperbaric exposure may be attributed to the suppression of insensible water loss (see above) which would tend to decrease the level of plasma osmolality. In fact, a slight decrease in plasma osmolality has been demonstrated in 3 dives (see Table 4). During the early hyperbaric exposure, the intrathoracic blood volume appears to increase (see above), which would also expect to inhibit the ADH system via the well-known Gauer-Henry reflex (7). However, contrary to this expectation, urinary excretion of ADH increased significantly during the early hyperbaric period in two dives (see above). Most likely, this early diuresis is not mediated by ADH but could be induced by other factors such as prolactin, atrial natriuretic factor or the suppression of renal sympathetic activity (see below). Although high hydrostatic pressure has been shown to inhibit the hydroosmotic action of ADH in the toad urinary bladder, the level of pressure required to counteract the ADH action is much too high (534 ATA for 80-100% inhibition of ADH effect) (6) to be considered an important factor.

Renin-Aldosterone

The renin-aldosterone data obtained from different dives are summarized in Table 7. Although the database for plasma renin activity (PRA) and aldosterone (P_{aldo}) is rather limited, the results are consistent in that these parameters increased during the hyperbaric period. Urinary excretion of aldosterone during the hyperbaric period also showed an increase in 6 dives while it remained virtually unchanged in the remaining 3 dives. Such stimulation of the renin-aldosterone system during hyperbaric exposure tends to develop during the early phase after the development of hyperbaric diuresis and is maintained (although somewhat attenuated) throughout the dive. However, unlike the behavior of the ADH system (see above), activity of the renin-aldosterone system returns to the predive level during the postdive period (Table 7). The mechanism for this stimulation of the renin-aldosterone system under high pressure is not clear. The early increase in the intrathoracic blood volume during the compression phase would tend to suppress sympathetic tone as well as renin release. However, the urinary excretion of epinephrine remained unchanged while that of norepinephrine tended to increase only slightly (~20%) during hyperbaric exposure, suggesting that the sympathetic nerve activity does not seem to decrease (3,26,27). Nor does it appear that the enhanced sympathetic nerve activity could account for the elevation of the renin-aldosterone system. On the other hand, it may be speculated that the elevated renin-aldosterone system is a response to the dehydration induced by the early hyperbaric diuresis (see above). This is consistent with the measured renin response to upright tilt during hyperbaria and, combined with the decreased ADH response to tilt, suggests that decreased ADH response to thoracic volume receptor unloading may be important in the hyperbaric diuresis (30).

Regardless of the mechanism underlying the stimulation of the renin-aldosterone system during hyperbaric exposure, it is important to recognize that such a phenomenon serves to help maintain a body fluid homeostasis by preventing excessive urinary loss of Na (and water). The tubular reabsorption of Na appears to be inhibited by high pressure, as indicated by the increased fractional excretion of Na despite the stimulation of the renin-aldosterone system in several dives (Tables 4 and 5). This may be attributed to a direct inhibitory effect of high hydrostatic pressure on the active transport of Na, as recently demonstrated in the toad skin (a functional model for the distal nephron of the mammalian kidney) by Hong et al. (20) (see below). However, it should also be noted that the increased level of plasma aldosterone during hyperbaric exposure may have an adverse effect on K homeostasis. As stated above, the urinary excretion of K is increased in the majority of dives (Tables 4 and 5), which is most likely due to the elevation of plasma aldosterone.

Prolactin

Prolactin reduces renal excretion of water, Na and K in man and may in some way be involved in electrolyte balance (21). Although prolactin secretion is known to increase in response to physical and emotional stresses, Karmali et al. (23) found a significant reduction of the plasma prolactin concentration

Table 7. Plasma renin activity (PRA), plasma aldosterone concentration (P_{aldo}) and urinary excretion of aldosterone ($U_{aldo}V$) before (pre), during (press), and after (post) hyperbaric exposure.

Pressure (ATA)	PRA (ng A-I/ml·h)			P_{aldo} (pg/ml)			$U_{aldo}V$ (ug/day)			Reference
	pre	press	post	pre	press	post	pre	press	post	
4							11.9	11.4	5.9	Leach et al. (26)
7							6.3	5.8	8.7	Matsuda et al. (29)
18.6	0.57	0.57	0.33	118	152	135	12.2	16.7	12.6	Hong et al. (18)
25-30							6.2	6.1	4.3	Neuman et al. (34)
25-37							8.3	11.6	14.0	Leach et al. (27)
31	1.41	2.83	3.89	89	112	126	2.7	4.0	-	Claybaugh et al. (4)
31	4.0	6.7	4.0	135	210	125	7.0	13.4	8.0	Claybaugh et al. (5)
37-49.5							9.0	12.3	3.4	Leach et al. (27)
49.5							7.5	12.5	10.0	Raymond et al. (38)
$\bar{x}$	2.00	3.36	2.74	114	158	128	7.9	10.4	8.3	
SE	1.03	1.79	1.20	13	28	3	1.0	1.4	1.3	

after a 2-hr simulation dive at 2 ATA air, which they attributed to the high pressure *per se*, and speculated that this completely unexpected fall in prolactin level may contribute to the hyperbaric diuresis. This view has been further supported by the observation that the plasma prolactin concentration decreased significantly from the predive level of 4.6 ng/ml to 3.0 ng/ml during the early (2nd day at 18.6 ATA) hyperbaric period when the significant osmotic diuresis was observed in the face of the increased urinary excretion of ADH (18). In fact, Hong et al. (18) postulated that this early hyperbaric diuresis may be due to the reduction of prolactin during the compression phase. However, in subsequent dives at 25-30 ATA (33) and 31 ATA (4), such reduction of the plasma prolactin concentration was not observed. Therefore, the potential role of prolactin in the development of early hyperbaric diuresis cannot be clearly defined at present. In this regard, however, it is interesting to note that the plasma prolactin concentration was found to be significantly elevated toward the end of a 12-day decompression period after a 14-day exposure to 31 ATA (4). If prolactin plays an important role in Na and K retention, an increase in the prolactin level would be appropriate after a sustained loss of both ions during the hyperbaric period.

Prostaglandin E2 (PGE_2)

The hydrosmotic action of ADH across the renal collecting tubule is known to be inhibited in the presence of PGE_1 or PGE_2 (12). In order to see if PGE_2 plays any role in the development of the hyperbaric diuresis (and natriuresis), especially during the early hyperbaric phase, the urinary excretion of PGE_2 was determined during the course of a saturation dive at 31 ATA (4). The results indicated that the rate of PGE_2 excretion varied insignificantly between 1.1~2.5 ug/day despite the presence of a typical diuresis and natriuresis during hyperbaric exposure. It is, therefore, doubtful if PGE_2 plays any role in the development of hyperbaric diuresis and natriuresis. However, additional studies are needed before a more definite conclusion can be drawn about the role of PGE_2.

Parathyroid Hormone (PTH)

As stated above, hyperbaria often increases inorganic phosphate excretion (see Table 4) and plasma Ca concentration while it decreases plasma concentrations of inorganic phosphate (4,18). These observations are consistent with increased plasma PTH concentration. In order to test the hypothesis that increased plasma PTH concentrations causes the phosphaturia, Claybaugh et al. (5) measured plasma PTH in a 31 ATA dive but failed to observe any increase in plasma PTH concentrations during hyperbaric exposure despite the significant increase in the urinary excretion of inorganic phosphate (45). Therefore, the mechanism for the hyperbaric phosphaturia is still totally unknown. On the other hand, previously reported increases in plasma Ca, accompanied by decreased plasma phosphate, could be a response to the relative inactivity caused by chamber confinement, instead of hyperbaria *per se*.

Atrial Natriuretic Factor (ANF)

Atrial stretch causes ANF to be released from the atrial tissue into the circulation (8). For instance, an increase in the intrathoracic blood volume, induced by a head-out water immersion, approximately doubles the blood concentration of ANF in man (31,37). Although ANF induces a diuresis, natriuresis and kaliuresis through direct inhibition of the appropriate tubular transport mechanisms, it is also known to exert its effects on the vascular smooth muscle and on the endocrine system (8). Since it is thought that the intrathoracic blood volume increases at least during the early (compression) phase of the hyperbaric exposure, it is reasonable to expect that there may be an increased release of ANF during the dive. If so, it could account for the early hyperbaric diuresis as well as for the hyperbaric natriuresis which persisted in several dives despite the stimulation of the renin-aldosterone level and the absence of changes in the urinary excretion of PGE_2 (see above). Moon et al. (32) determined the plasma level of ANF during the compression phase of two dives (61 and 46 ATA with $He-O_2-N_2$ mixture) and found it to increase (from predive level of 16.1 pg/ml to 26.8 pg/ml on day 6) during the 61 ATA dive but to slightly decrease (from 16.5 pg/ml predive to 11.50 pg/ml during days 5, 6, and 7) during the 46 ATA dive, despite the presence of dehydration (as indicated by increases in hematocrit and hemoglobin concentration) and hyperbaric diuresis and natriuresis in both dives. These investigators concluded that inappropriate secretion of ANF is not the only factor which mediates the diuresis (and natriuresis) seen during the compression phase of deep saturation dives. In a recent 7-day dive at 31 ATA, Sagawa et al. (unpublished data) also determined the plasma ANF concentration in three divers. Although a significant diuresis and natriuresis was again observed in all divers during exposure to 31 ATA, the plasma ANF concentration determined in early morning blood samples was maintained at around 30 pg/ml throughout the dive. These observations also strongly suggest that the hyperbaric diuresis or natriuresis is not mediated by ANF.

CHARACTERISTICS OF HYPERBARIC NOCTURIA

During the course of studying renal functions of the Japan Marine Science and Technology Center (JAMSTEC) divers during exposure to 31 ATA, Nakayama et al. (33) unexpectedly observed a marked increase in overnight urine flow, which mostly accounted for the increase in 24-hr urine flow at 31 ATA. It was later pointed out by JAMSTEC scientists that they had observed the same phenomenon in previous dives at $\geqq$ 25 ATA. This is very interesting since French scientists did not observe such nocturia in their diving experiments at 50 ATA using French divers (41). Why this hyperbaric nocturia is observed in Japanese but not in French divers is not clear. Whatever the reason for this ethnic difference, this phenomenon is highly reproducible in JAMSTEC divers and has been the focus of intensive studies by U.S. and Japanese scientists in recent years (4,5,45).

The most comprehensive studies on the hyperbaric nocturia were conducted in the Seadragon VI dive (31 ATA $He-O_2$ dive with 7 days at depth) by Shiraki et al. (45) who compared the diurnal (daytime, 0700-2200 h) and nocturnal (nighttime, 2200-0700 h) urine flow and solute excretion patterns during various phases (predive, 31 ATA and postdive) of the dive. These studies indicate that, although both diurnal and nocturnal urine flows increased significantly during exposure to 31 ATA, the relative magnitude of the increase was much greater for nocturnal (150%) than for diurnal (50%). However, the endogenous creatinine excretion remained the same throughout the dive in both periods, indicating that the glomerular filtration rate is unchanged at pressure during both day and night.

Urine osmolality decreased to a comparable level at pressure in both periods, but the amounts of total osmotic substances excreted increased significantly only during the night. Overall, the diurnal excretion of K,

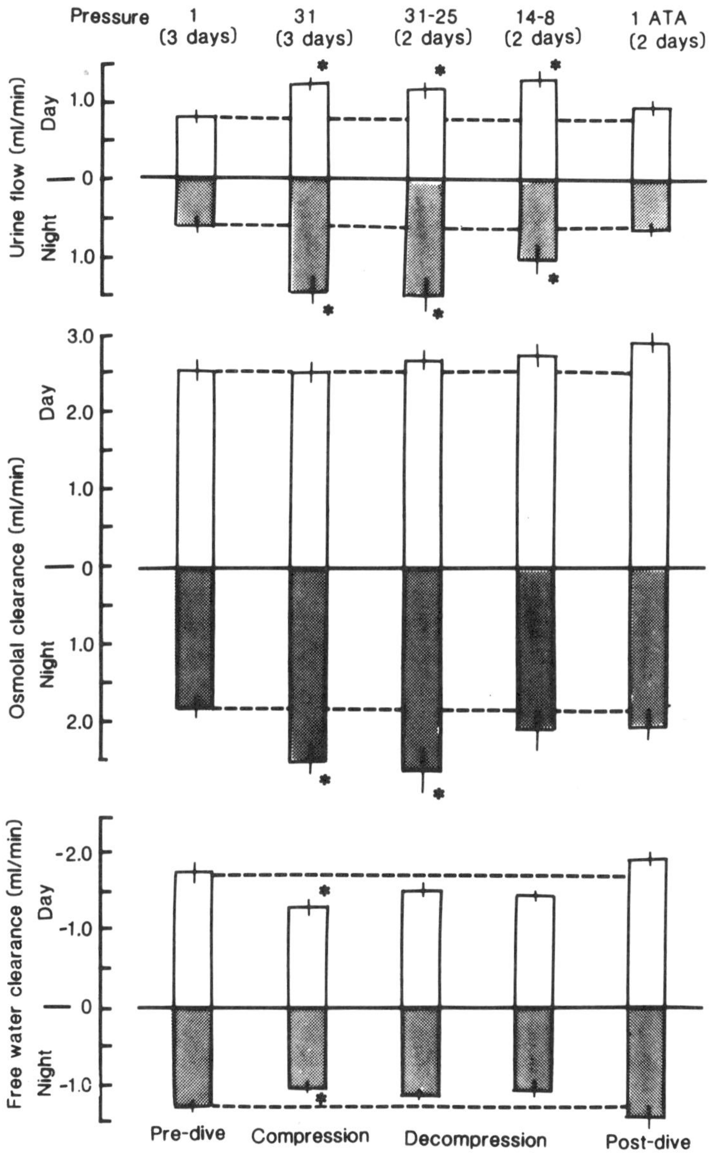

*Figure 8. Diurnal (daytime) and nocturnal (nighttime) urine flow and osmolal and free water clearances during various phases of a 31 ATA He-O_2 dry saturation dive (Seadragon VI). Vertical bars indicate ± 1 SE. * $P < 0.05$ as compared to the corresponding 1 ATA level. Adapted from Shiraki et al. (45) with permission.*

inorganic phosphate and urea increased while that of Na and Cl decreased significantly at 31 ATA, resulting in no net change in the excretion of total osmotic substances. Similarly, the nocturnal excretion of K and urea increased significantly at 31 ATA; however, in contrast to the diurnal pattern, the nocturnal excretion of both Na and Cl did not decrease but rather tended to increase while that of inorganic phosphate and Ca remained the same at pressure. Moreover, the smaller relative increase in diurnal urine flow at pressure was entirely due to the corresponding reduction in the negative free water clearance while nocturnal diuresis at pressure was accompanied by both an increase in the osmolal clearance (accounting for 80-90% of the nocturnal increase in urine flow) ánd a slight decrease in the negative free water clearance (Fig. 8). In other words, hyperbaric diuresis is basically a water diuresis during day and an osmotic diuresis at night. Increases in the excretion of Na, K, Cl and urea at night accounted for approximately 85% of the increase in the excretion of osmotic substances at 31 ATA.

Although the database is not as extensive as that in the above study conducted by Shiraki et al. (45), basically similar results on the diurnal and nocturnal excretion of water and osmotic substances during hyperbaric exposure

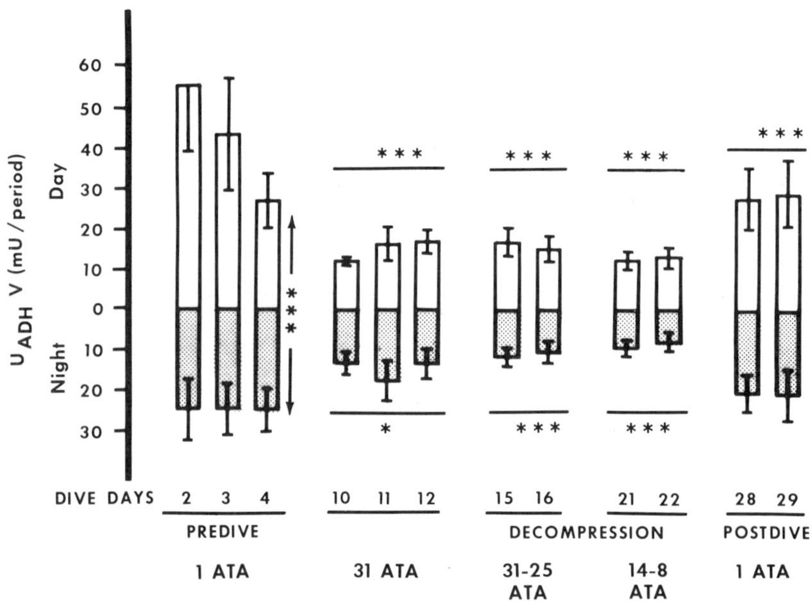

Figure 9. Diurnal (daytime) and nocturnal (nighttime) urinary excretion of antidiuretic hormone (ADH) during various phases of a 31 ATA He-O_2 dry saturation dive (Seadragon VI). Vertical bars indicate ± 1SE. Vertical arrows designate a significant ($P < 0.005$) difference between the daytime and the night time ADH excretion rates for dive Days 2, 3, and 4. Horizontal lines over the histogram bars indicate $P < 0.05$ (*), $P < 0.01$ (**) and $P < 0.005$ (***) as compared to predive Days 2 and 3. Adapted from Claybaugh et al. (5) with permission.

have been obtained from other JAMSTEC 31 ATA dives (4; unpublished data of Sagawa et al.).

In order to explore the endocrine mechanism underlying the above described hyperbaric nocturia, Claybaugh et al. (5) determined the diurnal and nocturnal excretions of ADH and aldosterone during the course of the Seadragon VI dive. As shown in Fig. 9, the urinary excretion of ADH decreased significantly at 31 ATA but, more importantly, the degree of inhibition was not different between day and night. As expected, the urinary excretion of aldosterone increased at 31 ATA but the degree of increase was again not different between day and night (Fig. 10). Therefore, neither ADH nor aldosterone seems to play any role in the development of hyperbaric nocturia. However, one can not rule out the possibility that the ADH and aldosterone receptor sensitivity may be altered at pressure (above 25 ATA) during night. Renal responses to head-out immersion are known to display a significant nocturnal attenuation, although the endocrine responses (such as ADH, renin-aldosterone and ANF) are not different between day and night (31,46). Superficially, it thus appears that the renal system is released at pressure from the state of nocturnal inhibition which exists under the normal 1 ATA condition. The rectal temperature which is kept lower while sleeping at night in the 1 ATA environment has also been shown to increase at 2-3 a.m. at 31 ATA (24). Obviously, the circadian rhythms for certain physiological functions are influenced by high pressure. Most likely, the central nervous system controls such alterations of the circadian functions.

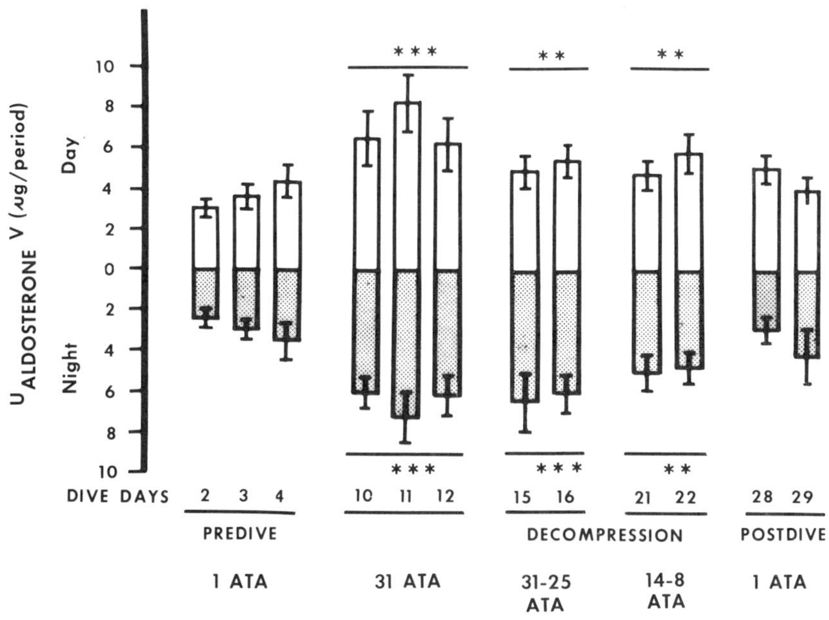

Figure 10. Urinary aldosterone excretion rate during daytime and nighttime. All symbols are as in Figure 9. Adapted from Claybaugh et al. (5) with permission.

HYDROSTATIC PRESSURE EFFECT ON ACTIVE Na TRANSPORT

As discussed above, urinary excretion of Na (or the fractional excretion of filtered Na) increased, as did the renin-aldosterone level, in many dives (see Tables 4, 5 and 7). This indicates the presence of a renin-aldosterone-independent mechanism which inhibits active tubular Na reabsorption under high pressure. Although the database is rather limited, it appears that neither PGE_2 nor ANF plays any role in modulating Na excretion during hyperbaric exposure (4, 32, 33; unpublished data of Sagawa et al.). Therefore, the possibility that a high hydrostatic pressure per se may affect active membrane transport of Na has been explored recently by several groups of investigators.

Goldinger et al. (10) showed that active Na efflux from human erythrocytes is inhibited reversibly by approximately 40% by pressure in the range of 30-150 ATA, with half-maximal inhibition found at ~20 ATA. This inhibition of active Na efflux under high pressure (up to 136 ATA) was demonstrated either in the absence of any changes in glucose utilization or in the face of increased intracellular levels of ATP and ATP/ADP; the NAD^+/NADH ratio also changed little at pressure, indicating that pressure does not seem to introduce any additional rate-limiting steps in glycolysis. These observations led Goldinger et al. (10) to conclude that high hydrostatic pressure exerts its inhibitory effect directly on the active Na transport mechanism. However, the mechanism whereby high pressure affects active Na transport across the membrane is entirely unknown. Nevertheless, these findings strongly suggest that high hydrostatic pressure may also affect the active Na transport across the renal tubular epithelium. This possibility was explored by Hong et al. (20) who studied the effect of high hydrostatic pressure (up to 300 ATA) on active Na transport across the toad skin, which is widely used as a functional model for the distal nephron of the mammalian kidney.

The net transport of Na across the isolated toad skin is known to be active and can be determined by simply measuring the short-circuit current (I_{sc}) at 1 ATA (50). Since the measurements of I_{sc} can be carried out rather easily even when the skin preparation is set up inside the hyperbaric chamber, this technique has been used in previous studies to investigate Na transport in hyperbaria. However, the equivalence of I_{sc} with the net Na flux across the epithelium under high pressure had not been validated until Goldinger et al. (9) demonstrated that I_{sc} across the toad skin can be wholly accounted for by net Na flux under pressures up to 100 ATA. Therefore, we can now interpret the I_{sc} data obtained from the toad skin exposed to high pressure in terms of the net Na flux.

During a steady-state exposure to high hydrostatic pressure, the baseline I_{sc} decreases in a pressure-dependent manner (~20% decrease at 50 ATA), leveling off at 200 ATA (20). In fact, the overall pressure-response relationship is not much different from that for active Na efflux from human erythrocytes (see above). These results strongly support the possibility that active transtubular Na reabsorption may also be subject to inhibition under high pressure, which in turn could lead to hyperbaric natriuresis. However, the cellular and/or molecular mechanism of such a pressure effect is not known.

According to the current cellular model for active Na transport across the toad skin, entry of Na into the epithelial cell across the outer (or apical) membrane is passive, while extrusion of Na from the cell across the inner (or basolateral) membrane is active and is mediated by Na-K-ATPase (28). Therefore, the inhibition of transepithelial Na transport observed under high pressure could be explained by a reduction of apical membrane Na permeability and/or an inhibition of the Na-K-exchange pump in the basolateral membrane. Wilkinson et al. (52) have indirectly determined apical membrane Na permeability at 100 ATA of hydrostatic pressure and concluded that it decreases under pressure and that the relative magnitude of the reduction is quantitatively similar to that of I_{sc}. However, their data do not provide information as to whether or not such a reduction of apical membrane permeability at pressure is due to a decrease in Na-channel conductance or in channel density.

The effect of high pressure on Na-K-ATPase is not clear cut. In agreement with the findings of earlier studies (11,15) in which pressure activation of Na-K-ATPase activity with cardiac, brain, and intestinal tissue homogenates was reported, Goldinger et al. (10) also observed a monotonic activation of Na-K-ATPase activity with human erythrocyte ghosts by pressure up to 150 ATA. As discussed above, the active Na efflux from human erythrocytes is clearly inhibited under pressure in the absence of any alteration in metabolism, indicating that the Na-K-ATPase activity must be inhibited under pressure. The reasons for this unexpected behavior of the Na-K-ATPase under pressure are not at all clear and the true effect of moderate hydrostatic pressure on the Na-K-ATPase activity is yet to be determined.

Studies on the toad skin also provided some evidence for the inhibitory effect of high hydrostatic pressure on the ADH action. In the amphibian (epithelial) preparation such as the toad skin, the I_{sc} is markedly stimulated (~100% increase in 30 min) in the presence of vasotocin (the amphibian ADH) in the medium bathing the inside (or serosal) surface. However, the magnitude of the peak response to vasotocin decreases at 200-300 ATA (20). Since vasotocin first interacts with adenylate cyclase located in the basolateral membrane to stimulate the synthesis of cAMP which serves as the intracellular mediator in increasing the apical membrane permeability (35), the direct effect of cAMP was then studied. The results indicated that the expected effect of cAMP was identical at both 1 and 300 ATA (20), suggesting that a hydrostatic pressure at 200-300 ATA might have interfered with one of the steps involved in the formation of cAMP. As discussed above, Coluccio et al. (6) showed that the hydrosmotic action of ADH in the toad urinary bladder preparation is inhibited by 107% under 544 ATA of hydrostatic pressure. Unfortunately, these investigators have not studied the dose dependence and hence we can not compare the inhibitory effect of pressure on ADH-induced water transport with that on ADH-induced Na transport. Moreover, because of the potential species difference we can not directly transfer the above information to human divers, although there is a possibility that the ADH action on tubular water and Na transport may be subject to some inhibition during hyperbaric exposure. Clearly, this possibility has to be experimentally proven inasmuch as ADH plays a central role in body fluid homeostasis.

SUMMARY

An increase in urine flow, often accompanied by increased excretion of osmotic substances such as Na, K and inorganic phosphate, is observed during a prolonged exposure of human divers to the hyperbaric environment. The magnitude of this diuresis is greater during the compression phase as compared to the subsequent steady-state hyperbaric phase. Moreover, the early diuresis is often accompanied by a greater increase in excretion of osmotic substances as well as by a transient mild dehydration. Typically, this hyperbaric diuresis develops in the absence of any increase in either glomerular filtration rate, daily fluid intake, or cold stress.

Fluid balance studies show that a significant reduction of insensible water loss in hyperbaria is most likely responsible for the hyperbaric diuresis. This view is supported by the fact that hyperbaric diuresis is accompanied by an increase in free water excretion and significant decreases in both plasma ADH level and urinary excretion of ADH.

The early hyperbaric diuresis may be triggered by the central pooling of blood, induced by breathing a denser gas which increases the intrathoracic negative pressure during inspiration; what role, if any, the gas osmosis plays in the development of early diuresis is not clear. The plasma renin activity, plasma aldosterone concentration and urinary excretion of aldosterone are all increased in hyperbaria in the face of natriuresis in many dives. Such stimulation of the renin-aldosterone system appears to be a response to the dehydration induced by the early hyperbaric diuresis.

Available information indicates that neither the urinary excretion of PGE_2 nor the plasma level of ANF show any significant changes in hyperbaria.

When environmental pressure exceeds 25 ATA, a marked nocturia (largely osmotic in nature) has been repeatedly observed in Japanese divers, which is not accompanied by any change in the pattern of urinary excretion of ADH or aldosterone.

In vitro studies indicate that active Na transport across the toad skin is indeed inhibited by high hydrostatic pressure, which may, at least in part, account for the osmotic component of the hyperbaric diuresis.

The opinions or assertions contained herein are the private views of the authors and are not to be construed as official or as reflecting the views of the Department of the Army or the Department of Defense.

REFERENCES

1. Alexander, W.C., C.S. Leach, C.L. Fischer, C.J. Lambertsen, and P.C. Johnson. Hematological, biochemical, and immunological studies during a 14-day continuous exposure to 5.2% O_2 in N_2 at pressure equivalent to 100 FSW (4 ata). Aerospace Med. 44:850-854, 1973.

2. Bennett, P.B., and M. McLeod. Comparative effect of compression rate and trimix ($He/N_2/O_2$) on performance at depth to 686m. In: Hyperbaric Medicine and Underwater Physiology, edited by K. Shiraki and S. Matuoka. Kitakyushu, Japan: Program Committee of III UOEH Symposium, 1983, p. 179- 188.
3. Buhlmann, A.A., H. Matthys, G. Overrath, P.B. Bennett, D.H. Elliott, and S.P. Gray. Saturation exposure at 31 ATA in an oxygen-helium atomosphere with excursions to 36 ATA. Aerospace Med. 41:394-402, 1970.
4. Claybaugh, J.R., S.K. Hong, N. Matsui, H. Nakayama, Y.S. Park, and M. Matsuda. Responses of salt and water regulating hormones during a saturation dive to 31 ATA (Seadragon IV). Undersea Biomed. Res. 11:65-80, 1984.
5. Claybaugh, J.R., N. Matsui, S.K. Hong, Y.S. Park, H. Nakayama, and K. Shiraki. Seadragon VI: A 7-day dry saturation dive at 31 ATA. III. Alterations in basal and circadian endocrinology. Undersea Biomed. Res. 14:401-412, 1987.
6. Coluccio, L.M., R.J. Brady, and R.H. Parsons. Pressure effects on the ADH-induced initiation of water flow in toad bladder. Am. J. Physiol. 244:F547-F553, 1983.
7. Gauer, O.H., and J.P. Henry. Neurohumoral control of plasma volume. Int. Rev. Physiol. Cardiovas. Physiol. II 9:145-190, 1976.
8. Goetz, K. Physiology and pathophysiology of atrial peptides. Am. J. Physiol. 254:E1-E15, 1988.
9. Goldinger, J.M., M.E. Duffey, R.A. Morin, and S.K. Hong. The ionic basis of short-circuit current in toad skin at high hydrostatic pressure. Undersea Biomed. Res. 13:361-367, 1986.
10. Goldinger, J.M., B.S. Kang, Y.E. Choo, C.V. Paganelli, and S.K. Hong. Effect of hydrostatic pressure on ion transport and metabolism in human erythrocytes. J. Appl. Physiol. 49:224-231, 1980.
11. Gottlieb, S.F., G.J. Koehler, and L.V.G. Rhodes. An oxygen and pressure-sensitive enzyme: Na-K adenosinetriphosphatase. In: Underwater Physiology V: Proceedings of the Fifth Symposium on Underwater Physiology, edited by C.J. Lambertsen. Baltimore, MD: Williams and Wilkins, 1976, p. 431-442.
12. Grantham, J.J., and J. Orloff. Effect of prostaglandin E_1 on the permeability response of the isolated collecting tubule to vasopressin, adenosine, 3'-5'-monophosphate and theophylline. J. Clin. Invest. 45:1154-1161, 1968.
13. Halsey, M.J., and E.I. Eger, Jr. Fluid shifts associated with gas-induced osmosis. Science 179:1139-1140, 1973.
14. Hamilton, R.W., J.B. MacInnis, A.D. Noble, and H.R. Schreiner. Saturation diving to 650 feet. Technical Memorandum B-411. Tonawanda, NY: Ocean Systems, Inc., 1966.
15. Hermick, S.K., and S.F. Gottlieb. Effect of increased pressures of oxygen, nitrogen, and helium on activity of a Na-K-Mg ATPase of beef brain. Aviat. Space Environ. Med. 48:40-43, 1977.
16. Hills, B.A. Gas-induced osmosis as a factor influencing the distribution of body fluid. Clin. Sci. 40:175-191, 1971.
17. Hong, S.K. Body fluid balance during saturation diving. In: International Symposium on Man in the Sea, edited by S.K. Hong. Bethesda, MD: Undersea Medical Society, 1975, p. 127-140.

18. Hong, S.K., J.R. Claybaugh, V. Frattali, R. Johnson, F. Kurata, M. Matsuda, A.A. McDonough, C.V. Paganelli, R.M. Smith, and P. Webb. Hana Kai II: A 17-day dry saturation dive at 18.6 ATA. III. Body fluid balance. Undersea Biomed. Res. 4:247-265, 1977.
19. Hong, S.K., J.R. Claybaugh, and K. Shiraki. Body fluid balance in the high pressure environment. In: Hyperbaric Medicine and Underwater Physiology, edited by K. Shiraki and S. Matsuoka. Kitakyushu, Japan: Program Committee of III UOEH Symposium, 1983, p. 223-234.
20. Hong, S.K., M.E. Duffey, and J.M. Goldinger. Effect of high hydrostatic pressure on sodium transport across the toad skin. Undersea Biomed. Res. 11:37-47, 1984.
21. Horrobin, D.F., P.G. Burstyn, I.J. Lloyd, N. Durkin, A. Lipton, and K.L. Muiruri. Actions of prolactin on human renal function. The Lancet, August 14, 1971, p. 352-354.
22. Johnson, P.C., T.B. Driscoll, W.C. Alexander, and C.J. Lambertsen. Body fluid volume changes during a 14-day continuous exposure to 5.2% O_2 in N_2 at pressure equivalent to 100 FSW (4 ata). Aerospace Med. 44:860-863, 1973.
23. Karmali, R.A., C.J. Weatherley, L. Parke, and D.F. Horrobin. Plasma prolactin levels during a simulated dive. Brit. Med. J. 2:237, 1976.
24. Konda, N., K. Shiraki, H. Takeuchi, H. Nakayama, and S.K. Hong. Seadragon VI: A 7-day dry saturation dive at 31 ATA. IV. Circadian analysis of body temperature and renal functions. Undersea Biomed. Res. 14:413-424, 1987.
25. Kylstra, J.A., I.S. Longmuir, and M. Grace. Dysbarism: osmosis caused by dissolved gas. Science 161:289, 1968.
26. Leach, C.S., W.C. Alexander, C.L. Fischer, C.J. Lambertsen, and P.C. Johnson. Endocrine studies during a 14-day continuous exposure to 5.2% O_2 in N_2 at pressure equivalent to 100 FSW (4 ata). Aerospace Med. 44:855-859, 1973.
27. Leach, C.S., J.R.M. Cowley, M.T. Troell, J.M. Clark, and C.J. Lambertsem. Biochemical, endocrinological and hematological studies. In: Predictive Studies IV: Work capability and physiological effects in He-O_2 excursions to pressure of 400-800-1200 and 1600 feet of seawater, edited by C.J. Lambertsen, R. Gelfand, and J.M. Clark. Institute for Environ. Med. Report 78-1: University of Pennsylvania, 1978, p. (E17) 1-59.
28. MacKnight, A.D.C., D.R. Dibona, and A. Leaf. Sodium transport across toad urinary bladder: A model "tight" epithelium. Physiol. Rev. 60:615-715, 1980.
29. Matsuda, M., H. Nakayama, F.K. Kurata, J.R. Claybaugh, and S.K. Hong. Physiology of man during a 10-day dry heliox saturation dive (Seatopia) to 7 ATA. II. Urinary water, electrolytes, ADH, and aldosterone. Undersea Biomed. Res. 2:119-131, 1975.
30. Matsui, N., Claybaugh, J.R., Tamura, Y., Seo, H., Murata, Y., Shiraki, K., Nakayama, H., Lin, Y.C., and Hong, S.K. Seadragon VI: A 7-Day Dry Saturation Dive at 31 ATA. VI. Hyperbaria enhances Renin but Eliminates ADH Responses to Head-up Tilt. Undersea Biomed Res 14:437-447, 1987.
31. Miki, K., K. Shiraki, S. Sagawa, A.J. Debold, and S.K. Hong. Atrial natriuretic factor during head-out immersion at night. Am. J. Physiol. 254:R235-R241, 1988.
32. Moon, R.E., E.M. Camporesi, T. Xuan, J. Holthaus, P.R. Mitchell, and W.D. Watkins. ANF and diuresis during compression to 450 and 600 MSW. Undersea Biomed. Res. 14(Supplement):43-44, 1987.

33. Nakayama, H., S.K. Hong, J.R. Claybaugh, N. Matsui, Y.S. Park, Y. Ohta, K. Shiraki, and M. Matsuda. Energy and body fluid balance during a 14-day dry saturation dive at 31 ATA (Seadragon IV). In: Underwater Physiology VII: Proceedings of the Seventh Symposium on Underwater Physiology, edited by A.J. Bachrach and M.M. Matzen. Bethesda, MD: Undersea Medical Society, 1981, p. 541-554.
34. Neuman, T.S., R.F. Goad, D. Hall, R.M. Smith, J.R. Claybaugh, and S.K. Hong. Urinary excretion of water and electrolytes during open-sea saturation diving to 850 fsw. Undersea Biomed. Res. 6:291-302, 1979.
35. Orloff, J., and J.S. Handler. The role of adenosine 3',5'-phosphate in the action of antidiuretic hormone. Am. J. Med. 42:757-768, 1967.
36. Paganelli, C.V., and F. Kurata. Diffusion of water vapor in binary and ternary gas mixtures at increased pressure. Respirat. Physiol. 30:15-26, 1977.
37. Pendergast, D.R., A.J. Debold, M. Pazik, and S.K. Hong. Effect of head-out immersion on plasma atrial natriuretic factor in man. Proc. Soc. Exp. Biol. Med. 184:429-435, 1987.
38. Raymond, L.W., N.S. Raymond, V.P. Frattali, J. Sode, C.S. Leach, and W.H. Spaur. Is the weight loss of hyperbaric habituation a disorder of osmoregulation? Aviat. Space Environ. Med. 51:397-401, 1980.
39. Raymond, L.W., E. Thalmann, G. Lindgren, H.C. Langworthy, W.H. Spauer, J. Croghers, W. Braithwaite, and T. Berghage. Thermal homeostasis of resting man in helium-oxygen at 1-50 ATA. Undersea Biomed. Res. 2:51-68, 1975.
40. Reid, R.C., and T.K. Sherwood. Properties of Gases and Liquids, 2nd Edition. New York: McGraw-Hill, 1966.
41. Rostain, J.C., R. Naquet, and A. Reinberg. Effects of a hyperbaric saturation (500 meter depth, heliox atmosphere) on circadian rhythms of two healthy young men. Internat. J. Chronobiol. 3:127-139, 1975.
42. Salzano, J.V., E.M. Camporesi, B.W. Stolp, and R.E. Moon. Physiological responses to exercise at 47 and 66 ATA. J. Appl. Physiol. 57:1055-1068, 1984.
43. Schaefer, K.E., C.R. Carey, and J. Dougherty, Jr. Pulmonary gas exchange and urinary electrolyte excretion during saturation-excursion diving to pressures equivalent to 800 to 1,000 feet of sea water. Aerospace Med. 41:856-864, 1970.
44. Shiraki, K. Diuresis in hyperbaria. In: Man in Stressful Environments - Diving, Hyper- and Hypobaric Physiology. Chapter 6, edited by K. Shiraki and M.K. Yousef. Springfield, Ill.: Charles Thomas, 1987, p. 93-114.
45. Shiraki, K., S.K. Hong, Y.S. Park, S. Sagawa, N. Konda, J.R. Claybaugh, H. Takeuchi, N. Matsui, and H. Nakayama. Seadragon VI: A 7-day dry saturation dive at 31 ATA. II. Characteristics of diuresis and nocturia. Undersea Biomed. Res. 14:387-400, 1987.
46. Shiraki, K., N. Konda, S. Sagawa, J.R. Claybaugh, and S.K. Hong. Cardiorenal-endocrine responses to head-out immersion at night. J. Appl. Physiol. 60:176-183, 1986.
47. Shiraki, K., S. Sagawa, N. Konda, and S.K. Hong. Hyperbaric diuresis and nocturia - a review. J. UOEH 7:61-72, 1985.
48. Shiraki, K., S. Sagawa, N. Konda, H. Nakayama, and M. Matsuda. Hyperbaric diuresis at a thermoneutral 31 ATA He-O_2 environment. Undersea Biomed. Res. 11:341-353, 1984.

49. Smith, R.M., S.K. Hong, R.H. Dressendorfer, H.J. Dwyer, E. Hayashi, and C. Yelverton. Hana Kai II: A 17-day dry saturation dive at 18.6 ATA. IV. Cardiopulmonary functions. Undersea Biomed. Res. 4:267-281, 1977.
50. Ussing, H.H., and K. Zerahn. Active transport of sodium as the source of electric current in the short-circuited isolated frog skin. Acta Physiol. Scand. 23:110-127, 1951.
51. Van Beaumont, W. Evaluation of hemoconcentration from hematocrit measurements. J. Appl. Physiol. 32:712-713, 1972.
52. Wilkinson, D.J., S.K. Hong, J.M. Goldinger, and M.E. Duffey. Hydrostatic pressure decreases apical membrane Na^+ permeability (P^a_{Na}) in K-depolarized toad skin. Fed. Proc. 46(4):1269, 1987.

5

HEAD-OUT WATER IMMERSION: A CRITICAL EVALUATION OF THE GAUER-HENRY HYPOTHESIS

J.A. Krasney[1], G. Hajduczok[2], K. Miki[3], J.R. Claybaugh[4], J.L. Sondeen[1], D.R. Pendergast[1] and S.K. Hong[1]

[1]Department of Physiology
School of Medicine and Biomedical Sciences
State University of New York at Buffalo
Buffalo, New York 14214

[2]Cardiovascular Center
University of Iowa College of Medicine
Iowa City, Iowa 52242

[3]Dept. of Applied Physiology
University of Occupational and Environmental Health
1-1 Iseigaoka, Yahatanishi-ku
807 Kitakyushu, Japan

[4]Dept. of Clinical Investigation
Tripler Army Medical Center
TAMC, Hawaii 96859-5000

INTRODUCTION

In recent years, there has been a renewed interest in the study of the physiological responses elicited during head-out water immersion (WI) in both humans and animals. This interest is based on the observation that WI leads to stereotyped cardiovascular, renal, fluid shift, and endocrine responses which develop rapidly. The homeostatic basis or rationale for this response pattern which involves the integrated responses of multiple systems is unclear at the present time. Therefore one goal of this chapter is to attempt to identify certain critical physiologic variables which may be regulated during the course of this complex response pattern which is generally elicited during the simple act of returning to the aquatic environment from whence we came. The major focus of this analysis will be on the hypothesis originally proposed by Gauer and Henry (34) concerning a physiologic link between heart and kidney and the particular role this link may play in governing the hormonal responses elicited during WI. In this regard, a number of excellent reviews representing several points of view related to this issue have been published (25,34,35,74).

Although Peters suggested in 1935 (77), based on a suggestion from Hartshorne (1847) (25), that the body possesses volume receptors which sense the "fullness of the blood stream", it was Gauer and Henry who first indicated that distention of one of the cardiac chambers could lead to a reflex diuresis. In their original experiments, using anesthetized open-chest dog preparations, they were able to demonstrate that elevating left atrial pressure resulting from mitral valvular obstruction by inflation of a balloon led to a diuresis which consisted primarily of an increase of free water clearance (34). In later experiments, they were able to show that the mitral obstruction water diuresis was associated with a depression of arginine vasopressin (AVP) secretion. This depression of AVP secretion was abolished by vagal section and thus it was demonstrated to be reflexly mediated (34). Although these receptors had been localized by Gauer and Henry to the left side of the heart, they emphasized in their hypothesis that blood volume is regulated by "intrathoracic stretch receptors" (34). The original Gauer-Henry hypothesis was therefore significant in that it identified the existence of a "heart-kidney link". Moreover, it stimulated further research in the field to the extent that, at present, the concept must be expanded to include additional receptor groups, other hormonal systems in addition to AVP, as well as neural responses. The expansion of the concept is related to later work by Gauer and Henry themselves (34), as well as to studies by other investigators. Thus, the essential point of the Gauer-Henry

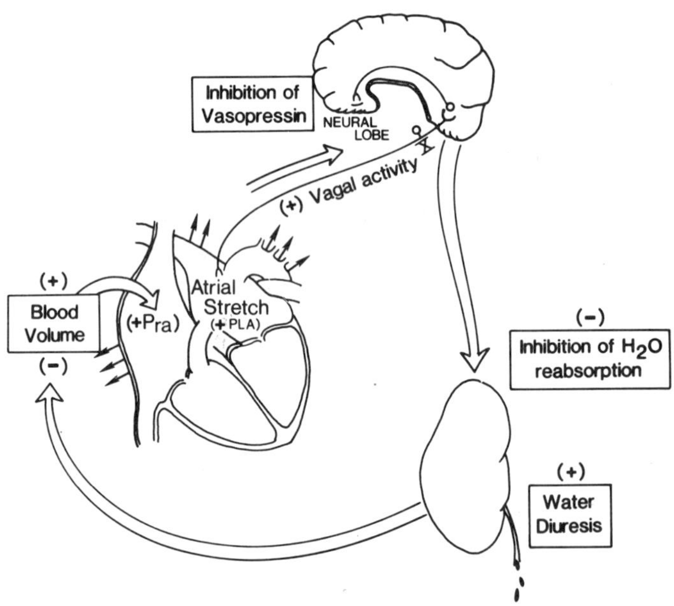

Figure 1 Early version of the Gauer-Henry hypothesis for blood volume regulation. Atrial stretch is envisaged to reduce vasopressin secretion which in turn evokes a water diuresis. (+) means increase; (-) means decrease.

hypothesis is that: an elevation of blood volume increases intrathoracic blood volume which engages cardiovascular mechanoreceptors, which in turn bring about a reflex reduction in blood volume via adjustments in secretion of volume regulatory hormones thus altering renal function and thereby lowering blood volume (Fig. 1). According to this view, then, it is blood volume which is the regulated independent variable. As will be developed, it has not always been clear that blood volume is being regulated in many studies of WI. In other words, a true correction of the plasma volume has not been demonstrated consistently.

The shift of blood into the thorax leads to an increase of the cardiac output (1,63). Since systemic O_2 consumption does not change in thermoneutral WI, the ratio of cardiac output to the systemic O_2 consumption is elevated significantly. This response represents an apparent violation of the autoregulation hypothesis where blood flow is normally considered to be regulated at a rate which is commensurate with local metabolic demands (41,55). It will be developed that the elevated cardiac output declines to pre-immersion levels after several hours in the water (15). Hence, the rationale for the systemic response may be to readjust blood flow down to a rate which is in accord with local metabolic demands. Therefore, blood volume may not be the primary regulated variable and instead the focus of the regulation may be on local O_2 delivery. It should be recognized that WI is a transient experience for terrestrial mammals. Hence, a net reduction of plasma volume would be expected to compromise function upon emersion from the water.

Water Immersion as a Model of Hypervolemia

Aside from the actual infusion of fluid into the vascular system, there are a variety of maneuvers which can be used to elicit hypervolemia in the region where the cardiovascular mechanoreceptors can be engaged, e.g. the thorax. These methods include negative pressure breathing (34) , assumption of the supine posture (34), lower body positive pressure (85), and WI. Of these methods, Gauer and Henry considered that WI under thermoneutral conditions was the "investigational tool of choice" (34) for the study of the responses to volume expansion. The reasons for this are that WI can be carried out in a non-invasive manner without modifying the composition of the plasma by the addition of exogenous fluid. In addition, it produces consistent central hypervolemia and highly predictable systemic responses when carried out under thermoneutral conditions. It should be added, however, that several investigators have demonstrated recently that another method, six or seven degree head-down tilt, may be of significant utility in eliciting central hypervolemia also (76). While central hypervolemia is a common feature of these maneuvers, it must be appreciated that each type of maneuver involves a different stimulus pattern. For example, WI is associated with a graded application of hydrostatic pressure which increases with water depth. On the other hand, application of lower body positive pressure involves a square wave increase of pressure on the lower extremities.

As may be seen in Fig. 2, thermoneutral WI of subjects in the erect posture, either standing or sitting, elicits a central translocation of blood into

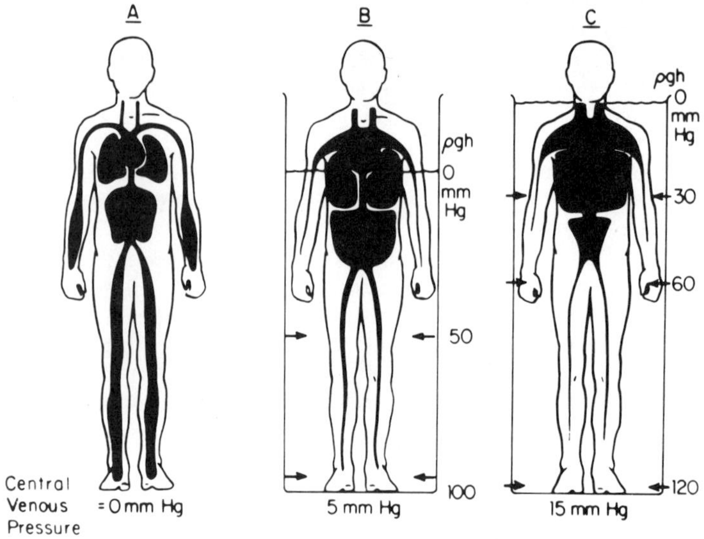

Figure 2 Head-out water immersion in humans under thermoneutral conditions offsets the relative pooling of blood in the dependent regions of the body and leads to a graded central shift of blood. Immersion to the mid-chest level causes a moderate rise of central venous pressure (B); immersion to the level of the neck (C) causes a marked elevation of central venous pressure. The hydrostatic pressure of the water column is indicated. Reproduced from Rowell, 1986, by permission of Oxford University Press (Ref 85).

the thorax which is graded, depending upon the depth of the WI, e.g. the pubic level, the level of the xiphoid, or the mid-cervical level. Thus, the systemic responses can be graded according to the level of WI. The shift of fluid into the chest is caused in large part by a differential pressure gradient on the surface of the body which leads to a decline of peripheral venous capacitance (54). In addition, WI to the mid-cervical level is associated with a negative-pressure breathing component (44).

The maintenance of thermoneutrality with no change in core temperature of the body or systemic oxygen consumption is an important experimental consideration in studies of WI. The thermoneutral temperature of man is between 34 and 35 degrees C. In early animal studies of WI using the dog, it was assumed that the thermoneutral temperature of the dog was the same as that of man (99). This has not proven to be the case as the thermoneutral temperature of the awake dog has been shown to be 37 degrees C. The awake dog will usually shiver after being in 34 degree water for about 20 minutes (55). In the other non-human species studied during WI, the monkey, the thermoneutral temperature is apparently similar to that of the human, 34-35 degrees (78,79,80), although a specific study addressing this question has not been performed in the primate model. WI at temperatures other than thermoneutral will lead to deviations from the usual stereotyped responses. For example, in cool water there may be a significant peripheral vasoconstrictor component which will alter the cardiac output as well as the renal and hormonal responses (16). This discussion will focus on the effects of thermoneutral WI partly for space considerations but also because there have been few comprehensive studies which have dealt with the renal and hormonal effects of deviating from the thermoneutral temperature in WI.

An important issue relative to making cardiovascular measurements during WI, especially measurements of hemodynamic pressures, is the location of the hydrostatic indifference point or HIP (85). Normally, in the human, the HIP is considered to be located at the mid-chest level, approximately at the level of the right atrium, and cardiovascular pressure measurements should be referred to this level. However, it is probable that the location of the HIP shifts during WI and the precise location of the HIP in WI remains to be determined. Some investigators simply assume that the HIP shifts to the surface of the water, for example, in WI to the level of the neck, cardiovascular pressures have been referenced to the water surface (51). This raises a problem when WI of lesser depths has been studied, for example to the level of the xiphoid. In the latter situation, the HIP undoubtedly shifts, but its location is unknown. Therefore, in some studies a pressure reference catheter has either been inserted into the esophagus (1) or implanted into the pleural space (55) in order to estimate the true distending or transmural pressures across the heart and great vessels in WI. The reference catheter allows for the quantitation of the effect of hydrostatic compression of the chest wall in WI. Therefore, it is important to be aware of the position of the pressure reference catheter. Although it will be shown later that central venous pressure is coupled to both tissue pressure and the water pressure, the transmural cardiac and vascular distending pressures must be known in order to define the level of stretch receptor stimulation.

Gauer and Henry originally equated the maneuver of thermoneutral WI to that of actual volume expansion (34). Indeed, Epstein has indicated that renal response to WI is the same as that produced by the infusion of 2 L of 0.9% NaCl solution (30). However, volume expansion (VE) is probably not equivalent to WI for a number of reasons. The central hypervolemia in WI is caused partly by hydrostatic compression of peripheral veins and a consequent decline of venous capacitance, whereas the central hypervolemia of VE is due to an elevation of mean circulatory filling pressure via the increased vascular volume (34). It is also commonly assumed that WI entails only a central hypervolemia without an accompanying peripheral hypervolemia while VE involves both a central and peripheral hypervolemia. This potential difference has been viewed as unimportant because what is supposed to matter is the presence of central hypervolemia. In fact, in WI there is also a peripheral hypervolemia as will be discussed below. Thus, in this respect, the two may be similar, however, in WI the vascular hypervolemia is due to an isotonic transcapillary fluid shift into the plasma compartment (66) , while in VE the plasma composition may be changed, and the transcapillary shift is likely to be in the direction of the interstitial compartment. Lastly, the buoyancy effect of WI unloads peripheral somatic postural and other receptors as well as altering the vestibulocerebellar input (23). In addition, the hydrostatic compression alters peripheral somatic inputs as well as afferent activity from the chest wall and the lung by an effect which resembles elastic respiratory loading (17). Moreover, WI causes an increase of pulmonary closing volume (81). These latter effects are not seen in VE and therefore VE should not be equated with WI.

It is also commonly assumed that WI can be equated to weightless or hypogravity states. While this is probably partly correct because of the buoyancy effect of water, there are a number of differences which may be critical. In both cases, there is a central hypervolemia, but it is caused for different reasons. In WI the peripheral tissues are compressed by a differential pressure gradient, whereas in hypogravity, venous pooling is minimal owing to the fact that dependent regions are absent. It is unclear whether there is a peripheral hypervolemia in hypogravity, in fact, the gradients for transcapillary fluid movement in this situation are uncertain. If anything, it might be predicted that fluid would tend to move out of the capillaries into the tissues in hypogravity states as tissue pressures would be reduced. In any case, the mechanoreceptor input profile from the peripheral tissues would clearly be different in the environment of space as compared to WI. That is, there would be hydrostatic compression of the legs in WI as compared to an absence of hydrostatic compression in hypogravity. Decreased peripheral tissue volume occurs in the lower limbs in both WI and hypogravity. This has been labeled the "bird legs" phenomenon in astronauts (43). Edema is common in the upper body and face during hypogravity (43).

Thus, while there are clear differences between WI, VE, and the hypogravic state, on balance, it would seem that the similarities between the three situations are significant enough to warrant continued study of the simple procedure of WI in order to obtain insights into the other two important situations. However, the differences between the three maneuvers may be critical and should be kept in mind when attempting to extrapolate from one circumstance to another (Table 1).

Species Effects on Water Immersion Responses

Extensive studies of the WI response have been carried out in the human because of the simple, non-invasive nature of the procedure. In particular, Epstein has attempted to standardize the renal and endocrine aspects of the human WI response (25). However, animal studies of WI have been carried out also because these preparations allow for invasive manipulations which have provided important insights into the mechanisms involved in WI. We have developed and standardized the conscious, trained instrumented dog model of WI (55) while Peterson and Benjamin in particular have focussed on the anesthetized, and then more recently, the conscious monkey preparation (78,79,80). Sheep, pigs, rats and rabbits have also been immersed (50, personal observations).

As was described for the thermoneutrality issue, species differences have to be kept in mind when comparing the results of various WI studies. In comparing humans versus other animals, it is important to note that the human in the upright position differs physiologically from quadruped mammals. The human has a larger vertical column of blood to be displaced centrally and,

Table 1. A comparison of water immersion (WI); volume expansion (VE); and hypogravity (HG)

	WI	VE	HG
Central hypervolemia	Yes	Yes	Yes
Peripheral hypervolemia	Yes	Yes	Unknown
Transcapillary fluid shift	Into plasma	Out of plasma	Unknown, out of plasma?
Somatic receptor input	Altered by differential pressure, tissue compression and buoyancy	Unaltered	Unloaded
Vestibulo-cerebellar input	Altered by buoyancy	Unaltered	Altered by hypogravity
Lower limb tissue volume	Decreased	Increased	Decreased, facial edema
Pulmonary input	Negative pressure breathing, elastic loading; increased pulmonary vascular volume	Increased pulmonary vascular volume	Increased pulmonary vascular volume

moreover, systemic vascular compliances differ among species (34,85). Thus, the potential for central translocation of blood, as well as the ability of the heart and great vessels to distend must be considered. In particular, potential differences between man as a biped and other species are important. Gilmore (35) has indicated that there are relative differences between the level of control of the kidney exerted via cardiac receptors and arterial baroreceptors through neural and hormonal mechanisms when species such as the dog and the primate are compared. Gilmore has argued that, in bipeds, the potency of cardiac receptors to influence the kidney has diminished and the importance of the high-pressure baroreceptors has increased owing to the assumption of the upright posture. For example, the rate of activity of atrial receptor discharge for a given level of left atrial pressure is diminished in the anesthetized monkey as compared to the anesthetized dog (98). While this assumption may be wholly or partly correct, the issue awaits further experimental clarification for several reasons: one, because some of the renal response patterns of the monkey may have been related to the use of the anesthetized, acutely operated, preparation; two, because most sub-human species comparisons have been done using the dog which shows a prominent Bainbridge cardiac accelerator response during WI, while other species, such as the pig do not (personal observation); and three, the monkey may not be as much of a biped as it as been assumed to be, and therefore its responses may not be quite as close to those of the human as is conventionally surmised. These issues will be elaborated on further in the section on specific cardiovascular reflexes which may contribute to the WI hormonal response. This presentation will attempt to utilize results from human, monkey, and canine investigations in order to arrive a synthesis of understanding about mechanisms controlling hormonal secretion during WI.

Methodological Considerations of the WI Model

The history of the use of WI as an investigational tool in both animals and man has been fraught with marked variations in experimental protocols which render interpretations from various studies difficult. Norsk and Epstein have described the air temperature, water temperature, type of water bath, and pre-hydration conditions used in their standardized human WI protocols (74). Animal studies have used varying water bath temperatures under anesthetized conditions with the animals spontaneously breathing (56); after acute closure of a thoracotomy (19) or with the chest intact (56); under artificial ventilation (73); totally immersed or with the head out of the water (73,99); in the erect position (56) or in the quadruped position (19); or conscious (55). Aside from water temperature differences, these varying experimental circumstances would be predicted to have marked influences on the results of these studies. For example, the use of positive pressure ventilation would interfere with or offset any tendencies for blood to shift centrally whether or not the head was out of the water. Also, the use of recent surgery including opening and closing the chest would be expected to markedly alter neural activity, plasma catecholamine levels, prostaglandin elaboration, and hormonal secretions (92). The use of the erect or sitting posture would elicit an important degree of venous pooling in species which are normally quadruped. If they are anesthetized, it might produce something resembling the "crucifixion response" with a profound level of venous pooling (99). On the other hand, the erect posture would allow for a greater volume of blood to be displaced centrally during WI. Since there is evidence in humans that pulmonary closing volume may increase in WI (81), some degree of arterial desaturation may occur which might engage the arterial chemoreflexes. Therefore, arterial blood gases and pH should be determined if possible. Finally, in terms of conscious animals, such as the dog, the amount and quality of training of the dogs to be immersed is very important as excitement will have a profound influence on hormonal secretory patterns (55).

In terms of the awake dog, we have found WI to be a very innocuous procedure providing enough effort is expended to ensure that the dogs are properly trained. We select dogs that are temperamentally amenable to undergo WI and then we train them to be immersed in the quadruped position to the mid-cervical level for one hour periods daily for one to two weeks prior to the study (Fig. 3). If the training is done properly, the dogs show no agitation upon entering the water. Plasma catecholamines are unchanged (41) and the investigator usually has to prevent them from going to sleep during the study. We use a sling frame assembly made from slotted angle which is lowered into

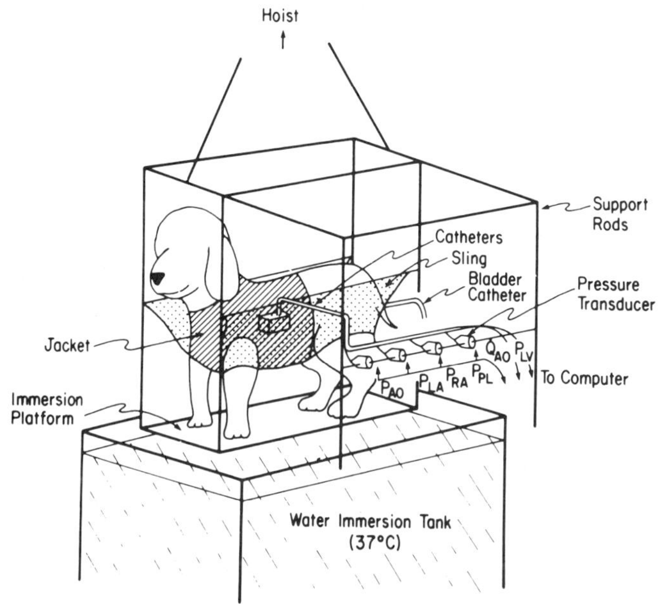

Figure 3 Experimental arrangement for study of the effects of water immersion in the awake, instrumented dog. QAO = cardiac output; PLV, PAO, PLA, PRA, PPL = left ventricular, aortic, left atrial, right atrial, pleural pressures, respectively. Reproduced by permission of the American Physiological Society (Ref 41).

the water via a boom and electric winch (Fig. 3). Monkeys can be trained to be seated in restraining chairs which are placed in a tank, which in turn can be filled (80).

CARDIOVASCULAR RECEPTORS

Cardiac Receptors

These receptors are sometimes referred to as the low-pressure receptors, or the cardiopulmonary receptors. They are generally divided into two groups; those receptor endings having myelinated afferents, and those having non-myelinated afferents. The more studied of these afferents course to the central nervous system via vagal pathways, while a group of non-myelinated afferents and myelinated afferents follows the sympathetic pathways (11).

Atrial receptors give rise to myelinated vagal afferent fibers. These receptors are believed to be located in unencapsulated nerve endings. The atrial receptors are mechanoreceptors which respond to cardiac volume changes which are transduced as stretch. It has been suggested that the actual stimulus for these receptors is atrial wall tension (11). Although receptors are distributed throughout the atria, in the dog, a group of receptors (Type B) with vagal myelinated afferents which has been studied in detail has been localized to the left atrial-pulmonary venous junctions. The receptors in this region are believed to be engaged during cardiac or left atrial stretch. In the dog, activation of these receptors is believed to elicit several effects: 1) cardiac acceleration, 2) depression of AVP secretion, 3) depression of renal sympathetic nerve activity, and 4) depression of renin, angiotensin II, and aldosterone secretion. The neural and hormonal effects in turn contribute to a diuresis and natriuresis (45,46,49,50) (Fig. 4). These effects then may lead either to a reduction of plasma volume or a return of blood volume to normal.

While the hormonal effects elicited by this reflex are generally agreed upon, the experimental conditions under which these responses have been studied have a marked influence on the quantitative nature of the renal response. As can be seen from an examination of Table 2, in anesthetized dogs, left atrial stretch generally has been shown to elicit primarily a water diuresis, whereas, in conscious, instrumented dogs, left atrial stretch generally elicits a striking natriuresis, with a minor free water excretion component. This observation supports the necessity for studying conscious preparations, if at all

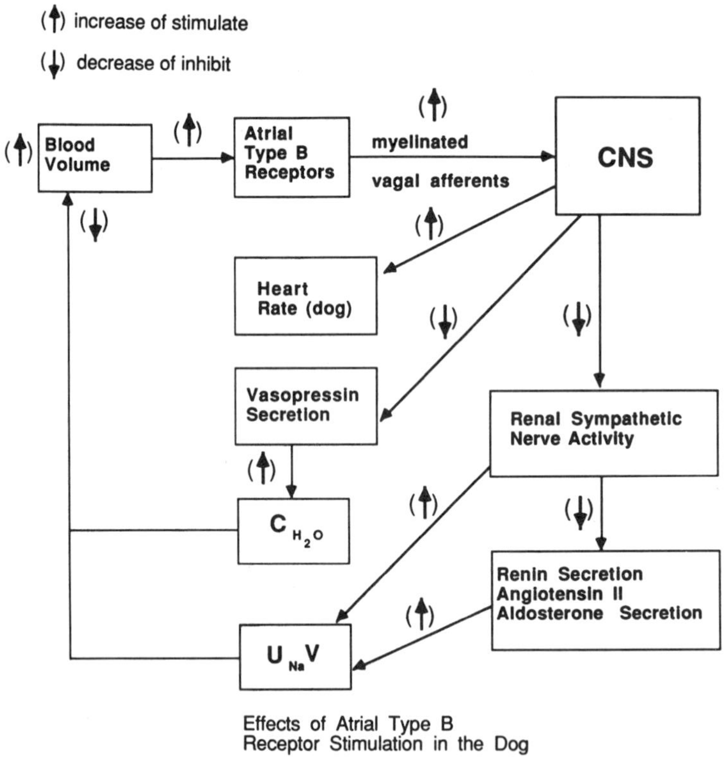

Figure 4 Expanded version of the Gauer-Henry hypothesis. Increased blood volume stretches the heart and activates type B receptors in the atria. The ensuing reflex effects return blood volume to control levels.

Table 2. Renal responses to elevation of left atrial pressure (balloon or snare)

Anesthetized dogs	Awake dogs
Ledsome, Linden, and O'Connor (61)	Lydtin and Hamilton (64)
Ledsome and Linden (60)	
Kappagoda et al. (49)	Kaczmarczyk et al. (45,46,47)
De Torrente et al. (20)	
Proznitz and Dibona (82)	Fater et al. (33)
Ledsome, Wilson, and Ngsee (62)	Goetz et al. (36)
Diuresis: +68 to 700% Mean: +258%	Diuresis: +64 TO 500% Mean: +314%
Natriuresis: 0 TO 182% Mean: +42%	Natriuresis: +217 TO 1000% Mean: +500%

possible, and implies that the vasopressin component is more prominent in anesthetized dogs, while the renal sympathetic-renin component is more important in awake dogs.

The bulk of the cardiac ventricular afferent input travels to the CNS via vagal non-myelinated C fiber afferents. The C fiber receptors can be activated by intracoronary injection of veratridine which elicits the Bezold-Jarisch or coronary chemoreflex. This reflex elicits bradycardia, hypotension, and apnea (8). Mechanical stimulation of these receptors presumably contributes to the regulation of ventricular volume. These receptors are likely engaged by cardiac distention during WI. From the standpoint of hormonal control during WI, this observation is important because, although the effects of C fiber stimulation on heart rate in the dog are opposite to those elicited by type B receptors, ventricular C fiber stimulation reflexly inhibits vasopressin secretion as well as renal sympathetic nerve activity (11,89). The latter effects could certainly contribute to the diuresis and natriuresis of WI. A recent study in the awake dog has suggested that ventricular receptors play a key role in the rise of AVP levels elicited during hypovolemic hemorrhage (96). Unfortunately, the extent to which afferent hormonal influences reflexly derived from ventricular C fiber afferents interact, or sum, with those derived from vagal myelinated afferents is unclear, particularly in conscious animals. It might be added that profound bradycardia, apnea, and hypotension are not typically observed during WI. To further complicate the issue, some evidence exists for vagal afferents which can increase, rather than inhibit, AVP secretion (72).

A portion of the ventricular afferent input travels via sympathetic myelinated and non-myelinated nerves. As these afferents are also of mechanoreceptor origin, they could conceivably be engaged during WI as well. At present, the effects of stimulation of sympathetic cardiac afferents on the control of the secretion of vasopressin and aldosterone, as well as renal sympathetic nerve activity are not entirely clear (11).

Therefore, there are powerful afferent inputs carried via four groups of afferent fibers emanating to the CNS from various parts of the heart. Clearly, activity from any or all of these groups of afferents could contribute potentially to cardiovascular, endocrine, and renal regulation during WI. The relative importance of each of these afferent groups in the WI response is uncertain. In terms of the atrial versus the ventricular input, the atria have received the major attention simply because the atria are more compliant. However, left ventricular transmural filling pressure increases in addition to atrial transmural pressures and the relative role of receptors responding to this influence in WI remains to be determined (11).

Arterial Baroreceptors

The high-pressure arterial baroreceptors, located in the carotid sinuses and aortic arch regions, aside from the well-known influence on arterial pressure by reflex modulation of cardiac function and total peripheral resistance, exert reflex control of the secretion of vasopressin and aldosterone. An increase of carotid sinus transmural pressure elicits a reflex inhibition of vasopressin secretion (86), a decline in renal sympathetic nerve activity (90), and decreases the secretion of renin and aldosterone (91). Although stimulation of aortic arch baroreceptors undoubtedly has similar influences on hormonal secretions, the relative effects of aortic arch versus carotid sinus stimulation on hormonal control remain to be determined, particularly in conscious, undisturbed animals.

The arterial baroreceptors are clearly engaged during WI. If anything, mean arterial pressure tends to increase in man and the monkey during WI (63,80) . In addition, stroke volume increases in humans which acts to raise arterial pulse pressure and this, in turn, also loads the baroreceptors (87). In the dog, as previously mentioned, WI leads to a cardiac acceleration and the rise in cardiac output is associated with the rise in heart rate as stroke volume is unchanged. Mean arterial pressure increases, but arterial pulse pressure is unchanged. In addition, total peripheral resistance is unchanged. Therefore, the rise in arterial pressure is related to the rise in cardiac output and the translocation of a volume of blood from the venous compartment into the arterial compartment (41). Thus, in the dog, there is a rapid resetting of the arterial baroreflex in WI such that the heart rate is elevated for any level of arterial pressure (97). Also, there is a decrease in the average gain or sensitivity of the baroreflex accompanied by an increase in the range over which the baroreflex controls heart rate. The reason the dog 'elects' to increase its heart rate during WI is unclear, but it may be because the canine left ventricle functions near the inflection point of the diastolic pressure-volume relation (13). In the intact dog, increases in cardiac filling pressure do not increase stroke volume because the increase in heart rate diminishes cardiac filling time (41). The potential contribution of a positive inotropic component to this response is uncertain. After cardiac denervation, however, the dog increases its cardiac output to exactly the same level during WI via an increase of stroke volume (41). The extent to which arterial baroreflex control of the circulation is modulated, or reset, during WI is important to determine, because the degree of modulation undoubtedly influences the regulation of the secretion of vasopressin, renin, and aldosterone, as will be discussed below. The monkey also shows baroreceptor resetting as arterial pressure increases, but heart rate is unchanged (80).

It is well to keep in mind that somatic and vestibular inputs are altered in WI and the potential effects of these altered inputs on hormonal control remain to be determined. At this point it is apparent that the relative importance of the different cardiac receptor inputs on hormonal regulation in WI is unclear, although the vagal inputs probably interact in some way to diminish vasopressin and aldosterone. Moreover, returning to the issue raised by Gilmore (35), the relative importance of cardiac receptors versus arterial baroreceptors in hormonal control is also unclear. As regards the biped versus quadruped question, it would seem prudent to reserve judgement on this matter since the bulk of Gilmore's argument is based on studies comparing anesthetized dogs with anesthetized monkeys. More conscious animal studies are needed to resolve this question, both in dogs and monkeys, as well as in other species which do not display a potent Bainbridge response, such as the pig. Several recent studies have indicated that the conscious monkey responds more like the conscious dog to volume expansion (93), and that vagal control of kidney function and vasopressin secretion is quite powerful in the awake monkey (93). Moreover, although type B afferent activity differs in the monkey as compared to the dog (98), little is known about species differences in the central processing of this afferent activity and how it is manifest in peripheral effector pathways.

With respect to the relative importance of cardiac receptors in the control of renal function during volume expansion, Fater et al. (33) were able to demonstrate that denervation of the heart in conscious dogs did not attenuate the diuresis and natriuresis which occurs during isooncotic volume expansion by dextran infusion. The interesting aspect of this study was that left atrial balloon inflation in intact dogs led to the expected cardiac acceleration and a natriuresis and diuresis. The responses to left atrial balloon inflation were abolished by cardiac denervation, but not the renal responses to VE. This study clearly implies that, although cardiac reflexes may contribute to the renal response to VE, these receptors are not essential to the response, and that other mechanisms, extra-cardiac in nature, may be of primary import. Whether the arterial baroreflexes are responsible for the persisting renal effects occurring during VE after cardiac denervation is not clear at present. This study also points out an important consideration which must be dealt with in attempting to derive meaningful conclusions about complex systems behavior from the results of removal of one set of inputs. In many instances, the body has been shown to have redundant mechanisms, which can be brought into play to achieve the same effect previously elicited by the ablated mechanism. Thus, removal of one mechanism may simply activate or reveal another mechanism which can take its place.

CARDIOVASCULAR EFFECTS OF WI

In humans, the immediate effect of WI to the mid-cervical level is to cause a rise in cardiac output, the magnitude of which has been shown to vary from +32% to +62% depending upon the method used to measure cardiac output or the experimental design (1,6,32,63). In the study by Farhi and Linarsson (32), the subjects were suspended in a harness during the air control period with the legs in the dependent position. Thus, their subjects may have had a greater degree of venous pooling in the dependent limbs, and thus more blood to shift centrally in WI. Mean arterial pressure may increase, but this is associated with an elevation of central transmural cardiac filling pressures of similar magnitude such that the arterial-venous pressure gradient is unchanged. Heart rate tends to slow or remain the same, therefore the cardiac stroke volume increases (32,63) along with arterial pulse pressure. Calculated total peripheral resistance decreases. The rise in cardiac output is graded according to the depth of immersion in the upright position (32). The increment in cardiothoracic blood volume is on the order of 700-800 ml with about 150 ml added to the diastolic cardiac volume (1,34,59). The increase of the cardiac output is sustained in a variable fashion if WI is carried out for several hours. The response pattern depends upon whether the subject is sedentary or has been athletically trained as a runner or a swimmer, and additionally on the hydration state of the subject and on the hydration protocol (15). In terms of the potential coupling between heart and kidney during WI, it is important to note that, in sedentary subjects, the elevated cardiac output decreases to pre-immersion levels within 2 hours, however, the diuresis and natriuresis persists for 2 to 4 hours. In trained runners and swimmers, the increase in cardiac output in WI is much greater and sustained for a longer period of time, yet the diuresis and natriuresis are markedly attenuated compared to responses of sedentary subjects (15,76). These experiments indicate that a potential exists for a dramatic dissociation to occur between the cardiac and renal responses in WI. This point of view is supported by the observation of Echt et al. (24) that the central venous pressure remains elevated for four hours of WI and the observation of Pendergast et al. (75) that plasma atriopeptin levels are also elevated for four hours of WI. The latter observations indicate that the cardiac stretch is maintained for four hours along with the renal response, yet the increased cardiac output is only maintained for two hours (76). Thus, the idea that the diuresis and natriuresis feedback to regulate cardiac filling pressure and cardiac output in WI (34) is probably incorrect. It is rather more likely that the renal response occurs to modulate vascular hypervolemia occurring as a result of a transcapillary fluid shift (see below).

As mentioned above, the dog responds to WI somewhat differently. The increase in cardiac output is about 25-30% above pre-immersion levels and this is associated with marked cardiac acceleration and a rise in ventricular inotropic state, while stroke volume is unchanged. The mean arterial pressure increases with no change of arterial pulse pressure or total peripheral resistance

(41,42). After total extrinsic denervation of the heart using the Randall method (41) with the additional modification of Fater et al. (33) to include dissection around the pulmonary veins, the rise in cardiac output during WI is identical in magnitude. However, the mechanism is entirely different in that, because heart rate does not change, stroke volume now is allowed to rise in response to cardiac stretch and activation of the Frank-Starling mechanism (41). In addition, the cardiac acceleration in response to left atrial balloon inflation is abolished. The mean arterial pressure rises in similar fashion, but in this situation, the arterial pulse pressure increases due to the increment of stroke volume. Total peripheral resistance is also unchanged during WI after cardiac denervation. Thus, while cardiac receptors are responsible for the rise in heart rate in the dog during WI, the peripheral resistance controlling limb of the baroreflex continues to be reset after cardiac denervation. Although both dog and man demonstrate elevated atrial and ventricular transmural pressures during WI, the stroke volume increases in the dog only after removal of the cardiac nerves. By comparison, then, the rise in cardiac output in normal humans is mediated via the Frank-Starling mechanism (63).

Hypervolemia in WI

The precise nature of the plasma volume response to WI apparently depends upon the experimental conditions. As indicated earlier, Gauer and Henry supported the view that central hypervolemia sets up reflex adjustments which ultimately lead to a true reduction of the plasma volume. However, the appearance of a reduction of plasma volume has not been reported consistently, which is at least partly because the hydration conditions in different experiments have varied. In addition, it takes time for a reduction in plasma volume to become manifest, if it occurs at all. Bazett reported significant reductions in plasma volume in humans based on elevations of hematocrit in dehydrated subjects (3,4). Gauer and Henry reported similar results (34). A reduction of plasma volume is less likely to be reported if the subjects are pre-hydrated before WI or not observed if the subjects are studied under volume repleted conditions (7).

Another reason for disparate observations concerning the plasma volume change in WI is that a transcapillary fluid shift occurs in WI in the direction of the plasma compartment. Von Diringshofen postulated in the late 1940's that this would occur (95) and the idea was reinforced experimentally later on by Davis and Dubois (19) in anesthetized dogs. Davis and Dubois (19) found in their acutely instrumented, splenectomized dogs that a decline of hematocrit occurred early in WI. They observed that the plasma osmolality decreased also and postulated that this was the mechanism whereby vasopressin secretion was diminished and a diuresis was brought about. Their data implied that WI caused a fluid shift out of the cells into the plasma compartment. In a later human study, Khosla and Dubois suggested that interstitial fluid pressure actually decreased during WI (51,52).

Subsequently, in our laboratory, Miki et al. were able to study conscious dogs during WI using an extracorporeal circuit to measure blood volume in a continuous fashion by means of ^{51}Cr labeled erythrocytes (66). The dogs were chronically splenectomized and studied in the non-replete state after food and water restriction overnight. They were mildly pre-hydrated to 2% of their body weight with 0.5% NaCl solution. WI led to a rapid increment of plasma volume on the order of +7% which peaked about 35 min into WI and then levelled off as the diuresis appeared about this time (Fig. 5). Following emersion, after 100 min in the water, plasma volume dropped very rapidly. This fluid shift was also reflected in the hematocrit and plasma protein responses. In contrast to the observations of Davis and Dubois (19), the plasma osmolality did not change, therefore, there was an isotonic fluid shift into the plasma. In other experiments, Miki et al. demonstrated that the plasma volume increased without an increase in thoracic duct lymph flow, further supporting the view that there is a transcapillary shift in WI (70). Measurements of tissue pressures via a wick method or a porous Guyton capsule indicated that, while calculated capillary hydrostatic pressure increases in WI, the rise in tissue pressure exceeds the rise in capillary pressure and net capillary reabsorption occurs. The decline in tissue pressure reported by Khosla and Dubois may have been related to their placing the reference pressure catheter at the water surface, whereas in our studies the pressure reference catheter was taped on the surface of the skin, overlying the capsule or the wick catheter (66). The effective pressure for transcapillary fluid movement is the absolute tissue pressure, not the transtissue pressure (wick pressure - atmospheric pressure).

During graded WI in the dog, peripheral tissue pressure in the forelimb increases as a function of the water depth, while pressure measured in the cephalic vein close to the capsule does not rise until the animal is immersed to the mid-chest level. Thus a pressure gradient between tissue and venous or end-capillary pressure is established (66). During deeper levels of WI, however, there is a linear coupling between tissue pressure, cephalic venous pressure, and central venous pressure.

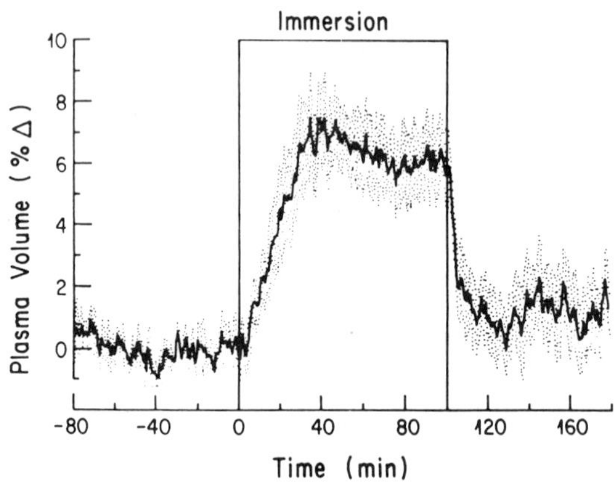

Figure 5 Water immersion leads to a rapid increase in plasma volume estimated by continuous recording of blood volume using ^{51}Cr labeled erythrocytes in the awake dog. The plasma volume peaks at about 35 min and levels off as the diuresis appears at that time. Reproduced by permission of the American Physiological Society (Ref 68).

Subsequently, in a chronic dog preparation where the kidneys were removed bilaterally, Miki et al. (68) demonstrated that the rise in plasma volume increased as high as 40% above the pre-immersion plasma volume. Since the interstitial fluid volume, which was obtained by subtracting plasma volume (^{51}Cr dilution method) from the extracellular fluid volume (^{125}I-dilution space), was not significantly changed, it was calculated that nearly 80% of the transcapillary fluid shift comes out of the cellular compartment. This view is reinforced by the fact that the fluid entering the plasma is rich in K^+. The mechanism of the fluid shift out of the cell is unclear, but it may simply involve the effects of mechanical compression of cells by the water pressure.

Therefore, early in WI, there is a major transcapillary shift of fluid into the plasma. The origin of this hypervolemia lies in the cellular compartment. The nephrectomized dog experiments indicate clearly that the kidney plays an important role in minimizing the increase in plasma volume by evoking a diuresis. Thus, in non-replete circumstances, WI may elicit a cellular dehydration and the hypervolemia is not selective, but occurs in the periphery as well as the central vascular compartment. The relative roles of the central hypervolemia and cardiac distention elicited by the central translocation of blood versus the general transcapillary fluid shift hypervolemia in contributing to the renal responses of WI are unclear. It is conceivable that the systemic hypervolemia could alter peritubular capillary dynamics and Starling forces in the kidney and thus contribute to a diuresis (66). Thus, there are three fluid shifts elicited during WI; these occur across the cell membrane, the capillary membrane, and the kidney. It is important to appreciate that this fluid shift may occur for the duration of the WI exposure with an ongoing influx of fluid into the plasma compartment.

Greenleaf (38,39,40) has confirmed that the fluid shift pattern which occurs in man follows that which occurs in the dog in both time course and magnitude as indicated by both hematocrit and plasma protein measurements, and Evans Blue dilution. Therefore, the renal response acts to minimize the hypervolemia in WI. However, the question remains as to whether plasma volume can actually be reduced below pre-immersion levels following renal elimination of the transcapillary shifted volume as a consequence of persisting central hypervolemia causing sustained cardiac distention if WI is continued. The early work of Bazett (3,4) and others (34) would suggest that this can occur over several hours, but some investigators report no change in plasma volume over several hours of non-replete WI (76). Theoretically, the degree of cardiac distention should be greater earlier in WI because of the combined effects of central translocation of blood and the volume shifted across the capillaries. Later on, as the shifted fluids are eliminated, the cardiac filling pressures should decline progressively. However, this correlation has not been observed in that central venous pressure (24) and plasma atriopeptin levels (75) remain elevated for four hours of WI, but the cardiac output declines to control levels after two hours of WI in sedentary man (76). It is more likely that, in view of the potential for a large volume of fluid to shift out of the cellular compartment during WI (68), the diuresis and natriuresis are sustained throughout WI, as long as four hours, because fluid is shifting into the plasma from the cellular compartment throughout this period. Thus, the kidney response acts to minimize elevations of plasma volume, rather than to bring about a net reduction of plasma volume. Measurements of fluid shifts and renal function during prolonged WI are required to establish the validity of this view. However, during 100 min of WI in the dog under non-replete conditions, the rise in central venous pressure is immediate. On the other hand, the plasma volume increases more slowly (Fig. 5) and the diuresis peaks about the same time as the plasma volume.

Regional Blood Flow in WI

Measurements of skeletal muscle blood flow in man by Balldin et al. using ^{133}Xe washout suggest that WI can lead to increased muscle flow after a short period in the water (2). In anesthetized, vertically immersed dogs, regional blood flows increase to skin, fat, respiratory and non-respiratory skeletal muscle, gastrointestinal tract, liver, spleen, pancreas, heart, and the kidney cortex (56). However, cerebral flow and flow to non-immersed facial muscles do not change as indicated by radiolabeled microsphere methods. By comparison, there is a time-dependent regional flow response as indicated by labeled microspheres in conscious dogs immersed in the quadruped position (42). While there are early sustained increases in skin and fat flows, as well as blood flows to heart and respiratory muscles, the cardiac output increase is directed into the gastrointestinal tract, liver, spleen, and pancreas, with no change in skeletal muscle flows (42). Renal cortical blood flow does not change. Later in WI, after 30 min, the increase in abdominal visceral flows subsides, and the increased cardiac output is redirected into skeletal muscles. There is a sustained increase in blood flow to the cerebellum. These response patterns are precisely the same after cardiac denervation,and therefore cardiac receptors do not contribute to the peripheral flow responses (42). The rise in skin and fat flows probably represents a response to superficial heating in 37 degree water, while the increases in coronary and respiratory muscle flows represent responses to increased cardiac work and respiratory loading, respectively. However, the reasons for the time - dependent redistribution of blood flow from viscera to muscle are unclear. Thus, increased flows to certain tissues can be accounted for on the basis of either thermal or metabolic requirements, but the flow responses in the abdominal viscera and skeletal muscle have an uncertain basis.

Since arterial pressure increases during WI, there is an early vasoconstriction in skeletal muscle, followed later by a vasodilation. Whatever the mechanisms for this vascular response, the early muscle vasoconstriction could drop muscle capillary hydrostatic pressure below the average estimated mean capillary pressure and thereby contribute to the fluid shift into the plasma (65). Later on, visceral vasoconstriction could have a similar effect. The time-dependent vasomotor responses could be related to temperature increases within the muscle or to relaxation of the tonus of postural muscles, actual alterations of sympathetic vascular tone, or to accumulation of products of metabolism (85). In any case, these responses may influence the primary locus of the transcapillary fluid shifts. Local blood flow responses occurring during WI periods longer than 100 min are unclear.

RENAL RESPONSES TO WI

As might be anticipated from the foregoing discussion, the nature of the renal response to WI depends upon the hydration state of the subject or animal. The typical response in a hydrated human is a diuresis, natriuresis, kaliuresis, and an increase of free water clearance (25,34). It takes 20 to 40 min for these responses to develop, and the period for which they are sustained depends upon whether volume repletion is carried out (7,25,34). In non-replete subjects, the responses begin to subside after 2 to 4 hours of WI (15). In replete subjects, the responses are well-sustained throughout WI (7). In hydrated subjects, Behn et al. (7) found that the diuresis was caused primarily by an increase of free water clearance (C_{H_2O}). By contrast, in dehydrated subjects the diuresis was caused mainly by an increase of sodium excretion ($U_{Na}V$) with minimal changes of the C_{H_2O} component.

The level of training also influences the nature of the renal response. Claybaugh et al. (15) found that the increase of urine flow rate and the natriuresis were significantly reduced in swimmers and runners during WI as compared to sedentary controls with similar hydration protocols despite greater and more sustained increases of cardiac output.

The time course and magnitude of the renal response of the conscious dog is similar to that of the human under hydrated and volume-replete conditions, with the exception that the kaliuresis tends to be less pronounced in the dog as compared to the human. In the non-volume replete state, the conscious dog shows a diuresis which has a smaller increase of C_{H_2O}. Therefore, the renal response of the awake dog is usually dominated by the natriuretic component. An exception to this generalization occurs in the awake, chronically splenectomized dog. In the experiments by Miki et al. (66) which measured blood volume continuously, the dogs were chronically splenectomized. It was surprising that, in these experiments, the dogs showed an attenuated natriuresis. In this case, the response consisted mainly of an increase of free water clearance. This peculiar observation implies that the spleen may play a permissive role in allowing the natriuresis to be expressed. The anesthetized dog also shows a large C_{H_2O} component during WI even under volume repletion, suggesting that anesthesia has an influence on the natriuretic mechanism (Table 2).

The anesthetized monkey shows responses similar to those of the awake human and dog under conditions of volume-repletion. The renal response of the monkey during WI differs markedly from the response elicited by VE. In particular, the onset of the WI diuresis and natriuresis is much faster during WI (79).

Therefore, in terms of hormonal contributions to the renal response during WI, it is well to keep in mind that the hydration and volume - replacement protocols can serve to dissociate the free water excretion component from the natriuretic component. In addition, the level and type of athletic training can modify the renal response pattern substantially (15).

In terms of the response of renal blood flow and glomerular filtration rate, most human studies suggest that both of these variables remain relatively constant during WI, or they may increase slightly (29). In anesthetized vertically immersed dogs, renal blood flow increases as measured by PAH clearance (99), and renal cortical flow increases as measured by labeled microspheres (56). By contrast, renal cortical blood flow and the distribution of renal cortical flow from inner to outer cortex does not change in the awake dog immersed in the quadruped position as measured by microspheres (42). In addition, GFR, as measured by creatinine clearance is unaltered. However, as arterial pressure rises during WI, renal blood flow must be held constant by renal vasoconstriction in the awake animal.

Hajduczok et al. (41) demonstrated that the input from cardiac nerves makes a profound contribution to the nature of the renal response to WI in the conscious, volume-repleted dog. Cardiac denervation was carried out by the one-stage intra-pericardial approach of Randall et al. (84) using an adventitial stripping procedure. Thus, the cardiac component of the Gauer - Henry hypothesis was experimentally tested for the first time. As mentioned, the intact dogs showed a diuresis which was osmotic in nature, having a primary natriuretic component. In fact, C_{H_2O} was unchanged. By comparison, the cardiac-denervated dogs had a diuresis response which was identical in time course and magnitude to that occurring in the intact dogs. However, the character of the diuresis was significantly altered in that there was now a significant increase of C_{H_2O}, and there was no significant alteration of sodium excretion or osmotic clearance (Fig. 6). Thus, the cardiac receptors clearly are responsible for the natriuretic response in the conscious dog. However, denervation of the heart acts to unmask a redundant mechanism which can eliminate the same volume of fluid by utilizing a different system. As will be discussed below, this system involves vasopressin suppression.

Since renal blood flow and GFR are usually unchanged in both humans and dogs, the natriuretic and diuretic responses to WI involve modifications of renal tubular functions. While it has been suggested that elevations of abdominal pressure could compress the kidney and elevate renal interstitial pressure and contribute to the diuresis, these effects occurred in both the intact and cardiac denervated dogs of Hajduczok et al., yet the nature of the diuresis was changed dramatically after cardiac denervation (41). Thus, the effects of kidney compression in WI are probably unimportant. Since arterial pressure is elevated in the dog in WI, this factor might have an influence on the kidney via a "pressure diuresis" mechanism (41). However, the rise in arterial pressure in the intact and cardiac-denervated dogs was identical during WI. In addition, preventing a rise in renal perfusion pressure by inflating a cuff on the suprarenal aorta does not influence the renal response to WI (personal observation). Thus, the contribution of a pressure diuresis response is doubtful. Lastly, the hypervolemia of WI accompanied by a reduction of plasma protein could alter peritubular Starling forces in the kidney and lead to a diuresis (66). However, for the reasons described above, the transcapillary fluid shift would not be expected to be altered by cardiac denervation, yet the character of the diuresis differed after denervation. Therefore, an alteration of peritubular Starling forces is clearly not a major factor in the renal response to WI.

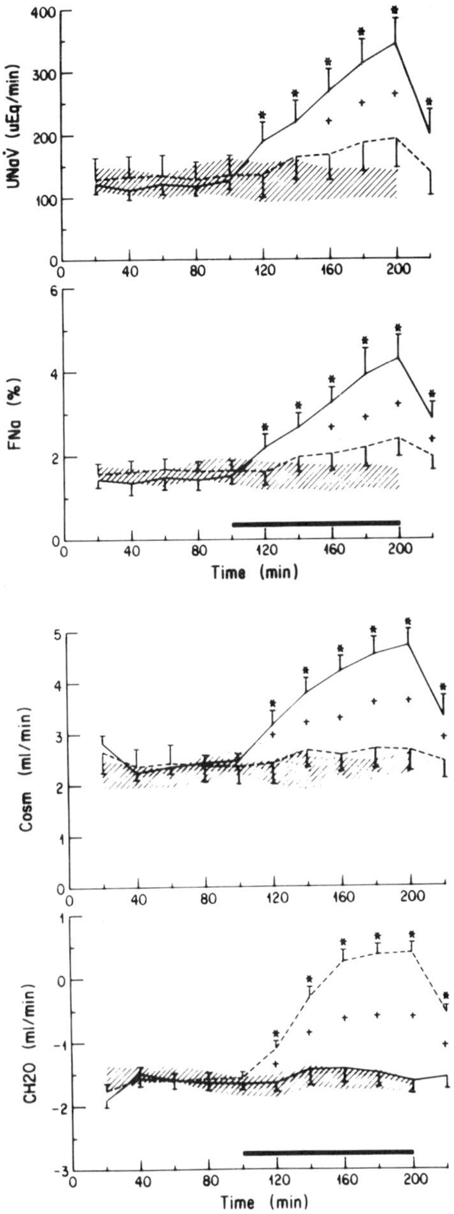

Figure 6 (upper panel) Effects of water immersion in the awake dog on sodium excretion ($U_{Na}V$) and fractional excretion of sodium (FNA). Immersion is at the horizontal black bar. Solid lines-intact dogs; dashed lines-cardiac denervated dogs; hatched line-timed control. Asterisks = significantly different from pre-immersion value; + = significantly different from corresponding immersion value. (Lower panel) Effects of water immersion on osmolar clearance (C_{osm}) and free water clearance (C_{H_2O}) in the awake dog. Symbols as in upper panel. Reproduced by permission from the American Physiological Society (Ref 41).

HORMONAL RESPONSES TO WI

Vasopressin

The major mechanisms for control of vasopressin (AVP) secretion during WI include increased vagal myelinated and non-myelinated afferent fiber activity resulting from activation of cardiac mechanoreceptors. In addition, elevations of mean arterial pressure and/or arterial pulse pressure may load the sino-aortic baroreceptors and reflexly inhibit AVP secretion (86,87). Osmotic stimuli could conceivably contribute to AVP regulation during WI, but, as described above, plasma osmolality is generally constant in WI as the fluid shifting into the plasma is isotonic. Therefore, the major input for control of AVP secretion in WI resides in the cardiovascular mechanoreceptors.

In humans, a recent review by Norsk and Epstein (74) indicates that a reduction of plasma AVP levels is generally responsible for the increase in free water clearance during WI, when it occurs in hydrated subjects. The problem in interpreting these studies is that AVP levels are quite low in hydrated subjects to begin with, and small reductions of circulating AVP are difficult to detect. Moreover, it is difficult to be certain whether small reductions of plasma AVP in humans are of physiological significance in contributing to the increase of C_{H_2O}. The paradox then is that generally AVP is modestly or not suppressed at all in WI in hydrated subjects where one is more likely to observe a water diuresis (74,57).

In dehydrated subjects, plasma AVP levels are quite high and they clearly decrease during WI. However, this decrease of AVP apparently has no effect on C_{H_2O}, as urine remains in the hypertonic range (74) and, moreover, it has no effect on the natriuresis.

Thus, a clear correlation between plasma AVP reductions and the appearance of an increase of C_{H_2O} in WI is not readily apparent. The primary evidence whereby the increase of C_{H_2O} in man is attributed to a decline in AVP secretion is based upon experiments where AVP was administered prior to WI and this maneuver was found to abolish the increase of C_{H_2O} (26). However, it must be emphasized that, while there is not a good correlation of C_{H_2O} with plasma AVP levels, other factors, such as prostaglandins and atriopeptin, could interact with AVP at the level of the kidney to influence C_{H_2O} in WI and these factors are discussed below. In addition, Bie et al. (9) have shown that the hydroosmotic response of the kidney is exquisitely sensitive to very small changes in plasma AVP levels.

In terms of cardiovascular mechanoreceptor influences upon AVP release in man, it has been found that plasma AVP does not always decrease when central venous pressure increases. On the other hand, a better correlation is usually observed between mean arterial and/or pulse pressure increases and plasma AVP decreases (74).

The monkey has been shown to demonstrate a consistent decrease of plasma AVP levels during both VE (79) and WI (80).

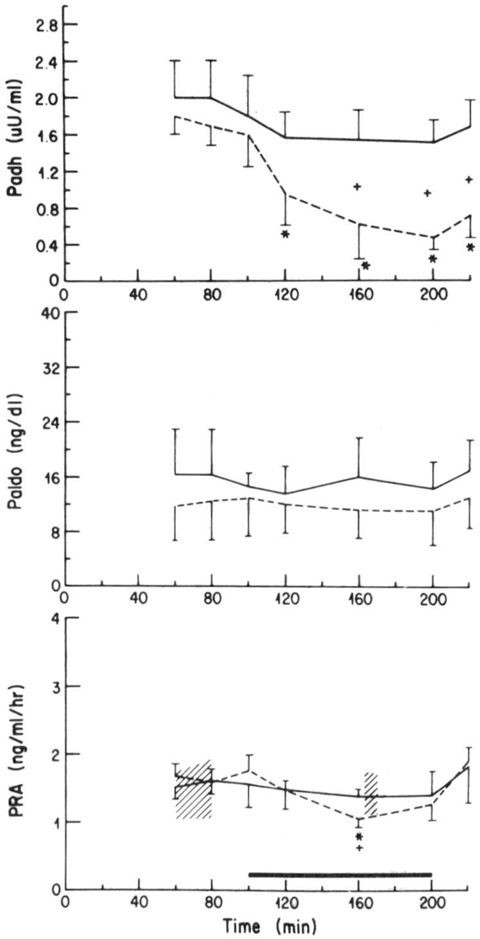

Figure 7 Effects of head-out water immersion in the awake dog on plasma vasopressin (P_{adh}), plasma aldosterone (P_{aldo}), and plasma renin activity in intact dogs (solid lines) and cardiac denervated dogs (dashed lines). Symbols as in Fig. 6. Reproduced by permission from the American Physiological Society (Ref 41).

As previously discussed, stretch of the left atrium in the anesthetized dog clearly elicits a vagally-mediated depression of AVP secretion and a rise in C_{H_2O} (60,61,62). In view of this observation, it was somewhat surprising that, in conscious dogs, where left atrial pressure increases markedly during WI, plasma AVP levels did not change significantly in the volume-replete state (41). Moreover, there was no change of C_{H_2O} (Fig. 6 and 7). By contrast, cardiac-denervated dogs show a significant depression of plasma AVP levels in parallel with a pronounced water diuresis (Fig. 6 and 7). Therefore, in the awake dog, a good correlation between plasma AVP and C_{H_2O} during WI is only apparent following elimination of the input from cardiac mechanoreceptors.

This implies that there is some sort of interaction occurring between cardiac mechanoreceptors and other systems to control AVP during WI. One interpretation is that cardiac receptors could be acting to keep AVP levels elevated in WI because in their absence, AVP decreases. This explanation does not seem plausible in view of the evidence from the wealth of literature which indicates that cardiac receptors act to depress AVP secretion. However, some evidence exists also which suggests that cardiac receptors may increase plasma AVP levels under certain conditions (72). A second possibility is that there is an interaction between cardiac and arterial mechanoreceptors in WI which interferes with the reduction of AVP secretion being manifest. In other words, cardiac receptors could inhibit an arterial baroreflex mediated reduction of AVP secretion. Another possibility is that a resetting of the arterial baroreflex control of AVP occurs during WI in the intact dog as is the case with baroreflex control of heart rate (97). Lastly, since heart rate increases in the intact dog, arterial pulse pressure does not change, even though mean arterial pressure increases. However, after cardiac denervation, the arterial pulse pressure increases as stroke volume increases along with the mean arterial pressure. Thus, the loading pattern on the baroreceptors is different in the denervated dogs, and this effect could clearly account for the fall in AVP levels. Whether this is a reflex effect (87) or a mechanical effect conveyed to the sella turcica from the rise in pulse pressure remains uncertain (83).

Additional studies have revealed that the blood flow to the neurohypophysis, as measured by radiolabeled microspheres, does not change during WI in the intact, conscious dog. However, by contrast, there is a significant reduction of neurohypophyseal blood flow in parallel with the reduction of plasma AVP levels during WI in cardiac-denervated dogs (42). Thus, a coupling between neurohypophyseal blood flow and secretion may occur during WI.

These experiments indicate that a complex interplay exists between the two major groups of cardiovascular mechanoreceptors for the control of AVP secretion in the conscious dog. The concept that emerges from these experiments is that the input from the arterial baroreceptors may be the primary determinant of the AVP response to WI in both humans and conscious dogs.

Lastly, in humans, the type and degree of athletic training has an influence on the urinary AVP response. Claybaugh et al. (15) demonstrated that WI resulted in significant decreases of urinary AVP excretion in mildly hydrated untrained subjects, but no changes were noted in swimmers and decreases were only noted during the second hour of WI in runners. It was concluded that trained men have a diminished sensitivity of the volume or mechanoreceptor control mechanisms for AVP control. Whether or not this is specifically related to altered arterial baroreflex function in trained individuals remains to be determined (5). In any case, these experiments emphasize the dissociation between the cardiac response and the endocrine response, because the elevation of cardiac output is greater and more sustained in the trained subjects (76).

Renin and Aldosterone Secretion

In general, renin and aldosterone secretion decline during WI in humans (28,31). These responses appear to be more consistently present than the AVP suppression, and less dependent upon the degree of hydration. However, the WI natriuresis usually is apparent within 40 min following immersion and this response is too fast to be mediated by a reduction of aldosterone secretion (25,74). Moreover, the diuresis of WI is not influenced by pre-treatment of subjects with the mineralocorticoid, desoxycorticosterone acetate (DOCA) (31). However, the natriuresis of WI is attenuated but not suppressed by DOCA in man (35). Therefore, it is probable that the natriuresis in man may be partly related to a suppression of renin and aldosterone secretion. Humans also show a consistent kaliuresis during WI and this may be related in large part to the natriuresis bringing about increased distal tubular flow and washout of K^+. Another possibility is that a increase in the filtered load of K^+ might occur as a consequence of a shift of K^+ out of the cellular compartment (6). The kaliuresis is in the opposite direction of what would be expected from aldosterone suppression.

The monkey also exhibits a suppression of plasma renin activity and plasma aldosterone during WI (68).

As indicated previously, the awake dog shows a diuresis which is largely osmotic and almost entirely related to a pronounced natriuresis (41). The presence of a kaliuresis is difficult to detect. Therefore, it is of interest that neither plasma renin activity nor plasma aldosterone activity are significantly altered during volume-replete WI (41). The lack of renin suppression is surprising in view of the elevation in arterial pressure which occurs (91). In addition, neither renin nor aldosterone are altered during WI following denervation of the heart (41). Thus, in the awake dog, the natriuresis is probably largely unrelated to alterations in renin or aldosterone secretion and other factors must be responsible for the striking natriuresis. While baroreceptor resetting may contribute to these apparent differences, more recent carefully controlled studies in our laboratory suggest that renin may decrease in the awake dog during WI under certain conditions (personal observations).

As is the case with AVP regulation, the degree of athletic training in humans influences the relation of the renal responses to the renin and aldosterone responses during WI (15). While both trained and untrained subjects responded to WI with similar decreases of renin and aldosterone, the trained subjects had attenuated natriuretic and kaliuretic responses along with depressed urine flow responses (15).

These studies collectively indicate that, in both humans and awake dogs, there is a poor correlation between suppression of plasma aldosterone levels and the natriuretic response. Therefore, it is likely that aldosterone suppression is not the major mechanism responsible for the natriuresis of WI. The kaliuresis, if present, may be secondary to the natriuresis or an increase of filtered load of K^+.

Atrial Peptides

Stretch of the atria releases peptides (atrial peptide, AP) which have been shown to exert both natriuretic and cardiovascular actions (37). Therefore, it is not surprising that WI elicits the release of AP in humans (75), awake dogs (67), and rats (50). Although AP levels in the plasma are promptly elevated after entry into the water, there are several issues which render its participation in the WI natriuresis ($U_{Na}V$) questionable. First, the time courses of the AP response and the $U_{Na}V$ response are different. AP levels rise rapidly within a few minutes to plateau at a constant elevated level throughout WI, whereas it takes 40 min for the natriuresis to appear and the sodium excretion rises progressively to peak after 2 hours or so (67). Second, it is not clear that the plasma levels of AP which are attained during WI are capable of initiating and sustaining a natriuresis (37). Third, in conscious dogs, Goetz et al. (36) showed that inflation of a balloon in the left atrium raises plasma AP levels and causes a diuresis and a natriuresis. However, in cardiac-denervated dogs, left atrial balloon inflation still elevated plasma AP levels, but the natriuresis was abolished. This study indicates that elevation of plasma AP is not enough by itself to elicit a natriuresis under these particular experimental conditions.

However, while elevations of AP may not contribute to the rapid natriuresis of atrial balloon inflation, there may be a time-dependent nature to the renal response to AP. In other words, there may be a period of time required for the renal response to AP to become manifest. In this regard, Bie et al. (10) have recently performed a study where small doses of AP were infused systemically into conscious dogs so as to produce modest, graded elevations of plasma AP. These modest AP elevations did not have immediate effects on $U_{Na}V$; however, after 45 min or so, the smaller doses did begin to increase sodium excretion. Therefore, a time-dependent contribution of AP to the natriuresis of WI cannot be ruled out at this time (10).

Another problem with assigning a role for AP to the WI natriuresis is that most studies have indicated that the AP natriuretic effect is associated with increased GFR and renal blood flow. Since the WI response is not generally associated with changes in renal hemodynamics, it has been difficult to envisage a role for AP in the natriuresis on this basis (67). However, the recent studies by Bie et al. (10) suggest that low doses of AP in conscious animals may elicit a natriuretic response in the absence of obvious changes in renal hemodynamics. Thus, a tubular effect of AP might contribute to the natriuresis (10).

It should be emphasized also that AP can interact with the other volume regulatory hormones in WI. For example, AP may interfere with aldosterone secretion (37). In addition, AP has been shown to suppress the hydroosmotic action of AVP (37). The potential role for these interactions in the renal response to WI is unclear.

AP has also been shown to bring about reductions of plasma volume and elevate hematocrit in the rat (37). This response is unrelated to any fluid elimination evoked by AP as it occurs after bilateral nephrectomy. The mechanism of this response may involve an elevation of the resistance to venous return and elevation of capillary hydrostatic pressure (37), as well as an increase of capillary permeability (37). These influences are compatible with the idea that AP may act to regulate cardiac filling (37). In addition, it has also been suggested that AP may alter arterial baroreflex sensitivity (67). Again, however, it is not known whether these effects can occur at the levels of AP which are observed in the plasma during WI. If these effects do occur, they could act to modulate the transcapillary fluid shift of WI as well as arterial baroreflex function.

Thus, a direct role for AP in the WI natriuresis is not readily apparent, although a more subtle, time-dependent influence of AP on the kidney may be present. The cardiovascular effects of AP may act to modulate the central hypervolemia in WI. In addition to AP, Epstein et al. (25,74) have identified a natriuretic factor present in the urine of subjects undergoing WI. The nature of this factor and its relative contribution to the WI $U_{Na}V$ response is unclear.

Renal Prostaglandins

A marked increase in urinary excretion of prostaglandin E (PGE) has been demonstrated to occur in both hydrated and dehydrated humans during WI (25). Prostaglandins have been shown to inhibit the action of AVP in stimulating cyclic adenosine monophosphate formation which in turn alters the permeability of the collecting duct (67). Therefore, increased PGE levels could interfere with AVP action within the kidney and contribute to the increase of C_{H_2O}. It has also been shown that indomethacin pretreatment may attenuate the WI natriuresis in man (35), suggesting that renal prostaglandins may play a modulating role in the sodium excretion response.

Circulating Catecholamines

Epstein (25) has shown that levels of circulating catecholamines are depressed in humans during thermoneutral WI (27). In addition, we have shown that plasma catecholamines are unchanged in the awake dog during WI (41). Therefore, influences from circulating catecholamines do not play a role in the renal or cardiovascular responses to WI.

ROLE OF THE RENAL SYMPATHETIC NERVES

The kidney receives a rich sympathetic innervation and all levels of the nephron are supplied with adrenergic nerve terminals. Dibona and others (21,22) have demonstrated that renal sympathetic neural activity can exert powerful effects on sodium excretion independent of any effects on renal hemodynamics. Stimulation of the renal sympathetic nerves at levels which do not alter renal blood flow or GFR cause significant reductions of renal sodium excretion (22). Conversely, suppression of renal sympathetic nerve activity (RSNA) elicits a natriuresis (82). Stimulation of left atrial vagal myelinated afferents or left atrial balloon inflation, as well as activation of vagal non-myelinated afferents from the heart have been shown to reflexly inhibit

RSNA (21,22). These experiments indicate that loading of cardiac mechanoreceptors may elicit a natriuresis via a reflex inhibition of RSNA. In addition, various experiments have indicated that loading of the high pressure arterial baroreceptors also leads to reflex inhibition of RSNA (21). However, the idea has been put forth that the cardiac receptors are more powerful in this regard (89). Whether or not this is true of conscious animals or humans remains to be clarified. The influence of RSNA on sodium reabsorption is mediated via alpha adrenergic receptors (22).

In our experiments (41), total extrinsic denervation of the heart abolishes the natriuresis occurring during WI in the volume-replete conscious dog. Therefore, the cardiac nerves play the major role in the natriuresis. Since it is difficult to ascribe a primary role for the natriuresis to the volume regulatory hormones as discussed in the previous section, by exclusion, it seems likely that the major mechanism for the natriuresis of WI in the awake dog involves reflex suppression of RSNA via cardiac receptors. In addition, because of the stroke volume increase after cardiac denervation, the central input derived from the arterial baroreceptors was greater than when the dogs were intact, yet the natriuresis was abolished. This suggests that the central mechanoreceptor input from the arterial baroreceptors is not adequate to initiate a natriuresis via reflex suppression of RSNA in this situation, although it likely plays an important role in AVP suppression (41).

While reflex suppression of RSNA is probably of critical importance in the WI natriuresis, further studies need to be done to clarify this issue. For example, if RSNA decreases, a decrease of plasma renin activity might be expected to occur as well (91). In fact, there is more often a reduction of plasma renin levels in man, an effect which is probably mediated by reduced RSNA. On the other hand, the lack of renin response in the conscious dog may be related to the renal vasoconstriction which occurs in WI. The renal vasoconstriction acts to keep renal blood flow constant in the face of an elevated arterial pressure, therefore, the renal vasoconstriction is likely an autoregulatory response. Since GFR is constant also, the vasoconstriction is likely occurring in the afferent arteriole and this influence might tend to unload the intrarenal baroreceptor (91) which, in turn, by itself tends to keep renin secretion up in the presence of reduced RSNA which would tend to lower renin secretion. Since arterial pressure does not increase very much in humans, the renal autoregulatory effect may be less pronounced (91), and thus renin secretion tends to diminish in WI in man.

Thus, the available experimental data indicates that the loading of cardiac stretch receptors elicits a natriuresis in WI via a reflex suppression of RSNA. Further experimental work is needed to support this hypothesis, but recent experiments in our laboratory indicate that renal denervation markedly impairs the WI natriuresis in the conscious dog (personal observations). Moreover, a recent study by Miki et al. (71) indicates that WI causes an immediate 45% reduction of RSNA in the conscious dog. In addition, renal denervation of these dogs abolished the natriuresis as well as the diuresis.

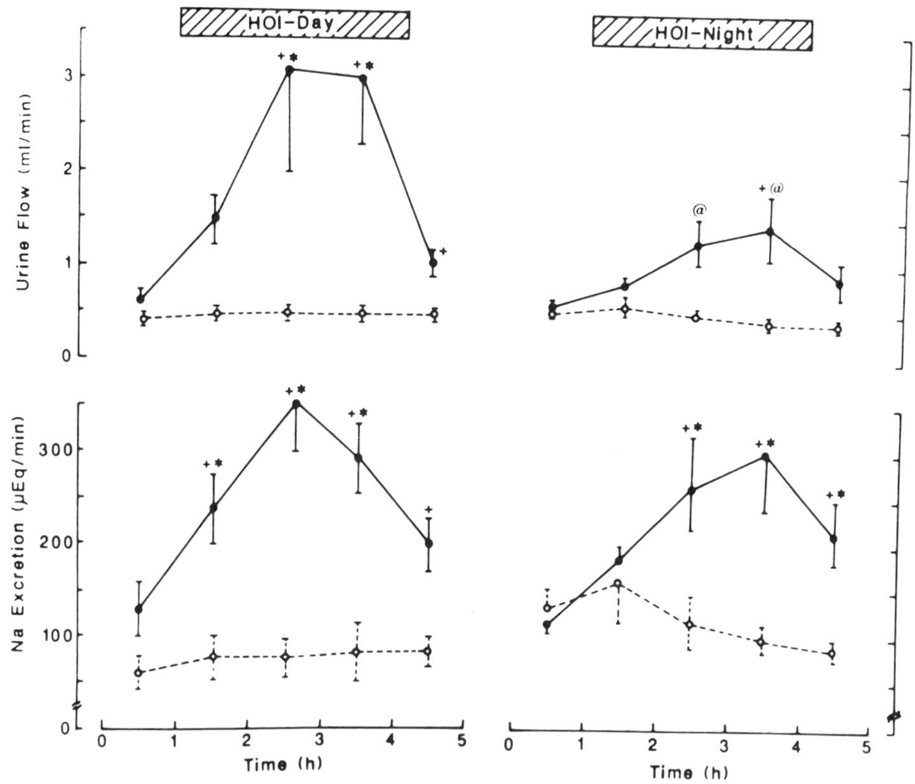

*Figure 8 Effects of head-out water immersion in the human on urine flow and sodium (Na) excretion during the day and during the night. Solid line-water immersion; dashed line-timed control. * $P < 0.05$ compared with corresponding 1 h value; + $P < 0.05$ compared with corresponding time control value; @ $P < 0.05$ compared with corresponding daytime value. The diuresis and natriuresis are attenuated at night. Reproduced by permission from the American Physiological Society (Ref 69).*

INFLUENCE OF CIRCADIAN RHYTHMS

The time of day the WI study is carried out can have a profound influence upon the nature of the renal response. Krishna and Danovitch (58) showed that in continuously hydrated subjects, the renal diuretic and natriuretic responses to WI were attenuated at night compared to the daytime despite similar reductions of aldosterone during the day and at night. Shiraki et al. (88) showed that when humans are subjected to WI after midnight, the diuresis and natriuresis responses are significantly attenuated also (88). The interesting feature of this study was that the suppression of renin, aldosterone, and AVP occurring during night-time WI was similar to that observed during daytime WI. Thus, the renal responses at night were dissociated from the hormonal responses. In a later study, Miki et al. (69) were able to demonstrate that plasma AP levels rose to a similar extent during the night in WI as they do during the day. Yet in this experiment, the WI natriuresis was significantly attenuated at night (Figs. 8,9). In both studies, the rise in cardiac output measured by impedance cardiography was identical during the day and night periods, therefore the input from cardiac mechanoreceptors was similar in both situations.

These studies provide further evidence for the view that the hormonal adjustments which occur during WI are not of primary importance, because the renal responses vary despite similar responses of AVP, aldosterone, and AP in man. This powerful circadian influence on the renal response to WI may not be present in all species.

Since control of RSNA by cardiac receptors appears to be of primary import in the WI natriuresis, it might be postulated at this time that the attenuated natriuretic and diuretic responses to WI at night in man may be related to a circadian influence on the cardiac receptor-RSNA reflex link. The influence of athletic training on the natriuresis in man may involve this particular link as well (15).

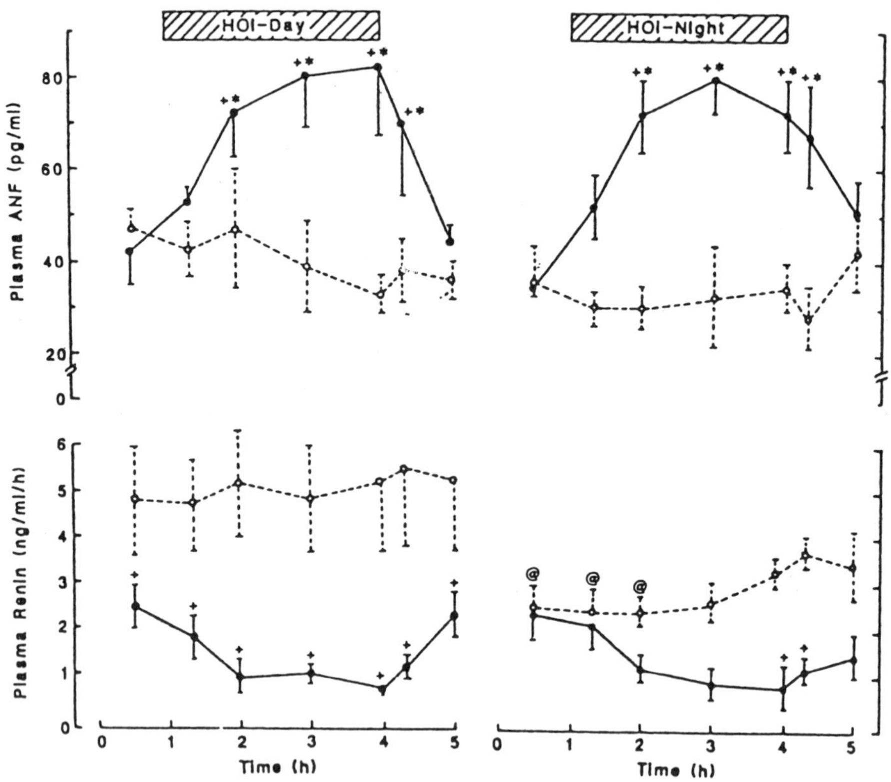

Figure 9 Effects of head-out water immersion on plasma atrial peptide levels (ANF) and plasma renin activity in humans during the daytime and at nighttime. Symbols as in Fig. 8. Resp^nses of atrial peptide and renin activity are similar during the day and night despite attenuated diuresis and natriuresis responses. Reproduced by permission from the American Physiological Society (Ref 69).

EFFECTS OF WATER TEMPERATURE

It is to be expected that variations of water temperature above and below the thermoneutral value will have profound influences on the cardiovascular, renal, and endocrine responses to WI. Unfortunately, there is little information available on this issue obtained from studies utilizing systematic observations based on deviations from standardized models in the thermoneutral state. Certainly, cool WI would be expected to be associated with cutaneous and deeper tissue vasoconstriction, with perhaps even decreased cardiac output responses and altered hormonal responses (16). Likewise, elevated water temperatures might lead to greater cardiac output increments along with vasodilation occurring in the insulative layers and differing patterns of hormonal responses (53).

CONCLUSIONS

WI has been used as a therapeutic modality for centuries, and we are only just now beginning to understand the physiological mechanisms which govern the complex response elicited by this simple and common maneuver. WI has been proposed as a non-pharmacologic therapeutic maneuver to promote fluid elimination in cirrhosis, nephrosis,and congestive heart failure (25,74). While WI might well prove to be effective in this regard, the precise effect of WI on plasma volume is unclear in light of the transcapillary fluid shift which occurs. It is well to keep in mind that the potential cellular dehydration and K^+ depletion which can occur in WI may be of clinical relevance as well as being important to the many people who use WI for recreational purposes. Moreover, the implications of WI studies for an understanding of the weightless state in space are obvious.

In terms of the original Gauer-Henry hypothesis, it would appear that the idea that there is a heart-kidney link is well supported. However, the original view that atrial receptors act on the kidney via AVP suppression has been added to by a wealth of experimental data. The importance of conscious animal studies has been emphasized and the idea that bipeds may differ from quadrupeds in the relative contribution of cardiac receptors versus arterial receptors needs further experimental support. The conscious monkey appears to possess powerful cardiac vagal AVP and renal control mechanisms (93).

At present, it may be concluded that, although WI can be associated with suppression of plasma AVP levels, depending upon the degree of hydration, as well as suppression of plasma renin activity and aldosterone secretion, along with increased AP levels, these hormonal changes are difficult to relate directly to the renal free water clearance and sodium excretion responses. AVP suppression clearly has the potential to contribute to free water excretion during WI. However, several lines of evidence point to a clear dissociation between cardiac responses, renal responses, and endocrine responses which is evident when the time courses of the responses are examined, along with the effects of physical training, and circadian rhythms.

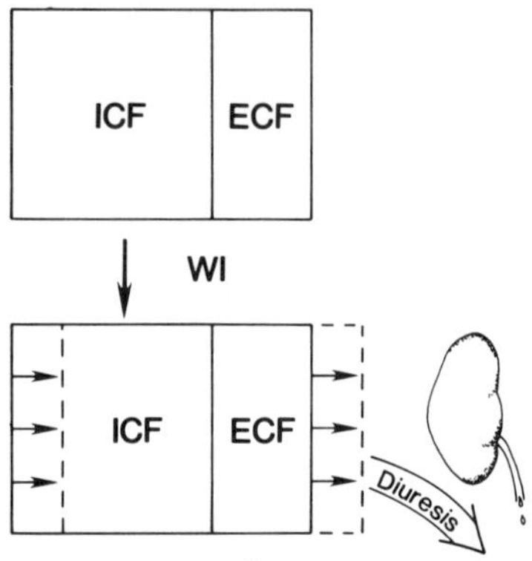

Figure 10 A fluid shift occurs from the intracellular compartment (ICF) into the extracellular compartment (ECF) during water immersion (WI). The kidney eliminates the shifted fluid.

It appears that the primary mechanism responsible for the natriuretic response to WI is a reduction of renal sympathetic nerve activity. The available data suggest that renal response to WI is largely dependent upon the loading of cardiac mechanoreceptors and that the loading of the cardiac receptors is the major mechanism whereby RSNA is suppressed. On the other hand, the primary mechanism for AVP suppression is likely to be loading of the high-pressure arterial baroreceptors. Further studies of WI should be directed to more precisely identifying the nature of the mechanoreceptor input patterns derived from cardiac inputs and arterial baroreceptor inputs in various species. In addition, factors which may contribute to altered arterial baroreceptor input patterns, either as the result of changed sensitivity such as might result from athletic training, or baroreceptor resetting should be investigated (5,15). Quantitation of the effects of the transcapillary fluid shift of WI per se on the kidney, exclusive of and added to the mechanoreceptor input, is needed. Lastly, the effects of circadian rhythms or physical training on RSNA responses to cardiac receptor stimulation need to be defined.

In summary, hormonal changes are elicited as part of the Gauer-Henry heart-kidney connection, however, these responses are of secondary importance compared to the powerful renal natriuretic effects evoked by the cardiac reflex reduction of renal sympathetic nerve activity. Thus, the primary heart-kidney connection in conscious animals and probably man which is engaged in WI involves renal sympathetic nerve pathways, and not hormones. Therefore, the basic idea put forth by Gauer and Henry which postulated a link between cardiovascular distention and the kidney is valid. Cardiac distention is clearly required for a renal response to occur (personal observations). However, the relative contribution of the endocrine component versus the renal adrenergic component has been redefined and the arterial baroreceptors should be included as inputs for this response in addition to cardiac receptors. Furthermore, the traditional concept that the kidney acts to reduce plasma volume below pre-immersion levels, thereby reducing cardiac filling pressures and cardiac output to normal is questionable (Figs. 1 and 4). Rather, it is more likely that

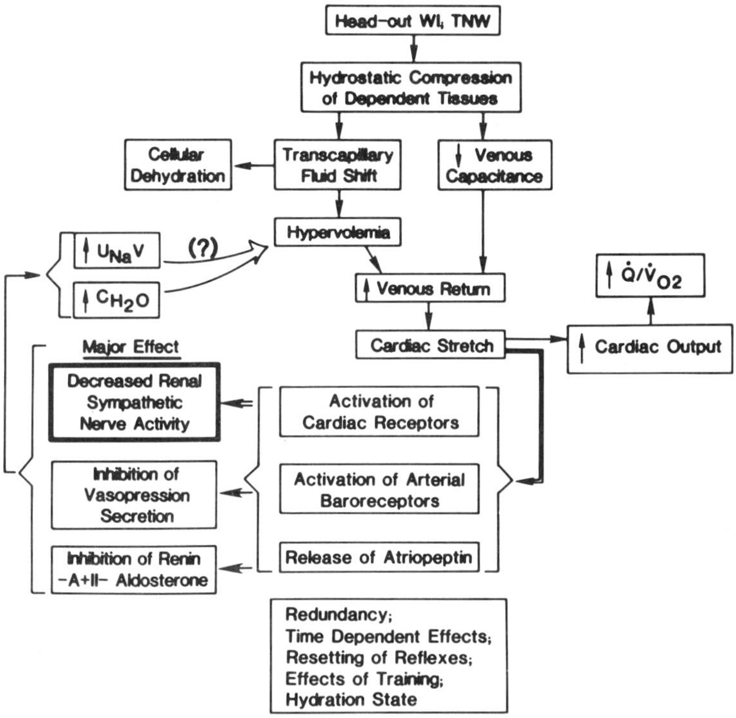

Figure 11 Current view of cardiovascular, renal, and endocrine responses which occur during thermoneutral (TNW) WI. WI is associated with a decline in venous capacitance which leads to a central translocation of blood into the thorax. In addition, fluid shifts out of the cells leading both to cellular dehydration and systemic hypervolemia. Stretch of the heart raises the cardiac output and the ratio of blood flow to metabolism in some tissues. In addition, cardiovascular reflexes are engaged and atriopeptin is released. The major consequence of activating cardiac receptors is a reduction of renal sympathetic nerve activity which promotes a natriuresis. Vasopressin may be reduced depending upon the degree of hydration contributing to an increase of free water clearance. Aldosterone decreases but this response is not well correlated with the natriuresis. The renal response consists of a major natriuretic component in human and dog, with a variable increase in free water clearance depending upon the degree of hydration. The renal response is also affected by circadian rhythms and athletic training. Further work is required to establish the relation between the renal response and the hypervolemia. It is unlikely that plasma volume is reduced below pre-immersion levels in euhydrated subjects during WI.

the renal response is directed toward minimizing hypervolemia occurring as the result of a sustained or continuing transcapillary fluid shift from the cellular compartment into the plasma compartment (Fig. 10). Thus, the regulated variable is plasma volume, but it appears to be regulated down toward pre-immersion levels, and not below pre-immersion levels, in the face of a ongoing influx of fluid into the plasma compartment. In other words, the renal response is unable to fully correct for the continuing leak of fluid into the plasma. This observation probably accounts for the maintained elevation of cardiac filling pressures during prolonged WI in the face of a prolonged diuresis. Mechanisms known to play a role in the cardiovascular - renal - endocrine response to WI are summarized in Fig. 11. The relation of this response to the cardiovascular regulation of regional O_2 delivery in WI remains to be determined.

ACKNOWLEDGEMENTS

The writing of this review and the research conducted by the authors which is cited in this review was supported by Program Project Grant PO1-HL- 28542 from the National Heart, Lung, and Blood Institute.

The opinions or assertions contained herein are the private views of the authors and are not to be construed as official or as reflecting the views of the Department of the Army or the Department of Defense.

REFERENCES

1. Arborelius, M.J., U.I. Balldin, B. Lilja, and C.E.G. Lundgren. Hemodynamic changes in man during immersion with head above water. Aerosp. Med. 43:592-598, 1972.
2. Balldin, U.I., C.E.G. Lundgren, J. Lundvall, and S. Mellander. Changes in the elimination of 133-xenon from the anterior tibial muscle in man induced by immersion in water and shifts in body position. Aerosp. Med. 42:489-493, 1971.
3. Bazett, H.C. Studies on the effects of baths on man. I. Relationship between the effects produced and the temperature of the bath. Am. J. Physiol. 70:412-429, 1924.
4. Bazett, H.C., S. Thurlow, C. Corwell, and W. Stewart. Studies on the effect of baths on man. II. The diuresis caused by warm baths, together with some observations on urinary tides. Am. J. Physiol. 70:430-452, 1924.
5. Bedford, T.G., and C.M. Tipton. Exercise training and the arterial baroreflex. J. Appl. Physiol. 63:1926-1932, 1987.
6. Begin, R., M. Epstein, M.A. Sackner, R. Levinson, R. Doughterty, and D. Duncan. Effects of water immersion to the neck on pulmonary circulation and tissue volume in man. J. Appl. Physiol. 40:293-299, 1976.
7. Behn, C., O.H. Gauer, K. Kirsch, and P. Eckert. Effects of sustained intrathoracic vascular distension of body fluid distribution and renal excretion in man. Pflugers Archiv. 313:123-135, 1969.
8. Bezold, A. Von, L. Hirt. Uber die physiologischen Wirkungen de essigsauren Veratrins. Unter Physiol. Lab. Wurzburg 1:75-156, 1867.
9. Bie, P., M. Mumksdorf, and J. Warburg. Renal effects of overhydration during vasopressin infusion in conscious dogs. Am. J. Physiol. 247:F103-F109, 1984.
10. Bie, P., B.C. Wang, R.J. Leadley, Jr., and K.L. Goetz. Hemodynamic and renal effects of low-dose infusions of atrial peptide in conscious dogs. Am. J. Physiol. 254:R161-R169, 1988.

11. Bishop, V.S., A. Malliani, and P. Thoren. Cardiac mechanoreceptors. In: Handbook of Physiology. The Cardiovascular System, edited by J.T. Shepherd and F.M. Abboud. Bethesda, MD: Am. Physiol. Soc., Sec. 2, Vol. III, Chapter 15, pp. 497-556, 1983.
12. Blomqvist, C.G., and H.L. Stone. Cardiovascular adjustments to gravitational stress. In: Handbook of Physiology. The Cardiovascular System, edited by J.T. Shepherd and F.M. Abboud. Bethesda, MD: Am. Physiol. Soc., Sec. 2, Vol. III, Chapter 28, pp. 1025-1063, 1983.
13. Boettcher, D.H., S.F. Vatner, G.R. Heyndrickx, E. Braunwald. Extent of utilization of the Frank-Starling mechanism in conscious dogs. Am. J. Physiol. 234:H338-H345, 1978.
14. Clark, J.H., D.R. Hooker, and L.H. Weed. The hydrostatic factor in venous pressure measurements. Am. J. Physiol. 109:166-177, 1934.
15. Claybaugh, J.R., D.R. Pendergast, J.E. Davis, C. Akiba, M. Pazik, and S.K. Hong. The effect of training on hormonal and urinary responses to supine posture and immersion. J. Appl. Physiol. 61:7-15, 1986.
16. Craig, A.B., Jr., and M. Dvorak. Thermal regulation during water immersion. J. Appl. Physiol. 21:1577-1585, 1966.
17. Craig, A.B., Jr., and M. Dvorak. Expiratory reserve volume and vital capacity of the lungs during immersion in water. J. Appl. Physiol. 38:5-9, 1975.
18. Crane, M.G., and J.J. Harris. Suppression of plasma aldosterone by partial immersion. Metab. 23:359-368, 1974.
19. Davis, J.T., and A.B. DuBois. Immersion diuresis in dogs. J. Appl. Physiol.: Respirat. Environ. Exercise Physiol. 42:915-922, 1977.
20. Detorrente, A., G.L. Robertson, K.M. McDonald, and R.W. Schrier. Mechanism of diuretic response to increased left atrial pressure in anesthetized dog. Kidney Int. 8:355-361, 1975.
21. Dibona, G.F. The functions of renal nerves. Rev. Physiol. Biochem. Pharmacol. 94:75-181, 1982.
22. Dibona, G.F. Neural regulation of renal tubular sodium reabsorption and renin secretion. Fed. Proc. 44:2816-2822, 1985.
23. Doba, N., and D.J. Reis. Cerebellum: role in reflex cardiovascular adjustment to posture. Brain Res. 39:495-500, 1972.
24. Echt, M., L. Lange, and O.H. Gauer. Changes of peripheral venous tone and central transmural venous pressure during immersion in a thermo-neutral bath. Pflugers Archiv. 352:211-217, 19974.
25. Epstein, M. Renal effects of head-out water immersion in man: implications for an understanding of volume homeostasis. Physiol. Rev. 58:529-581, 1978.
26. Epstein, M., A.G. Denunzio, and R.D. Loutzenhiser. Effects of vasopressin administration on diuresis of water immersion in normal humans. J. Appl. Physiol.:Respirat. Environ. Exercise Physiol. 51:1384-1387, 1981.
27. Epstein, M., G. Johnson, and A.G. Denunzio. Effects of water immersion on plasma catecholamines in normal humans. J. Appl. Physiol.:Respirat. Environ. Exercise Physiol. 54:244-248, 1983.
28. Epstein, M., J.L. Katsikas, and D.C. Duncan. Role of mineralocorticoids in the natriuresis of water immersion in normal man. Circ. Res. 32:228- 236, 1973.
29. Epstein, M., R. Levinson, and R. Loutzenhiser. Effects of water immersion on renal hemodynamics in normal man. J. Appl. Physiol. 41:230-233, 1976.

30. Epstein, M., D.S. Pins, R. Arrington, A.G. Denunzio, and R. Engstrom. Comparison of water immersion and saline infusion as a means of inducing volume expansion in man. J. Appl. Physiol. 39:60-70, 1975.
31. Epstein, M., and T. Saruta. Effects of water immersion on renin-aldosterone and renal sodium handling in normal man. J. Appl. Physiol. 31:369-374, 1971.
32. Farhi, L.E., and D. Linnarsson. Cardiopulmonary readjustments during graded immersion in water at 35°C. Respirat. Physiol. 30:35-50, 1977.
33. Fater, D.C., H.D. Schultz, W.D. Sundet, J.S. Mapes, and K.L. Goetz. Effects of left atrial stretch in cardiac-denervated and intact conscious dogs. Am. J. Physiol. 242:H1056-H1064, 1982.
34. Gauer, O.H., and J.P. Henry. Neurohumoral control of plasma volume. In: Cardiovascular Physiology II, edited by A.C. Guyton and A.W. Cowley. Baltimore, MD: University Park Press, Vol. 9, pp. 145-189, 1976.
35. Gilmore, J.P. Neural control of extracellular volume in the human and non-human primate. In: Handbook of Physiology. The Cardiovascular System, edited by J.T. Shepherd and F.M. Abboud. Bethesda, MB: Am. Physiol. Soc., Sec. 2, Vol. III., 1983.
36. Goetz, K.L., B.C. Wang, P.G. Geer, R.J. Leadley, Jr., and H.W. Reinhardt. Atrial stretch increases sodium excretion independently of release of atrial peptides. Am. J. Physiol. 250:R946-R950, 1986.
37. Goetz, K.L. Physiology and pathophysiology of atrial peptides. Am. J. Physiol. 254:E1-E15, 1988.
38. Greenleaf, J.E., J.T. Morese, P.R. Baines, J. Silver, and L.C. Keil. Hypervolemia and plasma vasopressin response during water immersion in man. J. Appl. Physiol.:Respirat. Environ. Exercise Physiol. 55:1688-1693, 1983.
39. Greenleaf, J.E., E. Schvertz, and L.C. Keil. Hemodilution, vasopressin suppression, and diuresis during water immersion in man. Aviat. Space Environ. Med. 52:329-336, 1981.
40. Greenleaf, J.E., E. Schvartz, S. Kravik, and L.C. Keil. Fluid shifts and endocrine responses during chair rest and water immersion in man. J. Appl. Physiol.:Respirat. Environ. Exercise Physiol. 48:79-88, 1980.
41. Hajduczok, G., K. Miki, S.K. Hong, J.R. Claybaugh, and J.A. Krasney. Role of cardiac nerves in response to head-out water immersion in conscious dogs. Am. J. Physiol. 253:R242-R253, 1987.
42. Hajduczok, G., K. Miki, J.R. Claybaugh, S.K. Hong, and J.A. Krasney. Regional circulatory responses to head-out water immersion in conscious dogs. Am. J. Physiol. 253:R254-R263, 1987.
43. Hargens, A.R. Introduction and Historical Perspectives. Tissue Fluid Pressure and Composition, edited by A.R. Hargens. Baltimore, MD: Williams and Wilkins, 1987.
44. Hong, S.K., P. Ceretelli, J.C. Cruz, and H. Rahn. Mechanisms of respiration during submersion in water. J. Appl. Physiol. 27:535-538, 1969.
45. Kaczmarczyk, G.A., W. Christe, R. Mohnhaupt, and H.W. Reinhardt. An attempt to quantitate the contribution of antidiuretic hormone to the diuresis of left atrial distension in conscious dogs. Pflugers Archiv. 396:101-105, 1983.

46. Kaczmarczyk, G.A., A. Krake, R. Eisele, R. Mohnhaupt, M.I.M. Noble, B. Singer, J. Stubbs, and H.W. Reinhardt. The role of cardiac nerves in the regulation of sodium excretion in conscious dogs. Pflugers Archiv. 390:125-130, 1981.
47. Kaczmarczyk, G.A., V. Unger, R. Mohnhaupt, and H.W. Reinhardt. Left atrial distension and intrarenal blood flow distribution in conscious dogs. Pflugers Archiv. 390:44-48, 1981.
48. Kappagoda, C.T., R.J. Linden, and H.M. Snow. A reflex increase in heart rate from distension of the junction between the superior vena cava and the right atrium. J. Physiol. 220:177-197, 1972.
49. Kappagoda, C.T., R.J. Linden, H.M. Snow, and E.M. Whitaker. Left atrial receptors and the antidiuretic hormone. J. Physiol. 237:663-683, 1974.
50. Katsube, N., D. Schwartz, and P. Needleman. Release of atriopeptin in the rate by vasoconstrictors or water immersion correlates with changes in right atrial pressure. Biochem. Biophys. Res. Com. 133:937-944, 1985.
51. Khosla, S.S., and A.B. DuBois. Fluid shifts during initial phase of immersion diuresis in man. J. Appl. Physiol.:Respirat. Environ. Exercise Physiol. 46:703-708, 1979.
52. Khosla, S.S., and A.B. DuBois. Osmoregulation and interstitial fluid pressure changes in humans during water immersion. J. Appl. Physiol.: Respirat. Environ. Exercise Physiol. 51:686-692, 1981.
53. Khight, D.R. and S.M. Horvath. Urinary responses to cold temperature during water immersion. Am. J. Physiol. 248:R560-R566, 1985.
54. Koubenec, H.J., W.D. Risch, and O.H. Gauer. Effective compliance of the total vascular system of man sitting in air and immersed in a bath. Pflugers Archiv. 355 (Sup.1):R24, 1975.
55. Krasney, J.A., G. Hajduczok, C. Akiba, B.W. McDonald, D.R. Pendergast, and S.K. Hong. Cardiovascular and renal responses to head-out water immersion in canine model. Undersea Biomed. Res. 11:169-183, 1984.
56. Krasney, J.A., D.R. Pendergast, E. Powell, B.W. McDonald, and J.L. Plewes. Regional circulatory responses to head-out water immersion in the anesthetized dog. J. Appl. Physiol.:Respirat. Environ. Exercise Physiol. 53:1625-1633, 1982.
57. Kravik, S.E., L.C. Keil, J.E. Silver, N. Wong, W.A. Spaul, and J.E. Greenleaf. Immersion diuresis without the expected suppression of vasopressin. J. Appl. Physiol.:Respirat. Environ. Exercise Physiol. 57:123-128, 1984.
58. Krishna, G.G., and G.M. Danovitch. Renal responses to central volume expansion in humans is attenuated at night. Am. J. Physiol. 244:R481- R486, 1983.
59. Lange, L., S. Lange, M. Echt, and O.H. Gauer. Heart volume in relation to body posture and immersion in a thermo-neutral bath. Pflugers Archiv. 352:219-226, 1974.
60. Ledsome, J.R., and R.J. Linden. The role of left atrial receptors in the diuretic response to left atrial distension. J. Physiol. 198:487-503, 1968.
61. Ledsome, J.R., R.J. Linden, and W.J. O'Connor. The mechanisms by which distension of the left atrium produces diuresis in anesthetized dogs. J. Physiol. 159:87-100, 1961.
62. Ledsome, J.R., J. Ngsee, and N. Wilson. Plasma vasopressin concentrations in the anesthetized dog before, during, and after atrial distension. J. Physiol. 338:413-421, 1983.

63. Lin, Y.C. Circulatory functions during immersion and breath-hold dives in humans. Undersea Biomed. Res. 11:123-138, 1984.
64. Lydtin, H., and W.F. Hamilton. Effect of acute changes in left atrial pressure on urine flow in unanesthetized dogs. Am. J. Physiol. 207:530-536, 1964.
65. Mellanger, S. Comparative studies on the adrenergic neurohormonal control of resistance and capacitance blood vessels in the cat. Acta Physiol. Scand. 50 (supp):176, 1960.
66. Miki, K., G. Hajduczok, S.K. Hong, and J.A. Krasney. Plasma volume changes during head-out water immersion in the conscious dog. Am. J. Physiol. 251:R582-R590, 1986.
67. Miki, K., G. Hajduczok, M.K. Klocke, J.A. Krasney, S.K. Hong, and A.J. Debold. Atrial natriuretic factor and renal function during head-out water immersion in conscious dogs. Am. J. Physiol. 251:R1000-R1008, 1986.
68. Miki, K., G. Hajduczok, S.K. Hong, and J.A. Krasney. Extracellular fluid and plasma volumes during water immersion in nephrectomized dogs. Am. J. Physiol. 252:R972-R978, 1987.
69. Miki, K., K. Shiraki, S. Sagawa, A.J. Debold, and S.K. Hong. Atrial natriuretic factor during head-out immersion at night. Am. J. Physiol. 254:R235-R241, 1988.
70. Miki, K., M. Pazik, E. Krasney, S.K. Hong, and J.A. Krasney. Thoracic duct lymph flow during head-out water immersion in conscious dogs. Am. J. Physiol. 252:R782-R785, 1987.
71. Miki, K., Y. Hayashida, S. Sagawa, and K. Shiraki. Role of sympathetic nerve activity in renal responses during head-out water immersion in conscious dogs. FASEB J. 2(5):A1319, 1988.
72. Mills, E., and S.C. Wang. Liberation of antidiuretic hormone: location of ascending pathways. Am. J. Physiol. 207:1399-1404, 1964.
73. Myers, J.W., and J.A. Godley. Cardiovascular and renal function during total body water immersion of dogs. J. Appl. Physiol. 22:573-579, 1967.
74. Norsk, P., and M. Epstein. Effects of water immersion on arginine vasopressin release in humans. J. Appl. Physiol. 64:1-10, 1988.
75. Pendergast, D.R., A.J. Debold, M. Pazik, and S.K. Hong. Effect of head-out immersion on plasma atrial natriuretic factor in man. Proc. Soc. Exp. Biol. Med. 184:429, 435, 1987.
76. Pendergast, D.R., A.J. Olszowka, M.A. Rokitka, and L.E. Farhi. Gravitational Force and the Cardiovascular System. In: Comparative Physiology of Environmental Adaptations, edited by P. Dejours. Karger, Basel, 1986.
77. Peters, J.P. Body Water: The Exchange of Fluids in Man. Springfield, Ill.: Thomas, pp. 287, 1935.
78. Peterson, T.V., J.P. Gilmore, and I.H. Zucker. Renal responses of the recumbent nonhuman primate to total body immersion. Proc. Soc. Exp. Biol. Med. 161:260-265, 1979.
79. Peterson, T.V., J.P. Gilmore, and I.H. Zucker. Initial renal responses of nonhuman primate to immersion and intravascular volume expansion. J. Appl. Physiol.:Respirat. Environ. Exercise Physiol. 48:243-248, 1980.
80. Peterson, T.V., B.A. Benjamin, and N.L. Hurst. Effect of vagotomy and thoracic sympathectomy on responses of the monkey to water immersion. J. Appl. Physiol. 63:2476-2481, 1987.

81. Prefaut, C., F. DuBois, C. Roussos, R. Amaral-Marques, P.T. Macklem, and F. Ruff. Influence of immersion to the neck in water on airway closure and distribution of perfusion in man. Resp. Physiol. 37:313-323, 1979.
82. Prosnitz, E.H., and G.F. Dibona. Effect of decreased renal sympathetic nerve activity on renal tubular sodium reabsorption. Am. J. Physiol. 235:F557-F563, 1978.
83. Rabischong, P., C. Clay, J. Vignaud, and R. Polierae. Approche hemohynamique de la signification fonctionelle due sinus cavernuex. Neuro-Chirurgie 18, n-7:613-622, 1972.
84. Randall, W.C., M.P. Kaye, J.X. Thomas, Jr., M.J. Barber. Intrapericardial denervation of the heart. J. Surg. Res. 29:101-109, 1980.
85. Rowell, L.B. Human Circulation Regulation during Physical Stress. New York: Oxford, 1986.
86. Share, L. Effects of carotid occlusion and left atrial distention on plasma vasopressin titer. Am. J. Physiol. 208:219-223, 1965.
87. Share, L., and M.N. Levy. Carotid sinus pulse pressure, a determinant of plasma antidiuretic hormone concentration. Am. J. Physiol. 211:721-724, 1966.
88. Shiraki, K., N. Konda, S. Sagawa, J.R. Claybaugh, and S.K. Hong. Cardiorenal-endocrine responses to head-out immersion at night. J. Appl. Physiol. 60:176-183, 1986.
89. Thames, M.D. Contribution of cardiopulmonary baroreceptors to the control of the kidney. Fed. Proc. 37:1209-1213, 1978.
90. Thames, M.D., B.D. Miller, and F.M. Abboud. Baroreflex regulation of renal nerve activity during volume expansion. Am. J. Physiol. 243:H810- H814, 1982.
91. Thames, M.D., M. Jarecki, and D.E. Donald. Neural control of renin secretion in anesthetized dogs: Interactions of cardiopulmonary and carotid baroreceptors. Circ. Res. 42:237-245, 1978.
92. Vatner, S.F., and E. Braunwald. Cardiovascular control mechanisms in the conscious state. N. Engl. J. Med. 293:970-976, 1975.
93. Vatner, S.F., W.T. Manders, and D.R. Knight. Vagally mediated regulation of renal function in conscious primates. Am. J. Physiol. 250:H546-H549, 1986.
94. Von Ameln, H., M. Laniado, L. Rocker, and K.A. Kirsch. Effects of dehydration on the vasopressin response to immersion. J. Appl. Physiol. 58:114-120, 1985.
95. Von Diringshofen, H. Die Wirkungen des hydrostatischen druckes des wasserbades auf den blutdruck in den kapillaren und die bindegewebsentwasserung. 7. Kreislaufforsch 37:382-390, 1948.
96. Wang, B.C., G. Flora-Ginter, R.J. Leadley, Jr., and K.L. Goetz. Ventricular receptors stimulate vasopressin release during hemorrhage. Am. J. Physiol. 254:R204-R211, 1988.
97. Yoshino, H., D.C. Curran-Everett, S.K. Hong, and J.A. Krasney. Altered heart rate-arterial pressure relation during head-out water immersion in the conscious dog. Am. J. Physiol. 254:R595-R601, 1988.
98. Zucker, I.H., and J.P. Gilmore. Responsiveness of type B atrial receptors in the monkey. Brain Res. 95:159-165, 1975.
99. Zucker, I.H., and J.P. Gilmore. Contribution of peripheral pooling to the renal response to water immersion in the dog. J. Appl. Physiol. 45:786-790, 1978.

6

FLUID AND ELECTROLYTE BALANCE AND HORMONAL RESPONSE TO THE HYPOXIC ENVIRONMENT

John R. Claybaugh[1], Charles E. Wade[2], and Samuel A. Cucinell[3]

[1]Department of Clinical Investigation
Tripler Army Medical Center
TAMC, HI 96859-5000

[2]Letterman Army Institute of Research
Division of Military Trauma Research
Presidio of San Francisco, CA 94129-6700

[3]Defense Nuclear Agency
Armed Forces Radiobiological Research Institute
Bethesda, MD 20814

INTRODUCTION

The effect of the hypoxic environment on body fluid regulating systems is influenced by both the direct and indirect effects of hypoxia. Regarding the direct physiological effects, for instance, hypoxemia can directly stimulate the carotid body chemoreceptors with subsequent stimulation of antidiuretic hormone (ADH) release (79), and by mechanisms still unclear, hypoxia reduces the secretion of aldosterone (15,16,39,57,62,81,84,85). In the natural setting, coincident environmental factors such as cold and exercise, discussed elsewhere in this text, and possibly hypobaria, may influence the responses to hypoxia. Additionally, the indirect effects of short-term hypoxia on respiration and cardiovascular reflexes also effect water and electrolyte regulating hormones, and the longer-term effects of decreased appetite impact on electrolyte balances which cause compensatory responses of these hormone systems. Finally, there are the poorly understood indirect consequences of "stress" on various hormonal systems, particularly those of ADH and glucocorticoids, that cannot be excluded from the mechanisms of hypoxia-induced effects on these systems.

In consideration of these complicating factors, it is not surprising to find reports that hypoxia stimulates (1,13,24,26,72,95), has no effect (4,7,12,25,30,36,37), and inhibits (12,68,88) ADH release, and stimulates (28,85,92), has no effect (15,81) or inhibits (39,50,90) renin release and similarly conflicting findings regarding aldosterone stimulation (27,40) and inhibition (e.g. 15,39,84,85,90). Most of these responses are, in fact, normal physiological responses to the hypoxic environment but differ because of time of exposure, dietary intake, and the other complicating factors mentioned. An attempt will be made to categorize these differences in the following discussion.

At this time there are too few studies to make a critical evaluation of the effect of hypobaria *per se*. Of those (23,37), the evidence suggests that hypobaria without hypoxia is accompanied by renin and aldosterone, ADH, cortisol, and prolactin responses that are similar to normobaric control values. Therefore, in the following discussion no distinction will be made between studies in which animals or human subjects breathed hypoxic gas mixtures or were exposed to hypoxic hypobaric chamber environments.

EFFECTS OF HYPOXIA ON WATER AND ELECTROLYTE BALANCE

The influence of the hypoxic environment on water and electrolyte balance has been the focus of extensive research for many years. However, the area has not been recently reviewed and it will be necessary to briefly cover this background in order to relate the endocrine responses to the various control mechanisms and the renal effects.

Evidence for Hypohydration at High Altitude

Although not without conflicting reports (33), most studies indicate that several days of exposure to hypoxia leads to a decrease in total body water. In many situations body weight is a simple method of assessing changes in total body water, but in the hypoxic environment this method is fraught with difficulties. Owing largely to a decrease in appetite, there are losses in fat, protein, and mineral stores that also contribute to the weight loss. In a study designed to account for these other routes of weight loss (46,53), losses attributable to fat, protein, and water were about 1.5, 0.4 and 1.8 kg respectively after 12 days at 14,100 ft. A similar, more direct approach to assessing body weight changes has also been done by carcass analysis in mice after three and seven days at two different altitudes, i.e., 14,100 ft and 20,000 ft. (32). In these studies there were also losses in lean body mass of 7 and 10%, and of body fat of 44 and 55% and of total body water of 10 and 14% at the two respective altitudes after seven days. Interestingly, the major losses were observed by the third day at both altitudes with only a slight additional loss in body fat during the next four days.

Indicator dilution methods of total body water also generally indicate a loss of approximately 2 liters of water in man during the first few days at high altitude (Table 1). There are other studies not included in this table in which statistically nonsignificant decreases were observed (e.g. 53), and some where increases (33) were observed with the D_2O method of total body water determination. In the former study (53), body density assessments of total body water indicated a 1.7 liter loss of body water after 12 days at 14,100 ft., which was statistically significant. Table 1 summarizes some studies in which

TABLE 1. Total body water determined by indicator dilution methods.

Body water volume (l) S L	H A	Diff	Altitude	Duration	Method	Ref.
40.8	39.8	1.0	17,500	5	4 AA	(27)
42.0	39.8	2.2	14,300	6	D_20	(52)
42.7	40.7	2.0	11,500	12	^3H_2O	(44)

S L = sea level, H A = High Altitude, Diff = S L - H A, 4 AA = 4-amino-antipyrine

statistically significant decreases in body water were observed with commonly used indicator dilution techniques.

In another method of assessing total body water, losses can be obtained through daily determinations of water balance. Though seldom measured, insensible water loss has been reported to be as high as 500 ml greater at a simulated altitude of 12,000 ft than at sea level (39). Thus, water balances determined with the omission of insensible water losses will underestimate the decrease in water balance at high altitude. Despite this underestimation, a limited period of about 4 days, including the day of transition, is accompanied by an immediate reduction in water balance as simply determined from water intake minus urine output (Table 2). By the fourth to fifth days at altitude the difference between water intake and urinary output are at sea level values. It should be pointed out that there are several other studies in which these parameters were measured, but interpretation is difficult because of superimposition of heavy exercise causing heavier sweating at sea level, or the ascents were not acute. However, if it is assumed that the subjects were in perfect balance during the control days, and if fecal water losses and metabolic water gains were unchanged, cumulative water losses not including additional insensible water losses would be about 0.3 to 3.0 liters over the first few days. It should also be noted that in the last study cited in the table below, Consolazio et al. (18) observed no difference between sea level and high

TABLE 2. Water Intake Minus Urine Output (l) After Acute Ascent to Altitude.

Sea Level		High Altitude							
day-2	day-1	ascent	day 1	day 2	day 3	day 4	n[1]	alt.(ft)	Ref.
1.6	1.5	0.3	0.8	0.8	0.9	1.5	10	14,100	(45)
	0.9	0.6	1.0				3	15,600	(90)
1.5	1.4	0.5	0.9	1.0	1.5		10	13,800[2]	
	1.2				1.3[3]		8	14,100	(18)

1. n = number of subjects; 2. unpublished observations (Claybaugh, Brooks and Cucinell); 3. This value was given for days 1-7 at high altitude.

altitude values when the first seven days at high altitude were pooled together. This lack of effect could be due to the averaging over such a long period; in addition, their study incorporated a liquid diet which may have influenced the response.

Effects of High Altitude on Electrolytes

Balances of Na and K have been determined in a number of studies in human subjects (17,39,45,46,51,84), and some have studied these electrolytes on a fixed food intake (17,39,45,51,84). With ad libitum food intake and the usual accompanying decrease in food consumption, Na and K intakes would be expected to decrease during hypoxic exposures and the urinary excretion of these electrolytes would also be expected to decrease (11,27,90). This effect of appetite, however, can be eliminated by a constant diet. In all such studies, summarized in Table 3, there is a consistent and statistically significant decrease in urinary potassium excretion, indicating potassium retention, and increases in plasma potassium have been reported (45). In the first three of these studies cited, there was a significant increase in sodium excretion. However, in general this renal response was not accompanied by changes in plasma sodium.

Studies on the effects of hypoxia on divalent cations are limited (11,34,35,46,69), and fewer have actually studied balances of intake and output (35,46). In human subjects at 12,400 ft altitude and on ad libitum and unmeasured dietary intakes, both Ca and Mg urinary excretion rates were reduced, but the serum concentrations of the two were affected differently. Thus, serum Mg increased and Ca decreased (11). Similarly, Hannon et al. (34) observed a tendency for serum Mg to increase during the first week at 14,100 ft in men on an ad libitum diet, but no changes in Ca were observed. However, in the only study in which Ca and Mg intakes and outputs were measured in

Table 3. Urinary excretion of Na and K (mEq/l) in subjects on a constant diet at high altitude.

Sea Level			High Altitude						
day-2	day-1	ascent	day 1	day 2	day 3	day 4	n	alt.(ft)	Ref.
135/67[1]				139/53[2]			10	12,000	(51)
127/59	150/64		148/56	176/36	182/52		10	12,000	(39)
88/86	68/88	63/52	56/32	93/50	115/52	98/65	5	11,500	(84)
	101/170[3]			125/137[3]			5	14,100	(17)
87/124	80/116	100/96	78/85	107/95	92/88	84/80	10	14,100	(45)

1. Na/K values, 2. average of 3 days at both sea level and high altitude, 3. average of 6 days. All other abbreviations are as in Table 2.

man on ad libitum diets, no differences in either Ca or Mg balances or serum concentrations of these cations were reported (46). Presently, therefore, we are without explanation for the suggestive evidence of increased serum Mg and decreased Ca levels at high altitude (11). Studies in rats in which the voluntary decrease in food intake at high altitude was matched in paired rats at sea level revealed decreases in urinary excretion of both Ca and Mg in both groups, but the decrease was greater in the pair fed sea level group than the hypoxic group, suggesting a more positive balance in the sea level group (35). This could be due to the diuretic effect of hypoxia, especially noticeable in the rat (88), which would promote general reduction in tubular reabsorption of most ions more at altitude than at sea level. The slight, albeit statistically significant, difference between sea level pair fed animals and those exposed to hypoxia was of little consequence to over all body stores (35). The major effect on divalent cations presently defined is the effect associated with decreased appetite. When intake is controlled little effect is observed in Ca excretion (69).

In summary, with the various methods used in different studies by different investigators there is general agreement that hypohydration is a consequence of ascent to high altitude. In man the volume of fluid loss is about 2 liters during the first week at altitude. The hypohydration is probably not only a consequence of short-term effects, but also the longer-term effects resulting in losses in lean body mass occurring up to two weeks (18,46). The studies in mice (46) would suggest an increased effect of hypohydration with more severe hypoxia, and in human subjects significant evidence for hypohydration has been observed even at the relatively moderate altitude of 11,500 ft (44), and in most studies at higher altitudes. Typically on an ad libitum food intake, the associated hypophagia would be expected to cause a reduction in the extracellular electrolyte content. In fact, this has been shown with reductions in Na, K, and Ca (34). If, however, the effect of dietary intake is minimized by administration of a controlled diet, high altitude is consistently associated with positive K balance (17,45). The mechanisms underlying these imbalances will be discussed below.

MECHANISMS OF HYPOXIA-INDUCED HYPOHYDRATION

It would seem probable that the lower atmospheric density and increased ventilation occurring at high altitude would promote an increased insensible water loss. Although this has been reported to account for up to a liter of additional water loss at 12,000 ft (39), other systems that are under physiological control, i.e., thirst and urine flow, are also major contributors to the body fluid deficit in a majority of other studies. In addition to increased insensible water loss, decreased thirst, and increased urine flow, decreased appetite also leads to a loss in body water as a consequence of the loss in lean body mass (e.g. 18,32,46,53). Both the decreased thirst drive and the decreased food intake recover toward sea level values as exposure is extended to one to two weeks (32). The focus of the following sections will deal with those aspects of water balance that are under physiological control by mechanisms responsive to the state of body hydration.

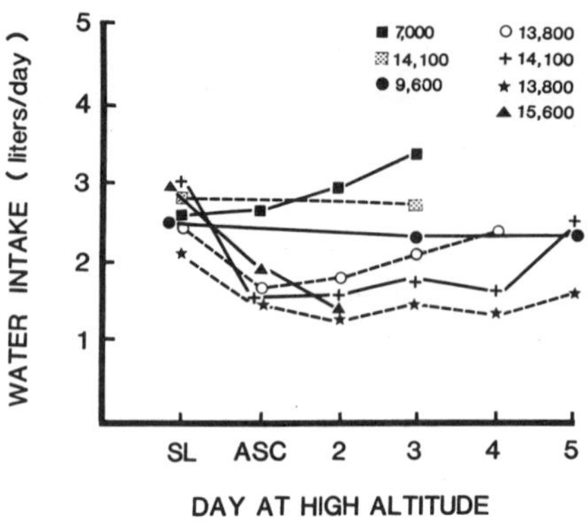

Figure 1. Water intake in human subjects at high altitude. 7,000 and 13,800 ft studies (unpublished observations, Claybaugh, Wade, Brooks, and Cucinell, n = 8 at 7,000 ft, and 10 at both 13,800 ft studies); 14,100 ft, indicated by stippled square (ref. 18, n = 10), 14,100 ft indicated by "+"sign (ref. 45, n = 10); 9,600 ft (ref. 27, n = 5), 15,600 ft (ref. 90, n = 4).

Effects of Hypoxia on Thirst and Mechanisms of Control

A decrease in water intake of approximately one liter per day is often observed during the day of ascent and the following day at altitudes of about 14,000 ft (Figure 1) when water is allowed ad libitum and exercise is not a major portion of the study. The figure suggests several generalities regarding the decreased thirst at altitude. First, in all studies except the one at 7,000 ft, when daily assessments were obtained a decrease in water intake was observed. Second, often when assessments are made after the first 2 days this difference in balance may not be observed.

As previously suggested (32), this effect on thirst is probably independent of the hypophagia. For example, in human subjects normal water intake can be accompanied by a 30% reduction in food intake, while in rats the hypodipsic effects of hypoxia appear to be greater than the hypophagic effects (32). In Figure 1, the significant decrease in thirst observed in 10 men at 13,800 ft, indicated by open circles, returned to normal levels of thirst during the third and fourth days. Caloric intake in that study, however, was 2,780 kCal/day at sea level, 1,530 on the day of ascent, and 1,270, 1,320, and 1700 on subsequent days at altitude, i.e., was significantly depressed by approximately 30% throughout the four days (unpublished observations, Claybaugh, Brooks, and Cucinell) despite the recovery of thirst. Such evidence suggests independent control of appetite and thirst suppression during hypoxia, and that a decreased thirst drive could contribute to the hypohydration.

Surprisingly few studies have investigated the mechanism of the decrease in thirst drive associated with hypoxia. The response is particularly evident in rats and the mechanism has been extensively studied in this model by Jones et al. (48,49). A possible role of ADH in the thirst drive mechanism was ruled out because both normal rats and rats with hereditary diabetes insipidus showed a similar decrease in water intake (48). In addition, nephrectomy did not affect the suppression in thirst drive, an observation that would suggest a minimal role if any for circulating angiotensin II (49). A decreased central production of angiotensin II, however, may contribute to the decreased thirst drive. Thus, Arregui et al. (3) reported that angiotensin converting enzyme (ACE) concentrations in certain areas of the brain are decreased after three weeks of hypoxia (10% O_2) in rats. Fifteen days after this exposure, the ACE concentrations had returned to pre-exposure values. In rats, the osmotic threshold for thirst was increased with hypoxia, but the sensitivity of the osmotic-thirst relationship was not altered in the studies by Jones et al. (49), suggesting an additional inhibitory influence on thirst separate from osmoreceptor control. Lastly, they also studied the volume regulatory mechanisms of thirst by producing a hypovolemic state by subcutaneous injection of polyethylene glycol. In rats receiving polyethylene glycol the thirst drive was suppressed during hypoxia by about 29% compared to similarly treated rats during normoxia exposure (49). Further data on these experiments were, however, not shown (49). Whether hypovolemia was capable of stimulating thirst in the hypoxic situation and whether the sensitivity of this stimulus was altered were not investigated. There are, therefore, questions remaining regarding the effect of hypoxia on the volume receptor mediated thirst mechanisms.

More recent studies regarding atrial natriuretic factor (ANF), suggest another avenue of future research. It has been shown that ANF when administered intracerebroventricularly (icv), will inhibit the dipsogenic response to icv administered angiotensin II (42). Whether or not there is an increase in central ANF activity during hypoxia is not known. However, recent studies have shown hypoxic stimulation of ANF from isolated rat and rabbit hearts (5), and hypoxia induced elevations of plasma levels of ANF in rats (59) and humans (22). This poses the possibility of increased circulating levels of ANF affecting thirst centers in the brain, possibly gaining access via circumventricular sites. Clearly, this is speculative, but serves to point out the lack of understanding of the mechanisms involved in the hypoxia induced inhibition of thirst.

Effects of Hypoxia on Urine Flow

Urine flow is also affected by hypoxia. A diuresis associated with hypoxia was probably first reported 50 years ago by Armstrong (2). Human subjects exposed to a simulated altitude of 12,000 ft for four and seven hours excreted up to 300% more urine and with a lower specific gravity than at sea level. He also noticed that the diuresis was not only dilutional but osmotic in nature. Studies over the next ten years confirmed these studies in unanesthetized rats and also demonstrated that there was an increased chloride excretion during the early phases of the diuresis (94). Burrill et al. (10) also demonstrated the chloriduria, but also a natriuresis and kaliuresis associated with increased urine flow during 2 hour exposures to 18,000 ft in 6 men. About 20 years later, Ullmann (19,93) provided new information demonstrating that this diuretic response to hypoxia was probably nonspecific. Thus it was shown that not only hypoxia of 14 to 10% O_2 but also simple hyperventilation produced a diuresis (Figure 2). It was further demonstrated by these investigators that hypoxia, with

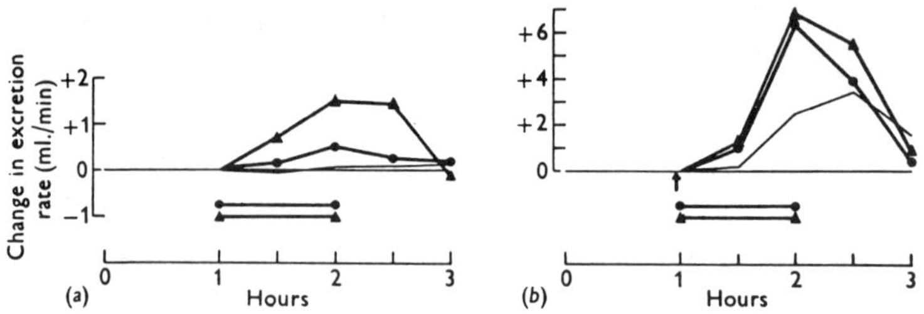

Figure 2. Changes in urinary excretion rate in response to hypoxia and hyperventilation. Each line represents average values for 6 subjects when dehydrated, panel a, and after drinking a standard volume of water, panel b. The thin line, bottom line in both figures, represents the control response. The circles indicate the response to breathing 14 - 10% O_2 in N_2 for one hour between hours 1 and 2. The triangles represent the response to 1 hour of forced breathing or hyperventilation. The time of experimental exposure is indicated by the two parallel lines beneath both panels of the figure. (Reproduced with permission, ref. 93)

or without hypocapnia, was associated with an equal magnitude of increased urine flow.

They further demonstrated that if hypoxia caused "distress" the subjects rapidly became oliguric. They concluded that "with acute anoxia the basal rate of secretion of antidiuretic hormone (ADH) may be diminished." However, they stated that the oliguria associated with distress "appeared to be the result of a sudden discharge of ADH from the neurohypophysis." In support of involvement of ADH in the hypoxia induced diuresis Ullmann reported unpublished observations that with no accompanying hypocapnia the response could be eliminated by the intravenous administration of ADH (unpublished observations cited in ref. 93). As will be discussed later, these conclusions appear to have been an accurate hypothesis regarding the ADH response to hypoxia.

It must be evident that the decreased thirst drive and increased urine flow cannot coexist very long. In fact, an increase in urine flow during the first 24 hours of hypoxic exposure is essentially never observed during ad libitum water intake (11,18,27,45,69,90). However, what is usually observed is probably best termed an inappropriate urine flow for the water intake. Thus, with a reduction of water intake of approximately 1 liter per day for the day of transition and the next 3 days at 14,100 ft, Janoski et al. (45) found urine flow to be reduced significantly only on 2 of those four days and only by an average of 600 and 500 ml on those days. The cumulative effect of this imbalance alone could account for a dehydration of over 3 liters during the first 4 days at altitude.

Inhibition of ADH in Response to Acute Mild Hypoxia

This inappropriate urine flow may be a reflection of the distinct diuresis observed in the acute setting. Few studies have investigated the possible role of ADH in this acute response despite the earlier suggestion (93). Over a decade later the first reports of reduced ADH in response to hypoxia were demonstrated in the rat (88) and human (12). Rats show this diuretic response even at quite severe hypoxia equivalent to 24,000 ft altitude. With this model Subramanian et al. (88) first reported a decreased plasma ADH concentration with hypoxia. At more severe hypoxia, i.e., equivalent to about 26,000 ft, oliguria accompanied by significantly increased ADH occurred. A similar response of ADH to hypoxia was reported in human subjects breathing hypoxic gas mixtures through a mouth piece (12). Figure 3 shows the response of eight subjects to mild and severe hypoxia. It is important to note that during this 20 minute exposure to the various gases, only the mild hypoxia elicited a reduction in plasma ADH concentration. With more severe hypoxia most of the subjects returned toward sea level values. This response of ADH to mild hypoxia was recently confirmed in a field experiment where 15 men involved in cable car construction made rapid ascents of about 6600 ft, worked for the week and returned to base for the week end (68). Blood samples taken before and after the ascent and descent revealed a reduced ADH concentration to about 25% of basal values when the subjects were at altitude. Although not statistically analyzed, an approximate 35% reduction in plasma ADH concentration was also reported during the first three days at 11,500 ft altitude in the field (8). Thus, of the few studies that have investigated this aspect of the ADH response to

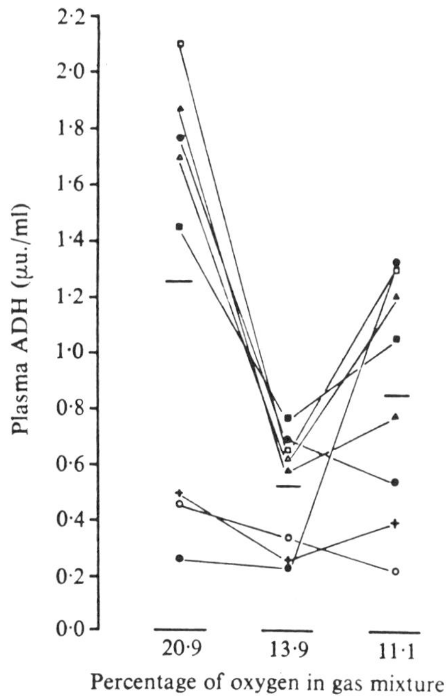

Figure 3. Effect of breathing various percentages of O_2 in N_2 for 20 min on the concentration of antidiuretic hormone (ADH) in the plasma of eight men. The horizontal bars are the mean values for the eight subjects designated by individual symbols. The order of exposures were randomized. (Reproduced with permission, ref. 12)

hypoxia, most have observed a decrease in plasma ADH concentration (8,12,68) with mild hypoxia, but with severe hypoxia of 11 to 10 %, accompanied by no symptoms of nausea or fainting, ADH concentration is unchanged during acute exposures (4,12,25,37). Additional support for a role of ADH in the diuresis of acute mild hypoxia was recently reported (29). These authors observed that hypobaric breathing increased urine flow in normal rats, but rats with diabetes insipidus exhibited a reduced urine flow and oliguria (29). The evidence, therefore, strongly favors a role of decreased ADH in the diuretic response to acute mild hypoxia for the following reasons: 1) administration of exogenous ADH inhibits the diuresis, 2) the diuresis does not occur in the absence of a functional ADH system, and 3) plasma ADH levels are significantly reduced by mild hypoxia.

One possible mechanism for the inhibitory effect of hypoxia on ADH release may involve the baroreceptors, but this has not been directly studied. The proposed mechanism argues that the increased ventilation causes a greater negativity in the intrapleural space, thereby increasing thoracic blood volume and atrial stretch (12,93). This is supported by the reports of increased thoracic fluid volume at high altitude as determined by transthoracic electrical impedance measurements (43,76). It must be taken into consideration, however, that impedance measurements cannot distinguish between intravascular and extravascular fluid. The fluid accumulation could, therefore, represent subclinical pulmonary edema as well as increased thoracic blood volume. A second mechanism potentially involved in the ADH inhibition with hypoxia is the apparent chemoreceptor response to CO_2. Philbin et al. (66) reported a stimulation of ADH with addition of CO_2 to inspired air in constantly hyperventilated, anesthetized dogs, with an associated decrease in urine flow. Conversely, they also showed an inhibition of ADH with hyperventilation and hypocapnia and an associated increase in urine flow compared to control conditions. Thus, with no change in ventilation rate the hypocapnia was associated with a decrease in plasma ADH concentration. Unfortunately, those studies were flawed by a lack of statistical analyses, but the stimulatory effect of CO_2 and acidosis has been confirmed in subsequent studies (72,97). Further studies of possible inhibitory effects of hypocapnia without changes in ventilation are apparently lacking. Thus, although the data implicating a reduction in circulating ADH as the underlying mechanism for the hypoxia induced diuresis is rather compelling, the control mechanisms explaining the reduction in ADH are not clear.

Stimulation of ADH Release by Hypoxia

Prior to any reports of a decrease in ADH in response to hypoxia, ADH had been shown to be stimulated during hypoxia. ADH stimulation by chemoreceptor mechanisms was first demonstrated by Share and Levy (79). In the intact organism, therefore, there are probably at least two effects of hypoxia on ADH, inhibitory and stimulatory. Studies regarding the stimulatory effects of hypoxia are abundant (1,13,14,24,26,72,73,75,79,95,97). At least part of this stimulatory effect would seem to be mediated through chemoreceptor stimulation. In Share and Levy's experiments, deoxygenated blood was perfused through an isolated carotid sinus of anesthetized dogs. They reported not only that ADH could be stimulated in this manner, but also observed that if the dogs were spontaneously breathing with the vagus nerves intact ADH was not increased (79). Thus, the conflicting input of baroreceptor and chemoreceptor responses to hypoxia were recognized over twenty years ago. The exact afferent pathway for the hypoxic stimulation of ADH via carotid sinus area stimulation is complicated by the presence of both baroreceptor and chemoreceptor afferents in the carotid sinus nerve. The stimulation of baroreceptor nerves would be expected to inhibit ADH release (80), where the stimulation of the chemoreceptor nerves would be expected to stimulate ADH release (79). Interestingly, when the carotid sinus nerve is electrically stimulated in the intact anesthetized dog, ADH, as assessed indirectly by urine flow changes with no changes in GFR, is stimulated (60), suggesting a dominance of chemoreceptor afferent input in this situation. In an attempt to specifically determine the afferent pathway, Anderson et al. (1) found that the antidiuretic response to hypoxic stimulation of ADH was retained after chemoreceptor but not baroreceptor denervation. Furthermore, their measured cardiovascular responses to hypoxia revealed no alteration in baroreceptor input. For instance, there was no change in cardiac output, mean arterial blood pressure, stroke volume, or GFR. Although they had measured increases in ADH in response to the hypoxia (10% O_2) in intact dogs, ADH was not measured in the denervation experiments. Instead, decreases in urine flow and increases urine osmolality with no changes in GFR were used as indirect evidence of ADH release.

For the most part, reports of ADH stimulation in response to hypoxia are of an acute design, that is, within two hours of exposure, and of fairly severe hypoxia, less than 11% O_2, and in a situation where hyperventilation is prevented (1,26,72,73,79,97) or cannot occur, such as in the fetus (20). In human subjects increases in plasma ADH concentration have only been reported in association with high altitude pulmonary edema (HAPE) (30,83) and during distress such as headache, nausea, or fainting (4,13,37). In animals exposed to hypoxia with no additional CO_2 in the inspired air, and allowed to spontaneously ventilate, stimulation of ADH has been reported with severe hypoxia, 10% O_2 in dogs (75,95) and 7% O_2 in goats (14). As yet unexplained increases in urinary ADH excretion during hypobaric exposures have been repeatedly observed at levels of hypoxia that do not lead to increased plasma concentrations of the hormone in the acute setting (13). When urinary ADH excretion was determined in human subjects over periods of days, as seen in Figure 4, the first 24 hours was associated with an increase in hormone excretion, which returns to sea level values during the next 24 hours. It should be noted that even at less severe hypoxia equivalent to 11,000 ft this response was still evident, albeit reduced.

The increased urinary excretion of ADH does not appear to occur if ascent is gradual (36). So it would seem likely that acute induction of hypoxia is necessary for the response.

The stimulation of ADH in association with hypoxia may be more complex than pure chemoreceptor mediated stimulation of the hormone. If the stimulation is due to only chemoreceptor mediated mechanisms, why does the response disappear so quickly? No studies have focused on the disappearance of

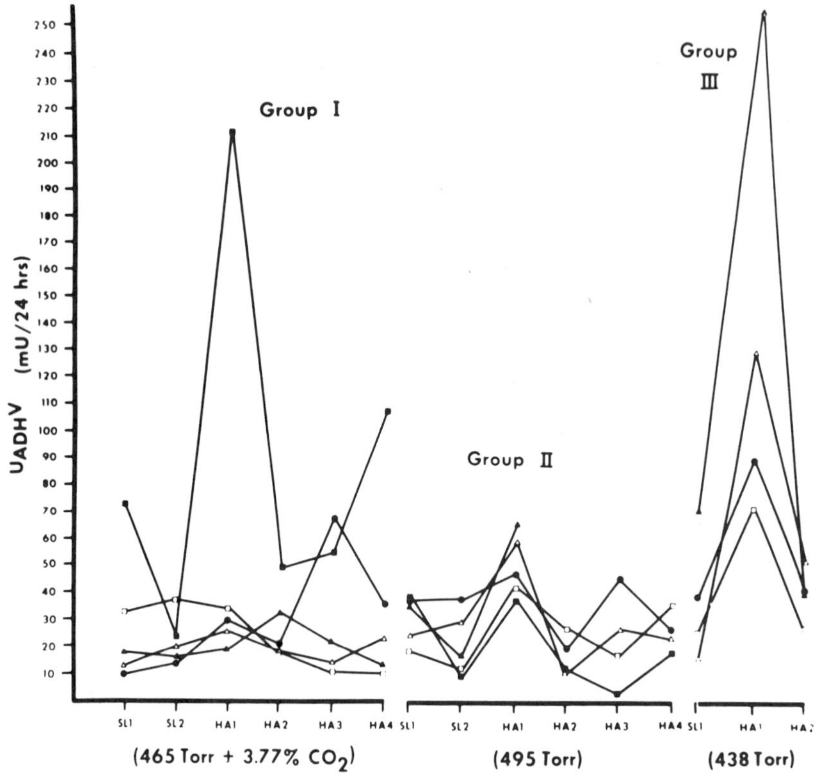

Figure 4. Urinary ADH excretion during hypobaric chamber exposure. For comparison, 495 Torr is approximately equivalent to 11,000 ft, and 438 Torr is about 14,000 ft. CO_2 was added to the inspired air in group I and the ambient pressure was lowered to produce equal levels of hypoxemia between groups I and II with eucapnia and hypocapnia respectively. Only groups II and III had statistically significant increases in the urinary excretion of ADH during the first 24 h of hypobaria. (Reproduced with permission, Ref. 13)

the response, and only two observations of stimulation and spontaneous recovery have been reported (13,14). Unfortunately, those may involve different mechanisms because of the different time frames of the studies, i.e., hours as opposed to days. Of possible importance regarding the increase in urinary excretion of ADH predominantly during the first day of exposure (13) is sleep apnea at high altitude. Sutton et al. (89) have reported the overnight arterial oxygen saturation in subjects at 17,600 ft. to be markedly reduced compared to daytime values or to values obtained from subjects taking acetazolamide. Thus, the hypoxemia is intensified at night, during which time plasma ADH levels have not been assessed. It is likely that the first night at high altitude is associated with greater effects of sleep apnea since there is less degree of acclimatization. Another interacting influence on ADH control may be the development of a reduced sensitivity of ADH to osmotic stimuli. Blume et al. (7) observed a remarkable increase in plasma osmolality which rose from

290 mOsm/kg to 302 mOsm/kg during ascent to 21,000 ft and after 26 days above 18,000 ft. Despite the increase in plasma osmolality, plasma ADH concentration and urinary ADH excretion remained unchanged. The nature of the time course of this change in osmotic sensitivity is unknown, but probably represents a separate inhibitory effect on ADH release such as hypocapnia which may persist after the recovery of hypoxemia (31). How these various factors interact in the control of ADH is unknown, but in combination or at different times of the acclimatization period they may account for maintenance of normal sea level values of ADH after one or two days at high altitude.

Acute hypoxia, unlike the studies of Blume et al. (7), has been shown by essentially all investigators to be unaccompanied by changes in plasma osmolality, ruling out osmoreceptor involvement in the regulation of ADH. In human subjects, acute exposure to less than 11% O_2 is usually accompanied by no change in ADH (4,12,37), but in the studies by Ashack et al. (4) and Heyes et al. (37) an increase in some of the subjects exposed to 10.5% O_2 was observed. In those subjects there was a coincident hypotension and nausea, either of which could stimulate ADH independent of chemoreceptor control. In animal experiments some of the stimulation may be due to "stress". In support of this idea is an alternative interpretation of some interesting studies by Raff et al. (73). In those studies, preinfusion with 2 ng/kg/min ACTH in anesthetized, artificially ventilated dogs caused a stimulation of endogenous glucocorticoid, which was elevated but waning during the imposition of hypoxia 80 minutes after stopping the ACTH infusion. The preinfusion of ACTH as compared to saline control greatly attenuated the increases in ACTH, cortisol, and ADH in response to hypoxia (Figure 5). The presence of glucocorticoids has been noted in previous work to apparently inhibit the response of ADH to nonspecific stress (70), and may be in part an explanation for the observations of Raff et al. (73). It should be emphasized that in these studies (73) the ADH response to hypoxia

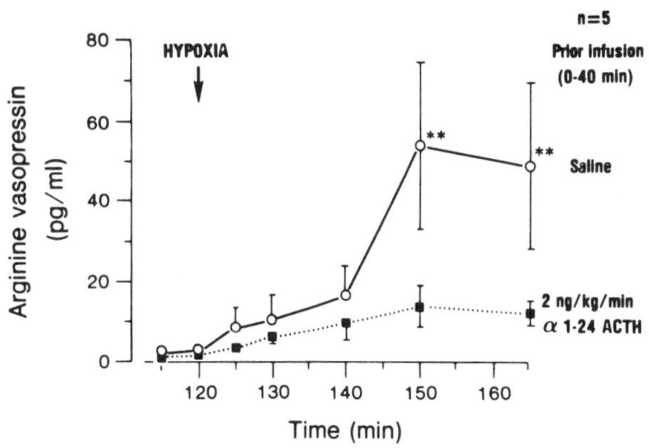

Figure 5. Plasma ADH (arginine vasopressin) responses in anesthetized artificially ventilated dogs inspiring 11% O_2 during hypoxia with and without prior ACTH infusion (2 ng/kg.min) for a 40 min period. Hypoxia was begun 80 min after cessation of ACTH infusion while glucocorticoid levels continued to fall. (Reproduced with permission, Ref. 73)

was not eliminated, and therefore does not rule out an independent role for chemoreceptor mediated ADH response. Such a stress response of ADH to acute hypoxia may also contribute to the transient increase in urinary ADH excretion upon rapid exposure to hypoxia (13), and may partially explain the transient increase in plasma ADH seen in the goat exposed to 7% O_2 (14). As mentioned previously, essentially all studies investigating hypoxia-induced stimulation of ADH are conducted within two hours. In this study on goats, ADH was assessed hourly during six hours of exposure and was found to be increased only during the first two hours.

As a final comment regarding ADH stimulation by hypoxia, it is important to point out that few studies have attempted to inhibit the response. We have mentioned the spontaneous disappearance (13,14) which needs further characterization, and the inhibition of the response by prior administration of ACTH (73). There is one other report of inhibition of hypoxia stimulated ADH release by inhibition of the prostaglandin system. Walker (95) demonstrated an inhibition of the acute response of ADH to hypoxia by iv infusion of meclofenamate (2 mg/kg bolus followed by 2 mg/kg/h) in conscious dogs while breathing 10% O_2. The exact means by which prostaglandins mediate the ADH response is unclear, but since meclofenamate does not cross the blood brain barrier, and since none of the measured cardiovascular parameters were altered, Walker concluded that central and cardiovascular effects of prostaglandins would not appear to be involved. This inhibitory effect of meclofenamate could not be demonstrated in newborn pigs during asphyxia, suggesting perhaps a different mechanism for the additional stimulatory effect of hypercapnia (56).

Effects of Hypoxia on Glucocorticoids

Aside from ADH effects on water balance, it has been proposed that increased glucocorticoids may also effect water balance at high altitude (8,83). It is beyond the scope of this review to discuss the proposed mechanisms for the interaction of glucocorticoids with ADH and water metabolism, but in the context of the present discussion it is important to recognize that with unchanging plasma ADH, infusion of cortisol can induce an increase in free water clearance (70). Thus, cortisol appears to have independent effects on water balance that can override the effects of ADH. The response of cortisol to hypoxia is somewhat similar to that of ADH. Thus, there are reports of no response (13,37), and stimulation (8,27,40,83,85,90) in man. In animals the response seems to be more consistently that of stimulation (e.g. 72,73), and has been shown to be dependent upon intact carotid sinus nerves (58). Interestingly, in the study conducted by Heyes et al. (37), 8 subjects were subjected to hypobaric hypoxia of 10.5% O_2, 4 of which responded with increases in ADH and also were more distressed by the hypoxia as mentioned earlier. Only those 4 subjects also showed similar increases in cortisol. Under such circumstances there may not be an antidiuretic response to the increased ADH. Brahmachari et al. (8) observed a slightly elevated plasma ADH level in subjects after a week of exposure to 11,500 ft. Regardless of the direct cause of the ADH response, there was nearly a doubling in urine flow associated with a 240% increase in plasma cortisol. Subjectively, these data are compatible with a possible ameliorating effect of increased glucocorticoid activity on the antidiuretic response to ADH at high altitude.

MECHANISMS OF SALT IMBALANCES

As with water balance, salt balances are influenced by acute effects of hypoxia and also long term effects, and the two effects can be seen to cancel one another at times. For instance, acute exposure to 14 to 10% O_2 increases the excretion of Na, K and Cl (10,19,93,94). It would seem possible that the mechanism underlying this response may be similar to the presumed mechanism underlying the immersion induced natriuresis and kaliuresis, namely increased thoracic blood volume. As mentioned previously, hyperventilation could be causing an increased thoracic blood volume induced by the increased pleural cavity negativity. Such a proposed mechanism for the increased excretion of electrolytes is probably not the whole explanation. Unlike the diuretic responses which are similar during acute hypocapnic and eucapnic hypoxia, the natriuretic, kaliuretic, and chloriduria responses are attenuated during eucapnic hypoxia exposures as compared to hypocapnic exposures (93). Also, Ullmann (93) observed that both hypoxia with hypocapnia and hyperventilation with hypocapnia produced an increased Na and K excretion at the expense of hydrogen ion and ammonium, suggesting that the hypocapnia played a major role in the solute portion of this acute diuretic response.

Despite prolonged hypocapnia at high altitude (31), however, even when subjects are fed constant diets, excretion of K and Cl are not increased (45). Instead, excretion rates of both K and Cl are decreased and may result in increased plasma levels of these ions (45). Since circulating levels of bicarbonate remain low, it would seem that the more avid reabsorption of Cl anion by the kidney would be a consequence of less bicarbonate anion available to accompany the reabsorption of the cations. As originally proposed by Slater (84), the enhanced reabsorption of K may be due to the reduced circulating levels of aldosterone and, possibly during the first two days, to the effect of extracellular alkalosis in promoting a shift of K into the cells. Although Na excretion at high altitude is usually not greatly increased when subjects are on constant diets (18,45), there are some reports of significant increases (39,51,84) which serve to point out a tendency toward a slight natriuretic effect of the high altitude environment. This too is a typical renal response to reduced circulating levels of aldosterone and suggests a possible involvement of increased ANF.

Little information is available on the control of divalent cations except as discussed earlier in this chapter. We are aware of one study in which parathyroid hormone was measured in cattle during treadmill exercise at simulated high altitude. Although these investigators demonstrated that the hormone was stimulated under these conditions, no sea level control values were obtained (6).

Atrial Natriuretic Factor Responses to Hypoxia

As mentioned earlier in this chapter, acute exposure to hypoxia produces a diuresis accompanied by an increase in the excretion of most ions that can be mimicked by simple hyperventilation. Although hypocapnia is an important factor in this response the possible increased thoracic blood volume could also contribute. Such an increase in atrial stretch would be expected to stimulate the release of ANF. This response has been recently demonstrated in rats after 21 days of exposure to hypobaric hypoxia equivalent to 18,000 ft (59). There was also a 50% increase in plasma ANF levels after 3 days, but this was not statistically significant. More recently, a stimulation of ANF was reported in human subjects after 2h of breathing 10% O_2 and 4.5% CO_2 (22). The resulting blood gas analyses revealed hypoxemia with a slight hypercapnia; in addition, diastolic blood pressure was increased, thus complicating the interpretation of exact mechanisms involved in the stimulation. Also in that study, as disturbingly and frequently reported with ANF assessments, there was no accompanying increase in fractional sodium excretion. Although du Souich et al. (22) observed a significant correlation between diastolic blood pressure and ANF levels in their experiments, another mechanism for the release of ANF could be independent of or in addition to atrial stretch. Baertchi et al. (5) observed several fold increases in the release rate of ANF from the effluent of isolated perfused hearts of rats and rabbits within 10 minutes of exposure to hypoxia. The level of hypoxia employed dropped the PO_2 in the perfusate from 563 mmHg to 21 mmHg. After 8-11 min of reoxygenation the ANF release rates were restored to original control values. These data pose the possibility of direct effects of hypoxemia on the cardiac tissue in stimulating the release of ANF. Taken together, all of these studies indicate that hypoxia stimulates ANF release.

The role of increased ANF levels in the overall diuretic response to acute hypoxic exposures has yet to be determined, but the potential involvement of ANF in contributing to many of the responses discussed clearly will be the focus of further studies. For instance, aside from studies on hypoxia, ANF has been shown to effect Na excretion (21), to inhibit ADH release (41,55), to inhibit thirst (42) and to inhibit renin and aldosterone secretion (e.g. 9).

Inhibition of Aldosterone by Hypoxia

Regarding the decreased aldosterone secretion at high altitude, it is important to recognize that although most studies indicate a decrease in aldosterone secretion (15,16,84,85,90) a few have shown that aldosterone can be increased (27,40). The latter, as discussed earlier, is probably due to reduction in dietary sodium intake. The former, however, is an apparent direct effect of hypoxia which reduces aldosterone secretion. Thus, essentially all studies in which renin and aldosterone levels have been simultaneously determined report a decrease in the aldosterone to renin ratio associated with hypoxia (e.g. 15,16,6263,69,81,85), suggesting an independent effect of hypoxia on renin and aldosterone. It would appear that hypoxia has no direct effect on the release of renin. The experiments of Spath et al. (86) serve as a good example of the evidence. They perfused the in situ kidney of the dog with hypoxemic

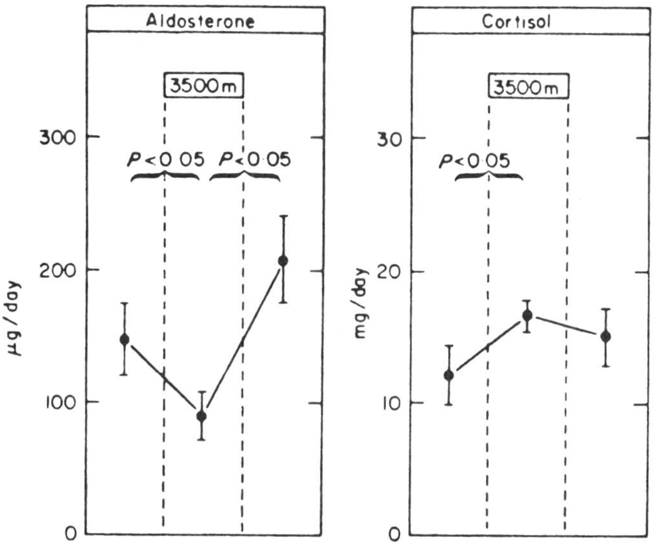

Figure 6. Aldosterone and cortisol secretion before, during, and after high altitude exposure. The values at high altitude were obtained during the third and fourth days after ascent, considering the day of ascent as the first day. (Reproduced with permission, ref. 85)

blood via an extracorporeal lung circuit allowing the rest of the blood of the animal to be at normal oxygen tensions. In this situation renin release, as detected in the renal venous blood, was unchanged as compared to control situations. The mechanism underlying the inhibition of aldosterone secretion by hypoxia has been an interesting and elusive area of research for several years.

Slater et al. (85) reported a decrease in aldosterone secretion at a mild level of hypoxia equivalent to about 11,500 ft altitude (Figure 6) which occurred in spite of increased plasma renin activity and increased cortisol secretion.

Several reports introduced evidence suggesting a possible role of decreased angiotensin converting enzyme (ACE) in the reduced aldosterone secretion observed (e.g. 63,87). The reports of Milledge et al. (62,63) were based on assessments of plasma concentrations of ACE in human subjects and the assumption had to be made that possibly this reflected general ACE activity such as the conversion of angiotensin I to angiotensin II during the blood passage through the lungs. However, these studies have since been retracted (61), but more importantly, decreased aldosterone associated with similar circulating angiotensin II levels has been observed during hypoxia compared to normoxia during states of exercise in healthy subjects (57) and patients with chronic obstructive lung disease (71). Thus, despite several reports of decrease and no change (4,15) in plasma ACE, the end result is that even with similar angiotensin II levels aldosterone secretion is decreased. However, Colice and Ramirez (16) dispelled the next logical explanation, i.e., that perhaps the adrenal gland was less responsive to angiotensin II. Figure 7 shows the

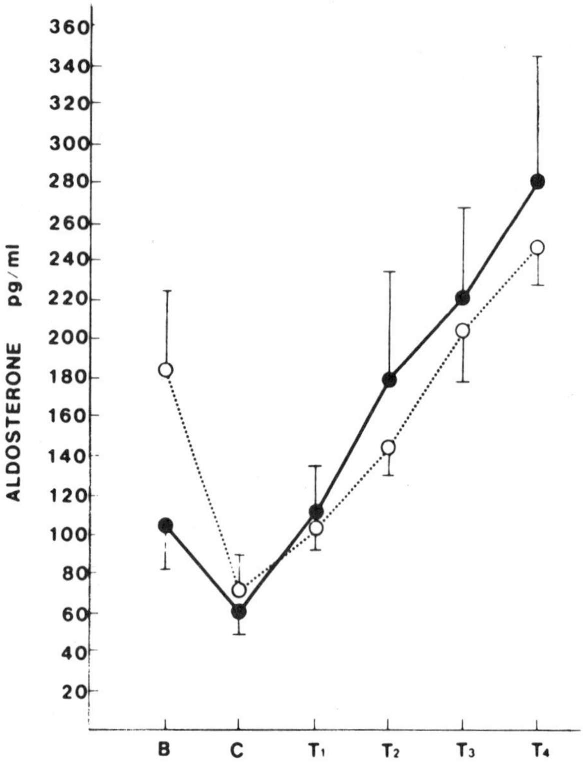

Figure 7. Open circles designate the hypoxemic state achieved by nitrogen inhalation sufficient to maintain 90% hemoglobin saturation. Closed circles designate the normoxic state. "B" is the baseline value followed by 30 min of rest until the control value "C". T1 through T4 are 20 min intervals with doses of infused angiotensin II increasing from 2 to 4 to 8 and finally 12 ng.kg-1.min-1. (Reproduced with permission, Ref. 16)

responses of nine subjects to 4 successive 20-min periods of increasing angiotensin II infusion on plasma aldosterone concentration during normoxic and hypoxic conditions. The data do not support the hypothesis of decreased adrenal sensitivity to angiotensin II. Similarly, the work of Keynes et al. (50) and more recently of Colice and Ramirez (15) would suggest that the adrenal sensitivity to adrenocorticotropic hormone (ACTH) in the release of aldosterone or cortisol is also not altered by hypoxia.

A recent report suggests that the decrease in aldosterone secretion is not dependent upon systemic hypoxemia. Schmidt et al. (78) have found that in the anesthetized cat perfusion of the vascularly isolated carotid body with venous blood for 45 min reduced plasma aldosterone concentration. Return of arterial blood to the perfusate was accompanied by a rapid increase in aldosterone levels. Although these experiments do not rule out a complicating effect of hypercapnia, they clearly indicate a different approach for further studies on the mechanism of decreased aldosterone secretion with hypoxia.

HORMONES AND ALTITUDE SICKNESSES

For the purposes of this discussion acute mountain sickness (AMS) will be considered as the combination of headache, nausea, loss of appetite and dizziness often encountered at high altitude. These are the major manifestations of the sickness and are among over sixty items in a standard questionnaire (77). The degrees of symptoms can vary from absence to very severe and immobilizing. High altitude cerebral edema (HACE) may in fact be an extreme development of the underlying causes for the headache and nausea typically observed in AMS. However, the symptoms become very severe including severe papilledema, stupor, seizures, coma, paralysis and death (82). High altitude pulmonary edema (HAPE) is a consequence of increased pulmonary arterial pressure at altitude, probably greater in the victims who eventually become ill, and also seems to be associated with individual susceptibility (83). Along with HACE it too can be fatal.

Certainly among the most influential reports stimulating much research in the endocrinology of water and electrolyte balance at high altitude was that of Singh et al. (82). Among the clinical findings associated with AMS these investigators observed an antidiuresis in the individuals predisposed to illness during the lag time between the arrival at high altitude and the next 6 to 96 hours. Subsequently, several of the same investigators studied some of the hormonal responses of 10 HAPE-prone subjects. All of these subjects had developed HAPE within 3 to 4 months prior to the investigation. Of these, 4 developed HAPE in this study within the first 3 days at 11,500 ft. In 3 of the 4 there was a marked increase in plasma ADH concentration. Hackett et al. (30) confirmed this finding in 4 of 4 subjects who developed HAPE at about 14,000 ft. Since predisposed patients have an antidiuresis, and since improvement is preceded by a diuresis, Singh et al (83) proposed a possible causal role of increased ADH in the development of HAPE. They also suggested a possible blunting or overriding of the ADH effects by elevated cortisol levels which frequently occur.

AMS is not always associated with elevated plasma levels of ADH (13,30). In some instances it is, and urinary ADH excretion has been observed to be markedly elevated prior to the onset of severe headache symptoms in 2 of 2 individuals (13). Moreover, with continuation of symptoms the ADH excretion does not remain elevated but begins to decline. Pain and nausea are both potent stimuli for ADH release, but continuation of symptoms with decreasing urinary ADH excretion suggests other mechanisms for the release of ADH under these circumstances. In addition, increases in urinary ADH excretion during the first 24 hours of high altitude exposure occur with or without symptoms (13).

Regardless of the mechanism, ADH has been observed to be increased in association with both HAPE and prior to AMS. Is there a possible involvement of ADH in these illnesses? This becomes a very speculative hypothesis; however, certain evidence does suggest possible involvement. ADH, in addition to its antidiuretic effects, of course is a potent vasopressor hormone. Somewhat unique effects of ADH in inducing increases in pulmonary arterial pressure and pulmonary edema have been reported. Swies (91) demonstrated that administration of large doses of ADH to rats will cause a sequential increase in arterial, left atrial, pulmonary arterial, and finally right atrial pressure. The last event occurs with the development of pulmonary edema. In this regard, Nyhan et al. (65) demonstrated pulmonary vasoconstriction by administration of exogenous ADH to conscious dogs. If, on the other hand, ADH is administered during specific blockade of the vasoconstrictor effects of ADH by a V1 receptor block, pulmonary vasodilation occurs (64). The latter response may be due to a V2 vascular receptor mediated response. Thus, a role for ADH in affecting pulmonary arterial pressure, independent of its renal effects, is indeed possible. The effects of V1 blockade on the increases in pulmonary arterial pressure in response to hypoxia have not been assessed to our knowledge. However, in rats subjected to 8% O_2, equivalent to about 23,000 ft, administration of a V1 receptor blocker reduced total peripheral resistance and mean arterial blood pressure (96) suggesting a role of ADH in the maintenance of vascular resistance during hypoxia. Future experiments in this area are obvious, and hold promise of implicating ADH in the pulmonary hypertension associated with hypoxia and possibly HAPE.

ADH may also be involved in the development of cerebral edema during hypoxia. Raichle and Grubb (74) demonstrated in the rhesus monkey that intracerebroventricular injections of ADH increased the brain capillary permeability coefficient and surface area product by approximately 50%. The dose of ADH, 10 units, is exceedingly high, far higher than would normally be present in the CSF compartment, which brings on questions regarding the physiological significance. However, the effects of lower doses have not been studied to our knowledge, so lower doses could be effective. Additionally, the resulting concentration of ADH at the sites of action in their experiments may be physiologically relevant. If such an effect of ADH does exist, the experiments of Wang et al. (97) are particularly important. They have demonstrated release of ADH into the CSF compartment in response to inhalation of 10% O_2 in anesthetized dogs. Furthermore, one hour after the hypoxia exposure, plasma ADH levels had returned to baseline, but CSF ADH levels remained elevated to the same degree as was observed at 60 min of hypoxia. Extending these findings, it is possible that a transient increase in plasma ADH in response to a continuing hypoxic stimulus, as discussed above, may be accompanied by a more prolonged increase in CSF concentrations of the hormone. Thus, severe symptoms of headache and nausea may not be accompanied by increased plasma ADH, but could be a result of concurrently high CSF ADH concentrations or perhaps of previously elevated CSF ADH levels.

Finally, in regard to possible ADH involvement in AMS, is the report of prevention of AMS by dexamethasone (47). As discussed above (see Figure 5), it appears that when hypoxia follows greatly elevated circulating glucocorticoid levels, the stimulation of ADH release to acute hypoxia is blunted (73). There are no reports in which the ADH response to high altitude exposure is compared between groups receiving any prophylactic measure for AMS and a placebo.

Thus, it is presently unknown what effect acetazolamide, dexamethasone, or spironolactone have on the ADH response to hypoxia.

Over 10 years ago, there were two independent reports of a negative correlation between the plasma levels of aldosterone and the severity of AMS symptoms (39,67). Unfortunately, followup of these experiments with the administration of mineralocorticoid at high altitude has not been performed. The mechanisms whereby decreased aldosterone could be causal in the development of AMS, however, are difficult to speculate on in the face of evidence that spironolactone, a competitive inhibitor of aldosterone at the renal distal tubule and collecting duct, can alleviate the symptoms (54). Thus, the role of endogenous mineralocorticoids in the symptomatology of AMS is unclear. Hopefully in future studies symptomatology will be monitored with an attempt to confirm or deny the previous observed correlations so that the fact is established.

In addition, the rapidly accumulating information regarding ANF includes the potential influence of this hormone on pulmonary arterial pressure (38). These authors demonstrated that administration of ANF to rats breathing 10% O_2 reduced hypoxic vasoconstriction. Isolated perfused lungs from rats exposed to chronic hypoxia and from non-exposed rats were ventilated with anoxic gas (95% N_2, 5% CO_2) and normoxic gas (95% air, 5% CO_2). The hypoxia induced a pulmonary vasoconstriction in both groups that could be inhibited when ANF was added to the perfusate. The rats exposed to hypoxia were less sensitive to the ANF, possibly due to down regulation of the receptors. As mentioned previously, the evidence is convincing that hypoxia stimulates ANF release (5,22,38,59). This area of research will undoubtedly flourish, and with the probable development of competitive antagonists and human use approval of ANF administration may provide valuable information regarding HAPE therapy.

A final note of caution in the interpretation of the hormonal involvement in all of these high altitude sicknesses must be made. The mechanisms of these diseases are unknown. It is not meant to be inferred that disorders of hormone release or action are necessarily the underlying cause. As mentioned, these hypotheses are speculative, and at present represent the direction taken by some endocrinologists in an attempt to determine mechanisms of cause and cure of sicknesses of high altitude.

SUMMARY

High altitude exposure results in a negative water balance. This is in part due to increased insensible water loss, decreased thirst, an inappropriately maintained urine flow despite the decreased thirst, and a decreased appetite. The hormonal involvement in these responses is unclear. For instance, no clear cut role for any hormone system has been established for the decreased thirst. Similarly, the maintenance of urine flow despite decreased intake is not reflected in the short term by an alteration in the plasma osmolality to plasma ADH relationship. However, evidence after prolonged exposure suggests that the

ADH response to increased osmolality is reduced (7). Also, increased cortisol and ANF levels may be contributing to the relative diuresis.

When dietary intake is controlled, high altitude is associated with a retention of potassium and a tendency to lose sodium. These responses are consistent with the reduced aldosterone levels which in turn are a result of a reduced responsiveness of aldosterone to renin. The mechanism of the latter is still unresolved.

The responses of ADH to hypoxia are very complex and have led to considerable confusion. We have tried to describe the differences in experimental designs that probably account for the reports of different responses. Clearly, degree of hypoxia, time of exposure, and whether or not the experiment allowed for spontaneous hyperventilation, are important considerations in comparing ADH responses from different studies.

The potential for hormonal involvement in acute mountain sickness, high altitude pulmonary edema, and cerebral edema continues as an important avenue of research aimed toward prevention and cure of these diseases. Lack of an animal model displaying these responses, and the present inability to use certain drugs in human studies has impaired progress. With eventual development of ANF antagonists, and approval to use ADH antagonists, more insight into these high altitude afflictions will be obtained.

The opinions and assertions contained herein are the private views of the authors and are not to be construed as official or as reflecting the views of the Department of the Army or the Department of Defense.

REFERENCES

1. Anderson, R.J., R.G. Pluss, A.S. Berns, J.T. Jackson, P.E. Arnold, R.W. Schrier and K.M. McDonald. Mechanism of effect of hypoxia on renal water excretion. J. Clin. Invest. 62: 769-776, 1978.
2. Armstrong, H.G. Principles and Practice of Aviation Medicine. Chapter 18, Chronic Altitude Sickness. The Williams and Wilkins Co., Baltimore, pp 284-286, 1939.
3. Arregui, A., G.R. Barer and P.C. Emson. Neurochemical studies in the hypoxic brain: substance P, met-enkephalin, GABA, and angiotensin converting enzyme. Life Sci. 28:2925-2929,1981.
4. Ashack, R., M.O. Farber, M.H. Weinberger, G.L. Robertson, N.S. Fineberg and F. Manfredi. Renal and hormonal responses to acute hypoxia in normal individuals. J. Lab. Clin. Med. 106: 12-16, 1985.
5. Baertschi, A.J., C. Hausmaninger, R.S. Walsh, R.M. Mentzer, D.A. Wyatt and R.A. Pence. Hypoxia-induced release of atrial natriuretic factor (ANF) from the isolated rat and rabbit heart. Biochem. Biophys. Res. Comm. 140: 427-433, 1986.

6. Blum, J.W., W. Biancha, F. Naf, P. Kunz, J.A. Fischer and M. DaPrada. Plasma catecholamine and parathyroid hormone responses in cattle during treadmill exercise at simulated high altitude. Horm. Metab. Res. 11: 246-251, 1979.
7. Blume, F.D., S.J. Boyer, L.E. Braverman, A. Cohen, J. Dirkse and J.P. Mordes. Impaired osmoregulation at high altitude. JAMA 252: 524-526, 1984.
8. Brahmachari, H.D., M.S. Malhotra, K. Ramachandran and U. Radhakrishnan. Progressive changes in plasma cortisol, antidiuretic hormone and urinary volume of normal lowlanders during short stay at high altitude. Indian J. Exp. Biol. 11: 454-455, 1973.
9. Brands, M.W. and R.H. Freeman. Aldosterone and renin inhibition by physiological levels of atrial natriuretic factor. Am J. Physiol. 254(Regulatory Integrative Comp. Physiol. 23): R1011-R1016, 1988.
10. Burrill, M.W., S. Freeman and A.C. Ivy. Sodium, potassium and chloride excretion of human subjects exposed to a simulated altitude of eighteen thousand feet. J. Biol. Chem. 157: 297-302, 1945.
11. Chatterji, J.C., V.C. Ohri, K.S. Chadha, B.K. Das, M. Akhtar, S.C. Tewari, P. Bhattacharji and A. Wadhwa. Serum and urinary cation changes on acute induction to high altitude (3200 and 3771 meters). Aviat. Space Environ. Med. 53: 576-579, 1982.
12. Claybaugh, J.R., J.E. Hansen and D.B. Wozniak. Response of antidiuretic hormone to acute exposure to mild and severe hypoxia in man. J. Endocrinol. 77: 157-160, 1978.
13. Claybaugh, J.R., C.E. Wade, A.K. Sato, S.A. Cucinell, J.C. Lane and J.T. Maher. Antidiuretic hormone responses to eucapnic and hypocapnic hypoxia in humans. J. Appl. Physiol. 53: 815-823, 1982.
14. Claybaugh, J.R., W.K. Stokes, B.J. Freund and G.H. Bryant. Plasma vasopressin is increased only during the first two of six hours of severe hypoxia in conscious goats. Fed. Proc. 46: 796 (abstract 2804), 1987.
15. Colice, G.L. and G. Ramirez. Effect of hypoxemia on the renin-angiotensin-aldosterone system in humans. J. Appl. Physiol. 58: 724-730, 1985.
16. Colice, G.L. and G. Ramirez. Aldosterone response to angiotensin II during hypoxemia. J. Appl. Physiol. 61: 150-154, 1986.
17. Consolazio, C.F., H.L. Johnson, H.J. Krzywicki and T.A. Daws. Metabolic aspects of acute altitude exposure (4,300 meters) in adequately nourished humans. Am. J. Clin. Nutr. 25: 23-29, 1972.
18. Consolazio, C.F., L.O. Matoush, H.L. Johnson and T.A. Daws. Protein and water balances of young adults during prolonged exposure to high altitude (4300 meters). Am. J. Clin. Nutr. 21: 154-161, 1968.
19. Currie, J.C.M. and E. Ullmann. Polyuria during experimnetal modifications of breathing. J. Physiol. 155: 438-455, 1961.
20. Daniel, S.S., R.I. Stark, A.B. Zubrow, H.E. Fox, M.K. Husain and L.S. James. Factors in the release of vasopressin by the hypoxic fetus. Endocrinology 113: 1623-1628, 1983.
21. deBold, A.J., H.B. Borenstein, A.T. Veress and H. Sonenberg. A rapid and potent natriuretic response to intravenous injection of atrial myocardial extract in rat. Life Science 28:89-94, 1981.

22. du Souich,P., C. Saunier, D. Hartman, A. Sautegeau, H. Ong, P. Larose and R. Babin. Effect of moderate hypoxemia on atrial natriuretic factor and arginine vasopressin in normal man. Biochem. Biophys. Res. Comm. 148: 906-912, 1987.
23. Epstein, M. and T. Saruta. Effects of simulated high altitude on renin-aldosterone and Na homeostasis in normal man. J. Appl. Physiol. 33: 204-210, 1972.
24. Forsling, M.L. D.L. Ingram and M.W. Stanier. Plasma antidiuretic hormone during hypoxia and anesthesia in pigs. J. Endocrinol. 85: 253-259, 1980.
25. Forsling, M.L. and J.S. Milledge. Effect of hypoxia on vasopressin release in man. J. Physiol. 267: 22P-23P, 1977.
26. Forsling, M. L. and E. Ullman. Release of vasopressin during hypoxia. J. Physiol. 241: 35P-36P, 1974.
27. Frayser, R., I.D. Rennie, G.W. Gray and C.S. Houston. Hormonal and electrolyte response to exposure to 17,500 ft. J. Appl. Physiol. 38: 636-642, 1975.
28. Gould, A.B. and S.A. Goodman. Effect of hypoxia on the renin angiotensinogen system. Lab. Invest. 22: 443-447, 1970.
29. Guiol, C., P. Montastruc and M-C. Prevost. Renal effect of acute hypobaric pressure breathing in normal and diabetes insipitus rats. J. Physiol. Paris 81: 41-44, 1986.
30. Hackett, P.H., M.L. Forsling, J. Milledge and D. Rennie. Release of vasopressin in man at altitude. Horm. Metab. Res. 10: 571, 1978.
31. Hannon, J.P. Comparative altitude adaptability of young men and women. In: Environmental Stress: Individual Human Adaptations, eds. L.J. Folinsbee, J.A. Wagner, J.F. Borgia, B.L. Drinkwater, J.A. Gliner and J.F. Bedi. Academic Press, New York, pp.335-350, 1978.
32. Hannon, J.P. Nutrition at High Altitude. In: Environmental Physiology: Aging, Heat and Altitude, eds. S.M. Horvath and M.K. Yousef. New York, Elsevier/ North Holland, pp 309-327, 1981.
33. Hannon, J.P., K.S.K. Chinn and J.L. Shields. Effects of acute high-altitude exposure on body fluids. Fed. Proc. 28: 1178-1184, 1969.
34. Hannon, J.P., K.S.K. Chinn and J.L. Shields. Alterations in serum and extracellular electrolytes during high-altitude exposure. J. Appl. Physiol. 31: 266-273, 1971.
35. Hannon, J.P., L.F. Krabill, T.A. Woolridge and D.D. Schnakenberg. Effects of high altitude and hypophagia on mineral metabolism of rats. J. Nutr. 105: 278-287, 1975.
36. Harber, M.J., J.D. Williams and J.J. Morton. Antidiuretic hormone excretion at high altitude. Aviat. Space Environ, Med. 52: 38-40, 1981.
37. Heyes, M.P., M.O. Farber, F. Manfredi, D. Robertshaw, M. Weinberger, N. Fineberg and G. Robertson. Acute effects of hypoxia on renal and endocrine function in normal humans. Am. J. Physiol. 243 (Regulatory Integrative Comp. Physiol. 12): R265-R270, 1982.
38. Hill, N.S. and L-C. Ou. The possible role of atrial natriuretic factor in modulating the pulmonary hypertensinve response to hypoxia. Chest 93 (3 suppl): 95S-96S, 1988.
39. Hogan, R.P., T.A. Kotchen, A.E. Boyd and L.H. Hartley. Effect of altitude on renin-aldosterone system and metabolism of water and electrolytes. J. Appl. Physiol. 35: 385-390, 1973.

40. Humpeler, E., F. Skrabal and G. Bartsch. Influence of exposure to moderate altitude on the plasma concentration of cortisol, aldosterone, renin, testosterone, and gonadotropins. Eur. J. Appl. Physiol. 45:167-176, 1980.
41. Iitake, K.,L. Share, J.T. Crofton, D.P. Brooks, Y. Ouchi and E.H. Blaine. Central atrial natriuretic factor reduces vasopressin secretion in the rat. Endocrinology 119:438-440, 1986.
42. Itoh, H., K. Nakao, G. Katsuura, N. Morii, S. Shiono, T. Yamada, A. Sugawara, Y. Saito, K. Watanabe, K. Igano, K. Inouye and H. Imura. Atrial natriuretic peptides: structure-activity relationship in the central action - a comparison of their antidipsogenic actions. Neuroscience Letters 74: 102-106, 1987.
43. Jaeger, J.J., J.T. Sylvester, A. Cymerman, J.J. Bernerich, J.C. Denniston and J.T. Maher. Evidence for increased intrathoracic fluid volume in man at high altitude. J. Appl. Physiol. 47: 670-676, 1979.
44. Jain, S.C., J. Bardhan, Y.V. Swamy, B. Krishna and H.S. Nayar. Body fluid compartments in humans during acute high-altitude exposure. Aviat. Space Environ. Med. 51: 234-236, 1980.
45. Janoski, A.H., B.K. Whitten, J.L. Shields and J.P. Hannon. Electrolyte patterns and regulation in man during acute exposure to high altitude. Fed. Proc. 28: 1185-1189, 1969.
46. Johnson, H.L., C.F. Consolazio, L.O. Matoush and H.J. Krzywicki. Nitrogen and mineral metabolism at altitude. Fed. Proc. 28: 1195-1198, 1969.
47. Johnson, T.S., P.B. Rock, C.S. Fulco, L.A. Trad, R.F. Spark and J.T. Maher. Prevention of acute mountain sickness by dexamethasone. New Engl. J. Med. 310:683-686, 1984.
48. Jones, R.M., F.T. LaRochelle and S.M. Tenney. Role of arginine vasopressin on fluid and electrolyte balance in rats exposed to high altitude. Am. J. Physiol. 240 (Regulatory Integrative Comp. Physiol. 9): R182-R186, 1981.
49. Jones, R.M., C. Terhaard, J. Zullo and S.M. Tenney. Mechanism of reduced water intake in rats at high altitude. Am. J. Physiol. 240 (Regulatory Integrative Comp. Physiol. 9): R187-R191, 1981.
50. Keynes, R.J., G.W. Smith, J.D.H. Slader, M.M. Brown, S.E. Brown, N.N. Payne, T.P. Jowett and C.C. Monge. Renin and aldosterone at high altitude in man. J. Endocrinol. 92: 131-140, 1982.
51. Kotchen, T.A., R.P. Hogan, A.E. Boyd, T.-K. Li, H.C. Sing and J.W. Mason. Renin, noradrenaline and adrenaline responses to simulated altitude. Clin. Sci. 44: 243-251, 1973.
52. Krzywicki, H.J., C.F. Consolazio, H.L. Johnson, W.C. Nielsen and R.A. Barnhart. Water metabolism in humans during acute high-altitude exposure (4300 m). J. Appl. Physiol. 30: 806-809, 1971.
53. Krzywicki, H.J., C.F. Consolazio, L.O. Matoush, H.L. Johnson and R.A. Barnhart. Body composition changes during exposure to altitude. Fed. Proc. 28: 1190-1194, 1969.
54. Larsen, R.F., P.B. Rock, C.S. Fulco, B. Edelman, A.J. Young, and A. Cymerman. Effect of spironolactone on acute mountain sickness. Aviat. Space Environ. Med. 57:543-547,1986.
55. Lee, J., R.L. Malvin, J.R. Claybaugh and B.S. Huang. Atrial natriuretic factor inhibits vasopressin secretion in conscious sheep. Proc. Soc. Exp. Biol. Med. 185: 272-276, 1987.

56. Leffler, C.W., D.W. Busija, D.P. Brooks, J.T. Crofton, L. Share, D.G. Beasley and A.M. Fletcher. Vasopressin responses to asphyxia and hemorrhage in newborn pigs. Am. J. Physiol. 252 (Regulatory Integrative Comp. Physiol. 21): R122-R126, 1987.
57. Maher, J.T., L.G. Jones, L.H. Hartley, G.H. Williams and L.I. Rose. Aldosterone dynamics during graded exercise at sea level and high altitude. J. Appl. Physiol. 39: 18-22, 1975.
58. Marotta, S.F. Roles of aortic and carotid chemoreceptors in activating the hypothalamo-hypophyseal-adrenocortical system during hypoxia. Proc. Soc. Exp. Biol. Med. 141: 915-927, 1972.
59. McKenzie, J.C., I. Tanaka, T. Inagami, K. Misono and R.M. Klein. Alterations in atrial and plasma atrial natriuretic factor (ANF) content during development of hypoxia-induced pulmonary hypertension in the rat. Proc. Soc. Exp. Biol. Med. 181: 459-463, 1986.
60. Michaelis, L.L. and J.P. Gilmore. Renal effects of electrical stimulation of the carotid sinus nerve. Surgery 65: 797-801, 1969.
61. Milledge, J.S. and D.M. Catley. Angiotensin converting enzyme activity and hypoxia. Clin. Sci. 72: 149, 1987.
62. Milledge, J.S., D.M. Catlet, M.P. Ward, E.S. Williams and C.R.A. Clarke. Renin-aldosterone and angiotensin-converting enzyme during prolonged altitude exposure. J. Appl. Physiol. 55: 699-702, 1983.
63. Milledge, J.S., D.M. Catley, E.S. Williams, W.R. Withey and B.D. Minty. Effect of prolonged exercise at altitude on the renin-aldosterone system. J. Appl. Physiol. 55: 413-418, 1983.
64. Nyhan, D.P., P.W. Clougherty and P.A. Murray. AVP-induced pulmonary vasodilation during specific V1 receptor block in concious dogs. Am J. Physiol. 253 (Heart Circ. Physiol. 22): H493-H499, 1987.
65. Nyhan, D.P., H.S. Geller, H.M. Goll and P.A. Murray. Pulmonary vasoactive effects of exogenous and endogenous AVP in conscious dogs. Am. J. Physiol. 251 (Heart Circ. Physiol. 20): 1009-1016, 1986.
66. Philbin, D.M., R.A. Baratz and R.W. Patterson. The effect of carbon dioxide on plasma antidiuretic hormone levels during intermittent positive pressure breathing. Anesthesiology 33: 345-349, 1970.
67. Pines, A., J.D.H. Slater and T.P. Jowett. The kidney and aldosterone in acclimatization at altitude. Br. J. Dis. Chest 71: 203-207, 1977.
68. Porchet, M., H. Contat, B. Waeber, J. Nussberger and H.R. Brunner. Response of plasma arginine vasopressin levels to rapid changes in altitude. Clin. Physiol. 4: 435-438, 1984.
69. Purshottam, T., M.L. Pahwa and H.D. Brahmachari. Effects of 6 hours hypoxic and cold exposure on urinary electrolyte and catecholamine excretion. Aviat. Space Environ. Med. 49: 62-65, 1978.
70. Raff, H. Glucocorticoid inhibition of neurohypophysial vasopressin secretion. Am. J. Physiol. 252 (Regulatory Integrative Comp. Physiol. 21): R635-R644, 1987.
71. Raff, H. and S.A. Levy. Renin-angiotensin-aldosterone and ACTH-cortisol control during acute hypoxemia and exercise in patients with chronic obstructive lung disease. Am. Rev. Respir. Dis. 133: 396-399, 1986.
72. Raff, H., J. Shinsako, L.C. Keil and M.F. Dallman. Vasopressin, ACTH, and corticosteroids during hypercapnia and graded hypoxia in dogs. Am. J. Physiol. 244 (Endocrinol. Metab. 7): E453-E458, 1983.

73. Raff, H., J. Shinsako, L.C. Keil and M.F. Dallman. Feedback inhibition of adrenocorticotropin and vasopressin responses to hypoxia by physiological increases in endogenous plasma corticosteroids in dogs. Endocrinology, 114: 1245-1249, 1984.
74. Raichle, M.E. and R.L. Grubb. Regulation of brain water permeability by centrally-released vasopressin. Brain Res. 143: 191-194, 1978.
75. Rose, C.E., R.J. Anderson and R.M. Carey. Antidiuresis and vasopressin release with hypoxemia and hypercapnia in conscious dogs. Am. J. Physiol. 247 (Regulatory Integrative Comp. Physiol. 16): R127-R134, 1984.
76. Roy, S.B., V. Balasubramanian, M.R. Khan, V.S. Kaushik, S.C. Manchanda and S.K. Guha. Transthoracic electrical impedance in cases of high-altitude hypoxia. Br. Med. J. 3: 771-775, 1974.
77. Sampson, J.B., A. Cymerman, R.L. Burse, J.T. Maher and P.B. Rock. Procedures for the measurement of acute mountain sickness. Aviat. Space Environ. Med. 54: 1063-1073, 1983.
78. Schmidt, M., B. Wedler, C. Zingler, C. Ledderhos and A. Honig. Kidney function during arterial chemoreceptor stimulation II. Suppression of plasma aldosterone concentration due to hypoxic-hypercapnic perfusion of the carotid bodies in anesthetized cats. Biomed. Biochim. Acta. 5: 711-722, 1985.
79. Share, L. and M.N. Levy. Effect of carotid chemoreceptor stimulation on plasma antidiuretic hormone titer. Am. J. Physiol. 210: 157-161, 1966.
80. Share, L. and J.R. Claybaugh. Regulation of body fluids. Ann. Rev. Physiol. 34: 235-260, 1972.
81. Shigeoka, J.W., G.L. Colice and G. Ramirez. Effect of normoxic and hypoxemic exercise on renin and aldosterone. J. Appl. Physiol. 59: 142-148, 1985.
82. Singh, I., P.K. Khanna, M.C. Srivastava, M. Lal, S.B. Roy and C.S.V. Subramanyam. Acute mountain sickness. New Engl. J. Med. 280:175-184, 1969.
83. Singh, I., M.S. Malhotra, P.K. Khanna, R.B. Nanda, T. Purshottam, T.N. Upadhyay, U. Radhakrishnan and H.D. Brahmachari. Changes in plasma cortisol, blood antidiuretic hormone and urinary catecholamines in high-altitude pulmonary oedema. Int. J. Biometeor. 18: 211-221, 1974.
84. Slater, J.D.H., E.S. Williams, R.H.T. Edwards, R.P. Ekins, P.H. Sonksen, C.H. Beresford and M. McLaughlin. Potassium retention during the respiratory alkalosis of mild hypoxia in man: its relationship to aldosterone secretion and other metabolic changes. Clin. Sci. 37: 311-326, 1969.
85. Slater, J.D.H., R.E. Tuffley, E.S. Williams, C.H. Beresford, P.H. Sonksen, R.T.H. Edwards, R.P. Ekins and M. Mclaughlin. Control of aldosterone secretion during acclimatization to hypoxia in man. Clin. Sci. 37: 327-341, 1969.
86. Spath, J.A., R.M. Daugherty, J.B. Scott and F.J. Haddy. Effect of acute local renal hypoxia on renin activity in renal venous plasma. Proc. Soc. Exp. Biol. Med. 137: 484-488, 1971.
87. Stalcup, S.A., J.S. Lipset, P.M. Legant, P.J. Leuenberger and R.B. Mellins. Inhibition of converting enzyme activity by acute hypoxia in dogs. J. Appl. Physiol. 46:227-234, 1979.
88. Subramanian, R., B. Bhatia and H.H. Siddiqui. Urine output and blood ADH in rats under different grades of hypoxia. In: Selected Topics in Environmental Biology, Chapter 50, eds. B. Bhatia, G.S. Chinna, B. Singh, Interprint Publications. New Delhi. pp 325-332, 1975.

89. Sutton, J.R., C.S. Houston, A.L. Mansell, M.D. McFadden, P.M. Hackett, J.R.A. Rigg and A.C.P. Powels. Effect of acetazolamide on hypoxemia during sleep at high altitude. New Engl. J. Med. 301:1329-1331, 1979.
90. Sutton, J.R., G.W. Viol, G.W. Gray, M. McFadden and P.M. Keane. Renin, aldosterone, electrolyte, and cortisol responses to hypoxic decompression. J. Appl. Physiol. 43: 421-424, 1977.
91. Swies, J. Haemodynamic changes accompanying lung oedema produced by iv injections of adrenaline or vasopressin into rats. Pol. J. Pharmacol. Pharm. 28: 335-340, 1976.
92. Tuffley, R.E., D. Rubenstein, J.D.H. Slater and E.S. Williams. Serum renin activity during exposure to hypoxia. J. Endocr. 48: 497-510, 1970.
93. Ullmann, E. Acute anoxia and the excretion of water and electrolyte. J. Physiol. 155: 417-437, 1961.
94. Van Middlesworth, L., R.L. Banner, F. Lawson and E.M. Cox. Effects of acute intermittent anoxia upon urinary volume, specific gravity and chloride. Proc. Soc. Exp. Biol. Med. 69: 288-290, 1948.
95. Walker, B.R. Inhibition of hypoxia-induced ADH release by meclofenamate in the conscious dog. J. Appl. Physiol. 54: 1624-1629, 1983.
96. Walker, B.R. Role of vasopressin in the cardiovascular response to hypoxia in the conscious rat. Am. J. Physiol. 251 (Heart Circ. Physiol 20): H1316-H1323, 1986.
97. Wang, B.C., W.D. Sundet and K.L. Goetz. Vasopressin in plasma and cerebrospinal fluid of dogs during hypoxia or acidosis. Am. J. Physiol. 247 (Endocrinol. Metab. 10): E449-E455, 1984.

7

HORMONAL REGULATION OF FLUID AND ELECTROLYTES DURING PROLONGED BED REST: IMPLICATIONS FOR MICROGRAVITY

John E. Greenleaf

Laboratory for Human Environmental Physiology
Life Science Division
NASA, Ames Research Center
Moffett Field, CA 94035

INTRODUCTION

It is not clear whether humans have fully adapted to the bipedal upright posture. That we must assume a body position (horizontal) that minimizes the effects of eugravity when fainting is imminent, for sleeping about eight hours per day when healthy, and for longer periods during recovery from injury and disease suggests that sufficient rest in bed in the horizontal body position is necessary for health and well-being. Humans can acclimate (adaptation within one lifetime) within limits to most environmental stresses; dehydration and radiation exposure being notable exceptions.

Since the advent of the space program, investigation into the mechanism of acclimation to prolonged bed rest and exposure to microgravity (weightlessness) has intensified. Bed rest is a rather good simulation for microgravity, although the time course of most bed-rest physiological responses is somewhat slower. Results from bed rest studies can be applied not only to astronauts but also to the multitude of bed-rested patients in hospitals and elsewhere. Remember that bed-rest acclimation (deconditioning) progresses simultaneously with recovery from injury and disease in hospitalized patients.

The scope of the overall mechanism for the bed-rest deconditioning syndrome involves (a) reduction in the hydrostatic pressure gradient within the cardiovascular system, (b) essential elimination of longitudinal pressure on bones, (c) usually a reduction in energy expenditure, (d) changed psychological, dietary and environmental conditions if the patient is moved into a medical facility, and (e) interactions between these stimuli. However, one of the first stimuli that occurs when the body is moved from the upright to the horizontal position is a fluid (blood) shift from the lower extremities into the viscera and thorax that begins a series of responses to reduce total body water. Thus, the focus of this brief review will be a discussion of the hormonal regulation of body fluids and electrolytes during bed rest with and without exercise training and a concluding section of data concerning astronauts in microgravity. Other relevant reviews have been prepared by Gharib (7), Greenleaf (12-14), Johnson (20), and Vernikos (31).

BED REST

First day

With the advent of more intensive research in space physiology, bed rest studies are being conducted with the subjects' head tilted slightly downward (from 4° to 12°) from the horizontal position. This head-down tilting accelerates some of the physiological responses in eugravity to approximate more closely similar responses resulting from exposure to microgravity.

There are two periods during bed rest when significant fluid shifts occur; the first day, and throughout the first month and beyond. With assumption of the horizontal or head-down position, there is a reduction in hydrostatic pressure in the cardiovascular system below the apex of the heart (hydrostatic indifference point) (21). Fluid transfers from the thighs, legs, and possibly the arms to the viscera, thorax and head. The subjects report feelings of head fullness, nasal congestion, and head ache; they often exhibit buccal and gingival turgescence and facial and palpebral edema (17,18,25,33). Not all subjects report these symptoms (6), but most signs and symptoms peak at about 48 hours and disappear within 96 hours (17).

After 4 hr of head-down bed rest the fluid volume of the combined lower extremities (thighs, legs, feet) decreases significantly by about 900 ml (6%) (2), calf circumference is reduced by 1 cm (2.7%), and the lower leg volume is decreased by 160 ml (5%) (18). With the same percentage loss (5%-6%) of fluid in the lower legs and thighs, the absolute loss is about 180 ml and 750 ml, respectively.

The headward transfer of fluid is accompanied by an absolute increase in plasma volume (calculated from changes in plasma protein concentrations or the hematocrit) of 6% to 7% during the first 2 hr of horizontal bed rest (9,35), and by 14% during the first hr of -10° head-down bed rest (9). This increase is followed by a decrease in plasma volume of 125 ml (-4.3%) after 6 hr that reaches 153-310 ml (-5.3 to -9.7%) after 24 hr of bed rest (6,25,33). After 15 min of head-down bed rest there were significant increases in central venous pressure (from 8.6 to 12.6 cm H_2O), cardiac output (from 6.9 to 7.9 liters/min), and stroke vol (from 104 to 113 ml); all these variables returned to baseline within 20 hr during bed rest (Fig. 1). Tissue and interstitial fluid volume shifts to the vascular system accompany these cardiovascular responses. Interstitial fluid pressures (measured with wick catheters) decreased ($P<0.05$) from a baseline value (measured in the horizontal body position) of +4.6 mmHg to +1.8 mmHg and -2.8 mmHg at 4 hr and 8 hr of head-down bed rest in the

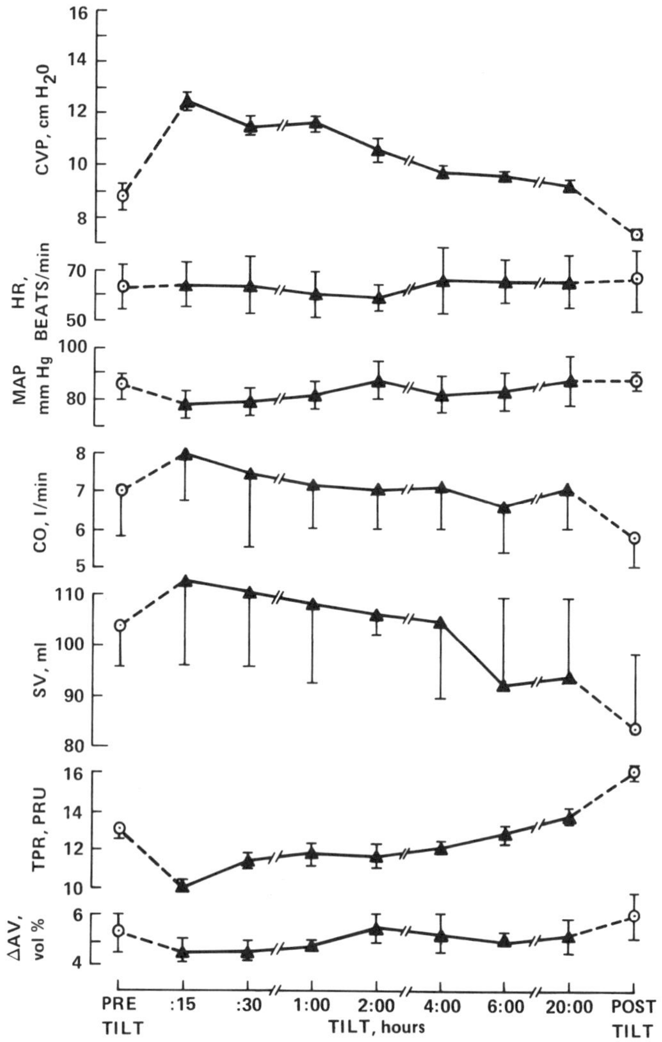

*Figure 1. Mean (±SD) central venous pressure (CVP), heart rate (HR), mean arterial pressure (MAP), cardiac output (CO), stroke volume (SV), total peripheral resistance (TPR), and arterio-venous O_2 difference (ΔAV) in 5 men before, during, and after 20 hr of -5° head-down tilt. *P < 0.05 from pre-tilt data. From ref. (6) with permission.*

anterior tibialis muscle, and from +0.6 mmHg to -2.1 mmHg and -3.8 mmHg, respectively, in the leg subcutaneous tissue (18). These progressive fluid shifts (dehydration) from the lower leg, and probably from the thigh muscles and subcutaneous tissue compartments, contributed only a small volume of fluid for the early absolute increase in plasma volume. Hargens (19) reported that only 100 ml of fluid shifted from the leg muscle and subcutaneous tissue interstitial space during 8 hr of head-down tilt (Fig. 2).

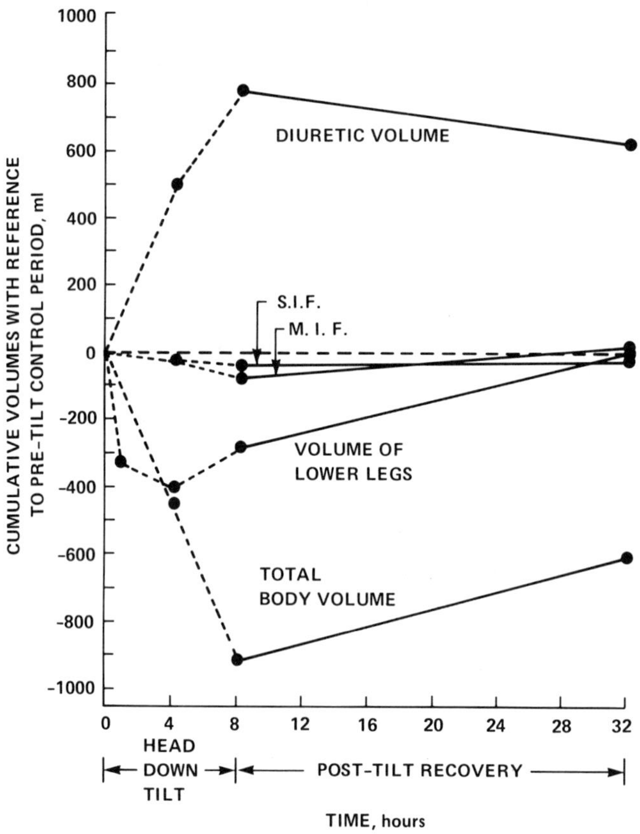

Fig. 2. Mean net cumulative fluid volumes, [and lower leg subcutaneous (S.I.F.) and muscle (M.I.F.) interstitial fluid volumes] from 8 men during 8 hr of -5° head-down tilt and for 24 hr of recovery in the horizontal position. From ref. (19) with permission.

Thus, most of the 900 ml of cephalic transfer fluid was venous blood. The 100 ml of interstitial fluid from both lower extremities can account for about half of the 6% to 7% (200-235 ml) increase in plasma volume. The other half must be derived from the interstitial compartment of the arms and trunk below the hydrostatic indifference point. This hypervolemia, coupled with the cephalic fluid transfer, combined to induce the increased central venous pressure and the other cardiovascular responses (Fig. 1). Concomitant with these fluid shifts and cardiovascular responses was a two-fold increase ($P<0.05$) in urinary flow and an accompanying significant increase in sodium and potassium excretion during the first 6 hr of tilt (6,15,18,19) that tended to decrease after 20 to 24 hr (Figs. 3 and 4). Voluntary fluid intake was unchanged after 4 hr of tilt (18) and tended to decrease thereafter (15,18). The cephalic fluid transfer appears to inhibit drinking similar to that during head-out water immersion; the mechanism is unknown but is probably related to the hypervolemia because plasma osmolality remains essentially constant during immersion (28).

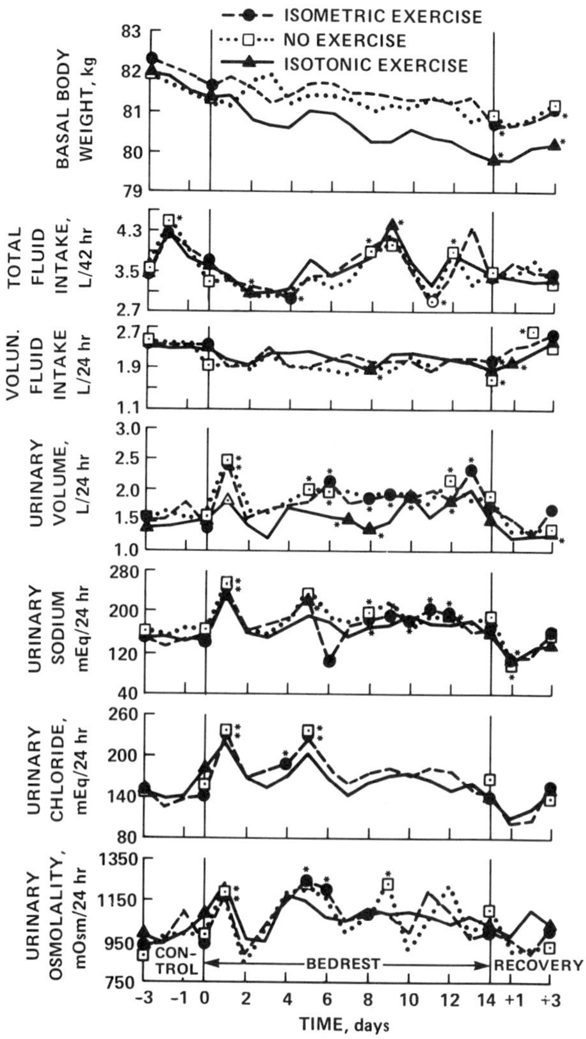

*Fig. 3. Mean body weight, fluid intake, and urinary volume and electrolyte excretion in 7 men during control, horizontal bed rest, and recovery periods for three regimens. *P < 0.05 from day minus 1 control value. From ref. (15) with permission.*

The early fluid-electrolyte response is to reduce the extracellular fluid volume via increased excretion of sodium chloride and water. It has been difficult to show statistically significant changes in various hormone systems early during bed rest or head-down tilt when the supine position was used for the control data. Gharib et al. (9) have recommended the sitting position as the pre-tilt control position. With this protocol the ensuing bed rest or head-down tilt hormone responses will be greater and this perhaps would facilitate understanding of these mechanisms. Considering the various control body

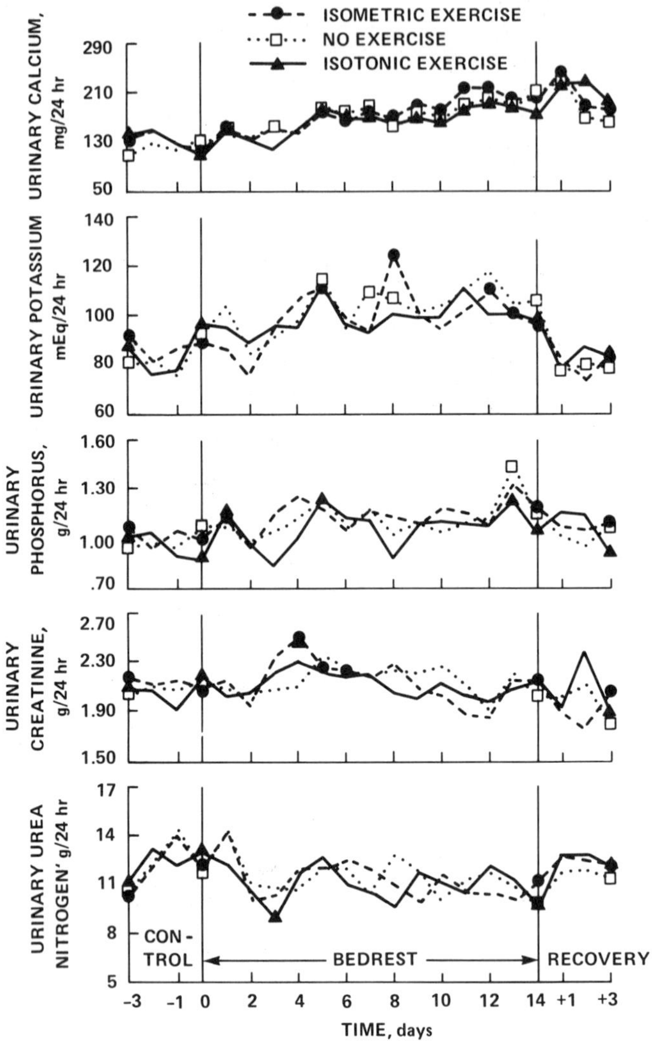

*Fig. 4. Mean urinary electrolyte and nitrogenous excretion in 7 men during control, horizontal bed rest, and recovery periods for three regimens. *P < 0.05 from day minus 1 control value. From ref. (15) with permission.*

positions, it is generally agreed that plasma renin activity and aldosterone concentration decrease (Fig. 5 and 6) during the first few hours of head-down bed rest (5,6,9,18,25). Renin is secreted by the juxtaglomerular (JG) cells located in the renal afferent arteriole. Major factors that increase renin release are reduced concentrations of sodium or chloride at the macula densa cells, decreased stimulation of vascular stretch receptors in the renal afferent arteriole, and increased sympathetic nerve and catecholamine activity on the JG cells which release renin via changes in calcium permeability. Decreases in

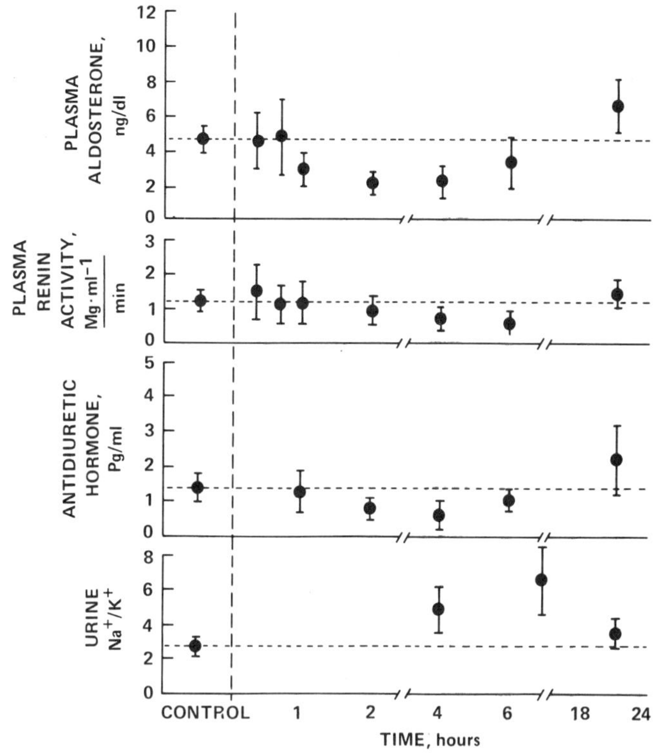

*Figure 5. Mean (±SE) plasma hormones and urinary sodium/potassium ratio in 5 men before and during 24 hr of -5° head-down tilt. *P < 0.05 from control level. From ref. (25) with permission.*

plasma and intracellular calcium concentrations by the action of parathyroid hormone may decrease renin release. Renin may stimulate secretion of aldosterone and antidiuretic hormone via an increase in angiotensin II (4). Aldosterone (mineralocorticoid) is an adrenal steroid derived from cholesterol with a half-life of about 30 min. It is released from the zona glomerulosa cells of the adrenal cortex by angiotensin II which, in turn, is stimulated by renin in response to a fall in blood pressure. Its only known physiologic action is to promote reabsorption of sodium chloride and excretion of potassium and hydrogen ions in kidney distal tubules and ducts of sweat glands, salivary glands, and the intestine. Its main function is to maintain extracellular fluid volume, potassium, and acid-base balance (4,11). A decrease in plasma aldosterone would account for the natriuresis and unchanged urinary potassium concentration associated with the diuresis occurring over the first day of bed rest.

It is difficult to ascribe the diuresis during bed rest only to inhibition of the antidiuretic hormone vasopressin (Figs. 5 and 6). Vasopressin, composed of nine amino acids in peptide linkage formed into a ring by a disulfide bridge connecting cysteine residues at positions 1 and 6, has a half-life of less than 5

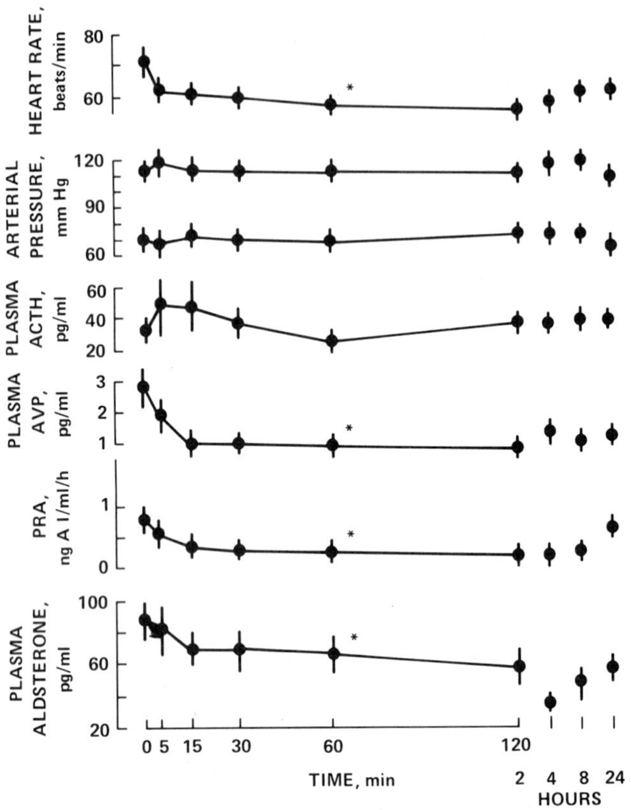

*Figure 6. Mean (±SE) cardiovascular and hormonal responses in 8 men during the first 24 hr of -6^{0} head-down tilt. *P < 0.05 decreases during first 2 hr. From ref. (5) with permission.*

minutes. Human vasopressin molecules contain arginine in position 8, hence the term arginine vasopressin. It is produced in the supraoptic nuclei of the hypothalamus and is transported down axons to the posterior pituitary gland where it is stored. At physiological concentrations its major function is to promote reabsorption of water in collecting ducts and distal tubules in the kidney. Vasopressin responds to less than a one percent change in plasma osmolality, and also to changes in the activity of volume pressure receptors in blood vessels and possibly in the heart. Its vasopressive activity (to increase blood pressure via increased constriction of vascular smooth muscle) usually occurs at very high concentrations. It is secreted in response to hypovolemic stressors: e.g., dehydration, exercise, ambient heat, acceleration, and upright posture. Secretion is inhibited by epinephrine, cold exposure, ethyl alcohol, and oral fluid consumption (4,11). In Nixon's (25) study (Fig. 5), control vasopressin concentration, measured with the subjects in the supine position, was well within the normal range (1.4 pg/ml) and tended to decrease to about 0.5 pg/ml following 4 hours of -5^{0} head down bedrest. In Dallman's study (Fig. 6), control AVP was about 2.8 pg/ml, measured with the subjects in the standing position, and decreased significantly to about 1.0 pg/ml after 60 min of -6° head down bed rest. So decreased AVP early in bed rest probably contributes to the diuresis, but the control body position is critical for establishing whether significant responses occur.

Catecholamines and atriopeptins can also influence urinary function. The catecholamines, epinephrine and norepinephrine, act to reduce renal blood flow with little change in glomerular filtration rate. Stimulation of renal sympathetic nerves increases renal tubular absorption of sodium chloride independently of changes in glomerular filtration rate, renal blood flow, and the actions of angiotensin II and the prostaglandins. Systemic administration of epinephrine and beta-1 agonists inhibits renal potassium excretion (4,11). Pequignot et al. (28) found no significant changes in plasma epinephrine, norepinephrine, or dopamine in young men during 10 hr of -6° head-down bed rest with or without leg cycle ergometer for 2 hr/day. When the seated position was used for control data, there were significant reductions in plasma epinephrine and norepinephrine concentrations during the first hr that remained depressed during 5 hr of -10° head-down tilt, while dopamine concentrations were unchanged (9). Attenuation of plasma catecholamine activity could result in decreased renin release, increased renal blood flow, and decreased tubular absorption of sodium and chloride.

Atriopeptins (AP) are found in the atria of the heart and the human molecule is a 28 amino acid peptide with a cysteinecysteine disulfide link forming a 17-residue ring. The hormone appears to be activated by the atrial pressure and induces a natriuresis when administered in pharmacological doses in animals and humans. While in large concentrations they have marked effects on glomerular filtration rate, sodium transport in the medullary collecting duct, fluid reabsorption in the proximal tubule via inhibition of angiotensin II, and natriuresis, it is not clear if the atriopeptins have a significant effect on fluid-electrolyte parameters in concentrations within the physiological range. From the very few data available, it appears that atriopeptin concentration increases significantly (2-fold) during the first 30 min of -9° head-down tilt (8). Goetz (10) has concluded that atriopeptins at normal physiological concentrations make minimal contributions to natriuresis and diuresis in humans. More important functions of atriopeptins are to induce cardiovascular changes including decreases in cardiac output, cardiac filling pressure, and atrial blood pressure; and to promote fluid shifts from plasma to the interstitial fluid space. They also may inhibit the sympathetic nervous system, reduce the rate of release of vasopressin, and also inhibit voluntary salt and water intake. Brain AP probably reduce the rate of release of vasopressin (10). But, like the prostaglandins, the actions of atriopeptins are so diverse that more work must be done to eliminate or confirm them as important factors for fluid-electrolyte homeostasis during bed rest.

First month and beyond

The reductions in plasma and interstitial fluid volumes that occur during the first day of bed rest continue for the next few days (Fig. 7). By the end of the second week the interstitial volume had returned to or increased slightly above control levels so that the extracellular volume had also returned to control

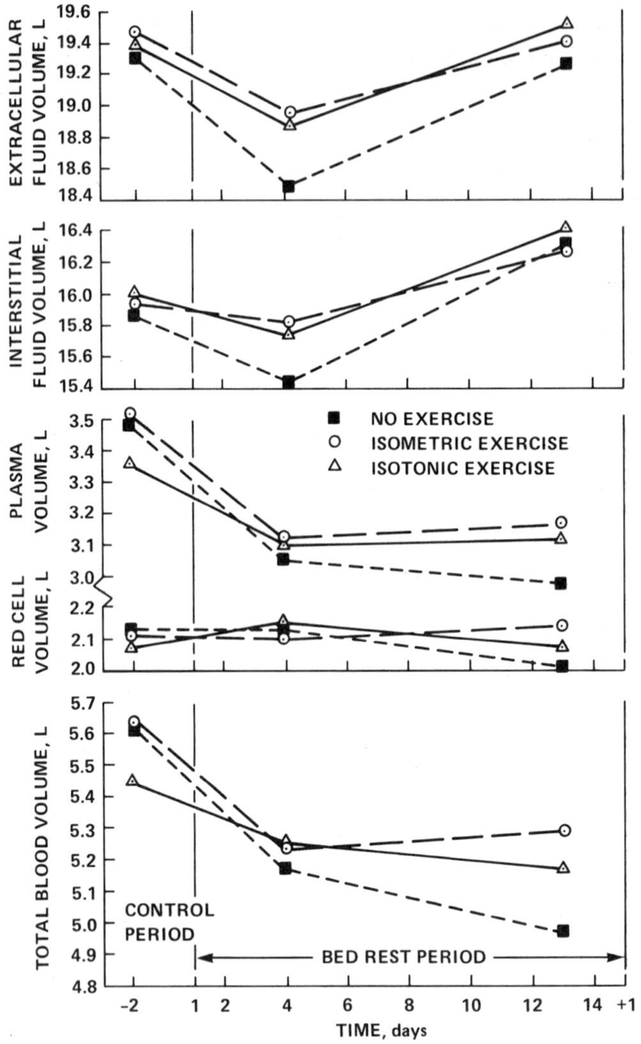

*Figure 7. Mean fluid compartment values in 7 men during ambulatory control and 14 days of horizontal bed rest for three regimens. *P < 0.05 from day minus 2 control value. From ref. (15) with permission.*

levels. Concomitantly, there were reductions in the contents of many plasma constituents (albumin, protein, sodium, potassium, chloride, calcium, phosphorus, glucose, osmolality) to maintain normal concentrations while the plasma volume decreased (15). After the first peak urinary excretion of water and electrolytes on day 1, there appears to be a somewhat attenuated second peak of sodium and chloride excretion and thus osmotic clearance about day 5 (Fig. 3). Thereafter, with the exception of urinary potassium and calcium, the urinary output of all constituents levels off (Figs. 3 and 4).

Smirnova et al. (29) measured sodium balance (intake, urine, feces, sweat) and body fluid compartment volumes before and after 120 days of -5° head-down bed rest (Table 1) without and with remedial procedures (drugs and exercise training). Exercise training during bedrest tended to exert an hypervolemic effect; compared with control levels plasma volume was +3.0% in the exercise group and -3.4% to -7.8% in the other groups after bed rest. The chronic hypervolemia was not due to a positive sodium balance. Changes in total body water, especially the increase in intracellular volume by 5.8% ($P<0.05$) with drug treatment (see Table 1 for details), followed the positive sodium balance. This finding confirms similar calculated fluid shifts from a water immersion-chair rest study (16). The compartmental fluid shifts during immersion were approximately in proportion to their normal ratios, while these fluid shifts during bed rest (Table 1) were not. There was a 2-3 fold greater loss (shift) of the extracellular (mainly interstitial) volume presumably into the intracellular fluid compartment during bed rest. Smirnova et al. suggested that the fluid was transferred from the interstitial space and stored intracellularly in connective tissue histocytes. But the mechanism of this transfer is not clear because it would require an increase in histocyte crystalloid or colloid osmotic

Table 1. Changes (±SE) in sodium balance and fluid compartment volumes during 120 days of -5° head-down bed rest.

	Δ Na+ Balance, mEq/120 d	Δ TBW, %	Δ ICV, %	Δ ECV, %	Δ PV, %	Δ ISV, %
Drug** Group (n=4)	4.9 ±1.8	-2.4 ±0.6	5.8 ±1.1	-15.0 ±2.4	-7.8 ±3.1	-16.7 ±3.3
Exercise*** Group (n=4)	-7.0 ±1.3	-8.5 ±1.3	-5.3 ±2.7	-13.8 ±3.2	3.0 ±9.6	-17.0 ±5.3
Drugs** plus Exercise (n=4)	-5.7 ±2.7	-5.0 ±1.7	-0.6 ±3.0	-12.0 ±2.5	-3.4 ±3.5	-14.7 ±3.0
Control Group (n=3)	-3.7 ±8.4	-6.3 ±1.2	-1.5 ±2.7	-13.2 ±0.7	-4.0 ±2.7	-14.3 ±0.9
	$*P_{2-1}$ $*P_{1-3}$	$*P_{2-1}$ $*P_{4-1}$	$*P_{4-1}$	NS	NS	NS

* $P<0.05$

** Drugs to prevent changes in mineral metabolism (xydiphone, glucamak), lipid metabolism and pancreatic function (solism, F-99), and to stimulate hemopoiesis (folicobalamin), plus UV irradiation.

*** High-speed forced, rapid-forced, and passive-active extension exercises for gravity muscle groups. From Ref. (29).

pressure to retain the fluid. Apparently the restoration of interstitial fluid volume after 2 weeks of bed rest does not continue during prolonged recumbency.

The hormonal responses during prolonged bed rest (throughout the first month and beyond) are more difficult to interpret because the homeostatic stimuli seem to be attenuated as acclimation (deconditioning) proceeds. Results from the most complete study of endocrine functions during 56 days of horizontal bed rest indicated uncoupling (reduced sensitivity) of (a) growth hormone secretion in response to hypoglycemia after 20 days of bed rest, (b) the glucose response to insulin after 30 days, and (c) the secretion of cortisol to ACTH between 30 and 54 days of bed rest (32). The most important conclusion from this and other studies (15,29) was that daily exercise of sufficient intensity and duration to compensate for the caloric deficit during bed rest without exercise, has no significant effect on fluid-electrolyte (except for plasma volume) or hormonal responses during bed rest for at least 120 days. This leaves reduction of hydrostatic pressure as the major stimulus change to activate the recumbent acclimation responses. The implication is that changes in hydrostatic pressure from daily changes of body position is the stimulus that maintains the hormonal coupling in normal, ambulatory humans.

As bed rest extends into months it is clear that a new equilibrium is being approached, if not actually reached, because people can survive continuous bed rest for many years. In this context the aging process accompanies the acclimation deconditioning process. Both probably have common physiological responses; for example reduced aerobic exercise power, muscle wasting, and bone demineralization. The Associated Press (1) has reported that Mr. Jonnie Richardson has undergone voluntary continuous bed rest since 1932 (when he was 16 years old) in his home in Laurel Springs, North Carolina. He is still in bed and, under the circumstances, doing rather well (J.E. Greenleaf, personal communication). According to the article he has not sat upright since 1942 nor rolled over into the prone position since 1960. He was diagnosed as having heart trouble and a goiter; his limbs are as thin as the legs of a "ladder-back chair". Remaining in bed is relatively easy, getting up is more difficult.

FLUID SHIFTS IN MICROGRAVITY

It is well-documented that most space travelers lose weight and body water during flight (20,24,30,34). The mean (±SE) weight loss in the nine Skylab astronauts was 2.6 ± 0.5 kg, while measured total body water (which normally constitutes 65% of body weight) decreased by only 0.8 liters; 31% of the total weight loss (Table 2, Fig. 8). Comparing data from Skylab III and IV, a similar loss of total body water was not in proportion to the large differences in body weight losses (Fig. 8). Mean body weight was still depressed by 1.3% on recovery day 10. The Skylab IV crewmembers on the longest flight (84 days) had the least loss of weight and the most rapid recovery (Table 2). By comparison, the two Soviet cosmonauts lost 3.5 kg and 5.7 kg of body weight, during the 150 day Salyut 7-Soyuz-T flight, that was restored by the ninth day of recovery.

Table 2. Body weight of Skylab astronauts before and on the first (Rec. 1), fifth (Rec. 5), and tenth (Rec. 10) recovery days.

	Launch	Rec.1	Δ,kg	%Δ	Rec.5	%Δ	Rec.10	%Δ
			Skylab II (28 days)					
Commander	61.9	60.1	-1.8	-2.9	61.5	-0.6	61.3	-1.0
Pilot	79.9	76.2	-3.7	-4.6	77.5	-3.0	77.3	-3.2
Scientist Pilot	77.4	74.4	-3.0	-3.9	75.0	-3.1	75.0	-3.1
$\bar{X}$	73.1	70.2	-2.8	-3.8	71.3	-2.2	71.2	-2.4
±SE	5.6	5.1	0.6	0.8	5.0	0.8	5.0	0.7
			Skylab III (59 days)					
Commander	68.6	64.7	-3.9	-5.7	66.8	-2.6	67.1	-2.2
Pilot	88.5	84.2	-4.3	-4.9	86.8	-1.9	87.7	-0.9
Scientist Pilot	62.0	58.3	-3.7	-6.0	60.3	-2.7	60.8	-1.9
$\bar{X}$	73.0	69.1	-4.0	-5.5	71.3	-2.4	71.9	-1.7
±SE	8.0	7.8	0.2	0.3	8.0	0.2	8.1	0.4
			Skylab IV (84 days)					
Commander	68.1	68.0	-0.1	-0.2	68.4	+0.4	68.6	+0.7
Pilot	67.8	66.3	-1.5	-2.2	67.4	-0.6	67.7	-0.2
Scientist Pilot	71.4	69.9	-1.5	-2.1	71.3	+0.1	71.4	0.0
$\bar{X}$	69.1	68.1	-1.0	-1.5	69.0	-0.1	69.2	0.2
±SE	1.2	1.0	0.5	0.6	1.2	0.3	1.1	0.3
Σ $\bar{X}$	71.7	69.1	-2.6	-3.6	70.6	-1.6	70.8	-1.3
±SE	2.9	2.7	0.5	0.6	2.8	0.5	2.8	0.5

Thornton and Ord (30) have shown a linear relationship between daily body weight loss and caloric intake per day/kg body weight in the Skylab astronauts. The linear equation is Wt. loss = -0.02 (kcal/day/kg) + 0.47 and the correlation coefficient (r) is 0.82, which suggests that 67% (r^2) of the average percent daily body weight loss can be accounted for by the deficit in daily caloric consumption. In general, caloric intake increased from 16-17 kcal/day/kg on Skylab II, to 18-21 kcal/day/kg on III, to 20-22 kcal/day/kg on IV (30). Greater food consumption usually promotes greater fluid intake, so the combination will aid in maintaining body weight in flight. Since daily exercise time increased from 0.5 hr/day on II, to 1.0 hr/day on III, and 1.5 hr/day on IV there was probably a chronic exercise-induced hypervolemia that would also attenuate the reduction in total body water (Fig. 8).

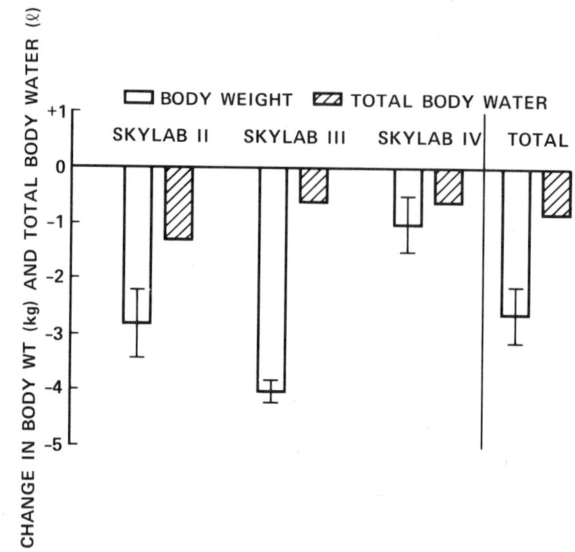

Figure 8. Mean (±SE) changes in body weight (kg) and total body water (liters) in the three astronauts in each of the Skylab flights. Total data N=9.

The mechanism of this total body water loss is not clear. A prominent hypothesis for the early loss in flight was the Gauer-Henry reflex where the postulated diuresis was caused by inhibition of vasopressin secretion from increased central (atrial) venous pressure due to a fluid shift from the legs to the thorax and head (27,28). Recent results indicate that men with no legs immersed to the neck in water still have a significant diuresis (K. Shiraki, personal communication). There is no evidence that astronauts have a diuresis early in microgravity (24). It has been reported that some astronauts have dehydrated themselves for a few days before flight in an attempt to reduce the in-flight cerebral edema. Since the astronauts lay on their backs with their legs elevated for a number of hours before lift-off, it is likely that any diuresis occurs there. The available data concerning atrial pressure and cardiac function during flight are equivocal. Ultrasonic measurements of jugular vein blood flow in one French astronaut indicated increased venous resistance (pressure) coupled with a 40% increase in resting cardiac output that persisted for 4 days of flight (8). Kirsch et al. (22) observed a decrease in peripheral venous pressure (as an estimate of central venous pressure) from 1 to 8 cm H_2O taken 22 hr after launch; too late to observe any potential early increase. Direct, continuous measurement of atrial venous pressure measured before, during launch, and during transition into microgravity would be necessary to answer this question.

One explanation for the reduction in total body water of astronauts in microgravity is that there was a moderate diuresis on the pad while awaiting launch in a recumbent head down position, assuming the astronauts were normally hydrated. Then, after entering microgravity, the excitement and stress of the launch coupled with nausea and vomiting (in some astronauts) would inhibit intake of food (anorexia) and fluid (involuntary dehydration). If the urine volume were normal or even slightly depressed, there would be a negative water balance and reduction in total body water. But there appears to be excess fluid in the head and thorax. Some interstitial fluid may have shifted into the vascular system early in flight, but the sustained increase in peripheral venous hematocrit (22) suggests it does not remain there. Plasma and interstitial fluid volumes probably decrease early in flight, but the latter appears to be restored by the second week of bed rest (15) and possibly during flight, so the 300-600 ml loss of extracellular volume during flight can be accounted for by the reduction of plasma volume (20). But it appears that the hypovolemia cannot account for the total shift or loss of fluid (Fig. 8). The splanchnic circulation could be a reservoir for fluid exchange during microgravity.

Perhaps the postulated increase in central venous pressure is too small or transient to cause a significant diuresis by means of vasopressin suppression, but it may be sufficient to release atriopeptins. The latter could stimulate some additional urine flow or just maintain normal flow accompanying the reduced drinking by increasing sodium loss in the urine (10). The result would be a more dilute plasma and interstitial fluid. This hyposmotemia plus the function of atriopeptins to shift fluid from plasma to the interstitial space (10) could account for the restoration and increased interstitial volume that appears to compensate for the chronic hypovolemia (15,20). Thus, the extracellular volume is restored while plasma volume remains depressed. If the interstitial volume were more hypotonic, this fluid could shift into the intracellular compartment contributing to the head edema which, in turn, could have an inhibitory effect on drinking as occurs during water immersion (23).

As flight duration lengthens to months, microgravity acclimation appears to return food and fluid intake to normal with restoration of body water and weight (20,34, Fig. 8). The crucial test of any limitation of acclimation to microgravity will come when daily exposures to prolonged, strenuous extravehicular activity are required during construction of the Space Station.

SUMMARY AND CONCLUSIONS

The first significant physiological change that occurs within the body when assuming the horizontal or head-down body position, and probably when first exposed to microgravity, is a loss of body water. The initial stimulus appears to be the change in hydrostatic pressure within the cardiovascular system. In spite of an apparent uncoupling of prominent hormonal interactions during bed-rest deconditioning (and possibly during microgravity), exercise-training induced hypervolemia probably helps to counter the hypohydrostatic induced dehydration. Thus, after nearly a year of spaceflight during which one cosmonaut exercised for about 4 hours per day, water balance and physiological functioning did not seem to be compromised significantly.

REFERENCES

1. Anonymous, Associated Press. Puzzling illness keeps man in bed 50 years. San Jose Mercury, May 26, 1982. p.12A.
2. Blomqvist, C.G., J.V. Nixon, R.L. Johnson, Jr., and J.H. Mitchell. Early cardiovascular adaptation to zero gravity simulated by head-down tilt. Acta Astronaut. 7:543-553, 1980.
3. Buckalew, V.M., Jr. and K.A. Gruber. Natriuretic hormone. In: The Kidney in Liver Disease, edited by M. Epstein. New York: Elsever, 1988, p.479-499.
4. Cox, T.C. Hormonal control of water and electrolyte metabolism. In: Handbook of Endocrinology, vol. II, part A, edited by G.H. Gass and H.M. Kaplan. Boca Raton, FL: CRC Press, Inc., 1987. p. 153-180.
5. Dallman, M.F., J. Vernikos, L.C. Keil, D. O'hara, and V. Convertino. Hormonal fluid and electrolyte responses to 6° anti-orthostatic bed rest in healthy male subjects. In: Stress: The Role of Catecholamines and Other Neurotransmitters, edited by E. Usdin, R. Ketnansky, and J. Axelrod, vol. II. London: Gordon and Breach Science Publishers, 1984. p.1057-1077.
6. Gaffney, F.A., J.V. Nixon, E.S. Karlsson, W. Campbell, A.B.C. Dowdey, and C.G. Blomqvist. Cardiovascular deconditioning produced by 20 hours of bedrest with head-down tilt (-5°) in middle-aged healthy men. Am. J. Cardiol. 56:634-638, 1985.
7. Gharib, C., G. Gauquelin, G. Geelen, M. Cantin, J. Gutkovska, J.L. Mauroux, and A. Guell. Volume regulating hormones (renin, aldosterone, vasopressin and natriuretic factor) during simulated weightlessness. Physiologist 28:S3O-S33, 1985.
8. Gharib, C., G. Gauquelin, G. Geelen, M. Vincent, F. Ghaemmaghami, and Ch. Grange. Levels of plasma atrial natriuretic factor (alpha hANF) during acute simulated weightlessness. Proc. 2nd Int. Conf. Space Physiol., ESA SP-237, 1985. p.173-176.
9. Gharib, C., G. Gauquelin, J.M. Pequignot, G. Geelen, C.-A. Bizollon, and A. Guell. Early hormonal effects of head-down tilt (-10°) in humans. Aviat. Space Environ. Med. 59:624-629, 1988.
10. Goetz, K.L. Physiology and pathophysiology of atrial peptides. Am. J. Physiol. 254:El-E15, 1988.
11. Goodman, H.M. Endocrine glands, Part XIII. In: Medical Physiology, vol. 2, edited by V.B. Mountcastle. St. Louis: C.V. Mosby Co., 1980. p.1459-1678.
12. Greenleaf, J.E. Physiological consequences of reduced physical activity during bed rest. In: Exercise and Sport Sciences Reviews, vol. 10, edited by R.L. Terjung. Philadelphia: Franklin Institute Press, 1982. p.84-119.
13. Greenleaf, J.E. Physiological responses to prolonged bed rest and fluid immersion in humans. J. Appl. Physiol. 57:619-633, 1984.
14. Greenleaf, J.E. Physiology of fluid and electrolyte responses during inactivity: water immersion and bed rest. Med. Sci. Sports Exerc. 18:20-25, 1984.
15. Greenleaf, J.E., E.M. Bernauer, H.L. Young, J.T. Morse, R.W. Staley, L.T. Juhos, and W. Van Beaumont. Fluid and electrolyte shifts during bed rest with isometric and isotonic exercise. J. Appl. Physiol. 42:59-66, 1977.

16. Greenleaf, J.E., E. Shvartz, S. Kravik, and L.C. Keil. Fluid shifts and endocrine responses during chair rest and water immersion in man. J. Appl. Physiol. 48:79-88, 1980.
17. Guell, A., L. Pourcelot, J.L. Mauroux, Ph. Dupui, and A. Bes. Interest of head-down tilt to simulate the neurocirculatory modifications observed during space flight. Proc. 35th Cong. Int. Astro. Fed., IAF-84-190, 1984. p.1-4.
18. Hargens, A.R., C.M. Tipton, P.D. Gollnick, S.J. Mubarak, B.J. Tucker, and W.H. Akeson. Fluid shifts and muscle function in humans during acute simulated weightlessness. J. Appl. Physiol. 64:1003-1009, 1988.
19. Hargens, A.R. Fluid shifts in vascular and extravascular spaces during and after simulated weightlessness. Med. Sci. Sports Exerc. 15:421-427, 1983.
20. Johnson, P.C. Fluid volumes changes induced by spaceflight. Acta Astronaut 6:1335-1341, 1979.
21. Kirsch, K., J. Merke, H. Hinghofer-Szalkay, and H.J. Wicke. Fluid volume distribution within superficial shell tissues along body axis during changes of body posture in man. Pfluegers Arch. 383:195-201, 1980.
22. Kirsch, K., A.L. Rocker, O.G. Gauer, R. Krause, C. Leach, H.J. Wicke, and R. Landry. Venous pressure in man during weightlessness. Science Wash. D.C. 225:218-219, 1984.
23. Kravik, S.E., L.C. Keil, J.E. Silver, N. Wong, W.A. Spaul, and J.E. Greenleaf. Immersion diuresis without expected suppression of vasopressin. J. Appl. Physiol. 57:123-128, 1984.
24. Leach, C.S., and P.C. Rambaut. Biochemical responses of the Skylab crewman: an overview. In: Biomedical Results from Skylab. chap. 23, edited by R.S. Johnston and L.F. Dietlein. NASA SP-377, 1977. p.204-216.
25. Nixon, J.V., R.G. Murray, C. Bryant, R.L. Johnson, Jr., J.H. Mitchell, O.B. Holland, C. Gomez-Sanchez, P. Vergne-Marini, and C.G. Blomqvist. Early cardiovascular adaptation to simulated zero gravity. J. Appl. Physiol. 46:541-548, 1979.
26. Pequignot, J.M., A. Guell, G. Gauquelin, E. Jarsaillon, G. Annat, A. Bes, L. Peyrin, and C. Gharib. Epinephrine, norepinephrine, and dopamine during a 4-day head-down bed rest. J. Appl. Physiol. 58:157-163, 1985.
27. Planel, H., and H. Oser. A Survey of Space Biology and Space Medicine. Noordvijk, The Netherlands: ESA Publ. Branch. 1984. Chap. 5 (Eur. Space Agency BR-17).
28. Shepherd, J.T., and P.M. Vanhoutte. The Human Cardiovascular System, Facts and Concepts. New York: Raven, 1979, chap. 6.
29. Smirnova, T.M., G.I. Kozyrevskaya, V.I. Lobachik, V.V. Zhidkov, and S.V. Abrosimov. Individual distinctions of fluid-electrolyte metabolism during hypokinesia with headdown tilt for 120 days, and efficacy of preventive agents. Kosm. Biol Aviak. Med. 20:21-24, 1986.
30. Thornton, W.E., and J. Ord. Physiological mass measurements in Skylab. In: Biomedical Results from Skylab, Chap. 19, edited by R.S. Johnston and L.F. Dietlein. NASA SP-377, 1977. p. 175-182.
31. Vernikos, J. Metabolic and endocrine changes. In: Inactivity: Physiological Effects, Chap. 5, edited by H. Sandler, and J. Vernikos-Danellis. New York: Academic Press, Inc., 1986. p. 99-121.

32. Vernikos-Danellis, J., C.M. Winget, C.S. Leach, and P.C. Rambaut. Circadian, endocrine and metabolic effects of prolonged bedrest: two 56-day bedrest studies. NASA Tech. Memo. X-3051, 1974. 42p.
33. Volicer, L., R. Jean-Charles, and A.V. Chobanian. Effect of head-down tilt on fluid and electrolyte balance. Aviat. Space Environ. Med. 47:1065-1068, 1976.
34. Vorobyev, Ye.I., O.G. Gazenko, Ye.B. Shulzhenko, A.I. Grigoryev, A.S. Barer, A.D. Yegorov, and I.A. Skiba. Preliminary results of medical investigations during 5-month spaceflight aboard Salyut-7-Soyuz-T orbital complex. Kosm. Biol. Aviak. Med. 20:27-34, 1986.
35. Widdowson, E.M., and R.A. McCance. The effect of rest in bed on plasma volume as indicated by haemoglobin and haematocrit levels. Lancet 1:539-540, 1950.

INDEX